D1565138

Series Editors:
Steven F. Warren, Ph.D.
Joe Reichle, Ph.D.

Communication
and Language
Intervention
Series

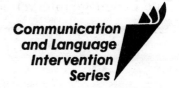

Volume 6

Assessment of
Communication and Language

Also available in the Communication and Language Intervention Series:

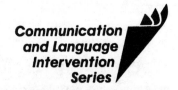

Volume 6
Assessment of Communication and Language

Edited by

Kevin N. Cole, Ph.D.
Research Faculty
Department of Speech and Hearing Sciences
University of Washington
Seattle, Washington

Philip S. Dale, Ph.D.
Professor
Departments of Psychology, Linguistics, and
Speech and Hearing Sciences
University of Washington
Seattle, Washington

and

Donna J. Thal, Ph.D.
Professor
Department of Communicative Disorders
San Diego State University
San Diego, California

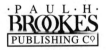

·P·A·U·L·H·
BROOKES
PUBLISHING C♀

Baltimore • London • Toronto • Sydney

Paul H. Brookes Publishing Co.
Post Office Box 10624
Baltimore, Maryland 21285-0624

Copyright © 1996 by Paul H. Brookes Publishing Co., Inc.
All rights reserved.

Typeset by Signature Typesetting & Design, Baltimore, Maryland.
Manufactured in the United States of America by
The Maple Press Company, York, Pennsylvania.

This book is printed on recycled paper. ✪

Library of Congress Cataloging-in-Publication Data

Assessment of communication and language / edited by Kevin N. Cole, Philip S. Dale,
  Donna J. Thal.
     p.   cm.—(Communication and language intervention series ; v. 6)
    Includes bibliographical references and index.
    ISBN 1-55766-193-6
    1. Language disorders in children—Diagnosis. 2. Communicative disorders in
children—Diagnosis. I. Cole, Kevin N. II. Dale, Philip S. III. Thal, Donna J.
IV. Series: Communication and language intervention series ; 6.
RJ496.L35L3665   1996
618.92'855075—dc20
                                           96-20950
                                            CIP

British Library Cataloguing-in-Publication data are available from the British Library.

Contents

Series Preface

T HE PURPOSE OF THE *Communication and Language Intervention Series* is to provide meaningful foundations for the application of sound intervention designs to enhance the development of communication skills across the life span. We are endeavoring to achieve this purpose by providing readers with presentations of state-of-the-art theory, research, and practice.

In selecting topics, editors, and authors, we are not attempting to limit the contents of this series to those viewpoints with which we agree or that we find most promising. We are assisted in our efforts to develop the series by an editorial advisory board consisting of prominent scholars representative of the range of issues and perspectives to be incorporated in the series.

We trust that the careful reader will find much that is provocative and controversial in this and other volumes. This will be necessarily so to the extent that the work reported is truly on the so-called cutting edge, a mythical place where no sacred cows exist. This point is demonstrated time and again throughout this volume as the conventional wisdom is challenged (and occasionally confirmed) by various authors.

Readers of this and other volumes are encouraged to proceed with healthy skepticism. In order to achieve our purpose, we take on some difficult and controversial issues. Errors and misinterpretations inevitably are made. This is normal in the development of any field and should be welcomed as evidence that the field is moving forward and tackling difficult and weighty issues.

Well-conceived theory and research on development of both children with and children without disabilities are vitally important for researchers, educators, and clinicians committed to the development of optimal approaches to communication and language intervention. For this reason, each volume in this series includes chapters pertaining to both development and intervention.

The content of each volume reflects our view of the symbiotic relationship between intervention and research: Demonstrations of what may work in intervention should lead to analyses of promising discoveries and insights from developmental work that may in turn fuel further refinement by intervention researchers.

An inherent goal of this series is to enhance the long-term development of the field by systematically furthering the dissemination of theoretically and empirically based scholarship and research. We promise the reader an opportunity to participate in the development of this field through the debates and discussions that occur throughout the pages of the *Communication and Language Intervention Series.*

Editorial Advisory Board

Volume Preface

ALMOST EVERY ASPECT OF LANGUAGE assessment of children is undergoing major changes. Language intervention professionals are being challenged to expand their thinking about who should be assessed, what behaviors should be evaluated, how to sample performance, and how to understand and make use of results. Several trends in demographics, legislation, and new knowledge about language development are responsible for these changes. Language intervention professionals are challenged to evaluate children at younger and younger ages, to accurately and fairly assess children who have cultural backgrounds that are different from the mainstream, to assess children who may speak English as a second language, and to assess a broader range of language structures, including discourse.

What is needed now is information about how to use new models in conjunction with current practices in order to provide the best services to children. Professionals need to know which new models appear promising and how to match the right tool to the right situation. This volume critically examines new models of intervention and reevaluates the usefulness of several traditional assessment tools. The focus here is on recent issues and advances, in contrast to a basic presentation of traditional models. Rather than a "menu" of what is available, chapters in this volume present a conceptual framing of the state of the art, including problems, issues, and "what works well."

This volume was designed to respond to assessment needs of children from diverse backgrounds. Chapters include information regarding multicultural applications, issues, and implications throughout all areas of language assessment. In addition, the volume includes a chapter by Gutierrez-Clellen (Chapter 2), which focuses specifically on concerns and ideas for assessing children from diverse linguistic and cultural backgrounds.

The new populations challenge professionals to expand their knowledge to a much broader range of children. This alone would be enough to occupy professionals' adaptive skills for some time. These challenges, however, are only the beginning. In addition to the expanding populations being served, language intervention professionals also face challenges in assessment driven by a more sophisticated understanding of communication development and disorders. Advances in the understanding of phonological development, for example, bring with them a need for new assessment approaches that are far different from and more complex than previous methods. As discussed by Stoel-Gammon in Chapter 4, professionals must consider not only a phoneme's position within a word but also factors such as word length, stress position, and phonetic environment in order to understand the rule system that children employ. New models are not limited to the area of phonological development; professionals' knowledge of semantic development, morphosyntactic performance, and pragmatic ability is expanding and increasing in complexity, driving changes in how they assess children's language ability. Chapter 5 of this volume, by Leonard and Eyer, for example, presents two children's language samples that, using traditional assessment methods, appear to be somewhat comparable. When a new transformational framework is applied to each, however, it becomes strikingly apparent that the samples are profoundly different in their complexity.

In addition to new populations and expanded models of the form, content, and use of language, language intervention professionals have new information about more global aspects of the process by which children learn language. For example, professionals' understanding that children learn and use language most effectively in environments other than clinical settings has motivated professionals to conduct assessments in naturalistic environments and to tie assessment closely to intervention in these settings. Similarly, professionals' knowledge of individual differences in children's learning has led to dynamic assessment practices that tell professionals about learning patterns and rates of progress, as well as current performance status. Even professionals' basic understanding of who has a language disorder is in a state of transformation. New ideas about how cognitive skills and communication skills influence each other require professionals to reconsider traditional assessment models.

With all of these changes in whom professionals serve and how they serve them, it is not surprising that service providers feel somewhat disoriented and dissatisfied with available assessment tools and procedures. This sense of unrest with the state of the art is reflected in the results of a survey by Huang, Hopkins, and Nippold (in press), who report that less than 25% of speech-language pathologists interviewed were satisfied with available assessment practices. Clearly, changes are needed in how professionals evaluate children's communication skills. The purpose of this volume is to address this issue by exploring new ideas and new methods of assessing communication development in children.

One of the first steps in reestablishing equilibrium between assessment challenges and existing methods is to clarify why assessments are conducted in the first place. What do we want to know from communication assessments? Once this question has been answered, it is possible to evaluate an assessment practice to determine whether it actually provides the information sought. At the most basic level, assessments have two broad and perhaps mutually exclusive goals. The first goal is to identify important skills and processes that the child must master in order to allow the professional to plan intervention and evaluate treatment efficacy. The second goal is to identify the child's ability in relation to same-age peers, providing information for diagnosis and program efficacy evaluation. Norm-referenced assessments are used to meet this second goal because they are designed specifically to confirm the presence or absence of a disorder, relative to the performance of same-age peers. This type of assessment is required for meeting funding requirements (insurance eligibility, state department of education service eligibility guidelines, etc.) and to provide information to parents to allow them to understand the relative severity of their child's delay. It also may help in arriving at a diagnostic label that may suggest causal factors or help predict future performance.

Norm-referenced measures must be used with caution, however, because they are designed specifically to show *differences* among children, rather than to show what a child might be expected to know at a certain age. For example, if a sample test item is answered correctly by most 4-year-olds, then distinguishing among them would not be likely, and, therefore, the item would not be used for the 4-year-old level, even if it represents an important skill for 4-year-old children. Thus, items on norm-referenced tests are not based on what most children *should* know at a given age but rather on which items can distinguish among children at a given age. As a result, skills tapped on norm-referenced tests may not be the skills that are central to communication ability at a given age level. In addition, norm-referenced tests can predict future status for groups of children but are less accurate in predicting for individual children (Taylor, 1994). Although they are useful in research with large groups of children, using them to identify an individual child's progress in intervention may be questionable.

Another concern with using norm-referenced tests is whether a sample of behavior can be generalized and assumed to represent the child's usual performance. All direct assessment rests on using a small sample of behavior, usually observed in a single context, to represent the child's underlying level of development. This assumption may be particularly problematic for normed tests because they tend to be formally administered using standardized procedures and materials, thus restricting the range of skills that may be observed. Validity of norm-referenced test results also is threatened by sampling limitations. The measures may not be normed on populations with which they will be used, especially children from various ethnic backgrounds.

While norm-referenced tests attempt to provide information about how a child performs relative to peers, the *standards* model, sometimes referred to as criterion-referenced assessment, is used to assess student performance in relation to some absolute standards. This type of measure addresses the first goal of assessment noted previously: identifying specific skills and processes that the child needs to develop. Professionals ask whether a child has mastered a skill rather than whether the child is better or worse at a skill than other children his or her age. Unlike norm-referenced testing, the standards model selects skills for assessment specifically because of their importance for communicative functioning, regardless of whether the test item distinguishes among children's performance. Thus, if a skill is important for 4-year-old children, then it would be included in the assessment even if knowledge of the child's ability to complete the task did not inform about whether the child was a relatively higher-functioning 4-year-old or a relatively lower-functioning 4-year-old.

The standards model also lends itself to flexible assessment procedures. Because the goal is to determine whether (and, with some measures, under what conditions) a child can perform a skill, behavior can be sampled in a variety of ways over a range of contexts at different times. The goal is to find out what the child can do rather than whether the child is better or worse at the task than other children. Thus, it is not essential to assess performance using highly controlled procedures to ensure that all children tested are responding to the same stimuli. In fact, a few standards models incorporate dynamic assessment procedures that allow the tester to probe a variety of conditions that may influence the child's performance. The purpose of altering the testing conditions is to identify whether language-learning impairments are content based or process based and how best to approach instruction (see Peña, Chapter 12).

The standards model, like all approaches to assessment and intervention, is based on a set of assumptions that are important to recognize. First, the model assumes that professionals know at least some of the key skills that a child should have at certain ages or the sequence in which specific skills should emerge and that professionals can use this information to plan intervention. Second, it assumes that somewhat different child performances can reflect the same standards. For example, a child might demonstrate the pragmatic intent of "refusal" using a variety of communicative forms. Finally, and perhaps most challenging, the model assumes that service providers and researchers can learn to be fair and consistent judges of diverse student performances (Taylor, 1994). This last assumption is especially important because the lack of standard administration procedures increases subjectivity in interpreting results.

It might be easy to conclude from these descriptions that the norm-referenced model is less desirable and the standards model is more informative. This is not the intent of the contrastive descriptions provided and would, in fact, be an erroneous inference. Each model serves a very distinct set of purposes. When norm-referenced tests are used to meet state and federal eligibility requirements, to document overall program efficacy, or to verify the level of delay for a child, they can be appropriate and informative. When they are used to develop intervention plans for a student or are used to assess progress for an individual child, they have much less to offer. Unfortunately, speech-language pathologists frequently attempt to use norm-referenced tests in this way and are predictably less than satisfied with the results (Huang et al., in press). Standards-model assessments are much more useful for determining whether the child has mastered the skills and may provide some useful information for setting intervention goals.

Standards-model assessments also have limitations. The model often relies on somewhat subjective judgments of child performance, which can be a potential threat to test reliability. Because of this element of subjectivity, organizations that fund intervention (e.g., state and federal funding agencies, insurance providers) generally require the use of norm-referenced measures as well as standards-model assessments. In addition, standards assessments often do not lend themselves easily to psychometric standardization, so information about a child's performance along the typical distribution curve is not obtainable. The standards-model assessment cannot inform professionals about how much better or worse a child's performance is relative to peers. Only performance in specific ability areas can be measured. This provides little information about how much delay or advance a child might be experiencing in relation to same-age peers. This is not trivial information for parents and professionals who must plan for the child's future and allocate resources. In addition, most standards models, like most norm-referenced measures, do not provide a great deal of information about the child's specific processes of learning. Dynamic assessment procedures, however, have been incorporated in some standards-model assessments, and this direction is promising in gathering important information about the nature of the child's ability to benefit from intervention.

As noted previously, it is essential to know what information you want to gather from your assessment. This knowledge will lead to selecting the appropriate tool. To meet the assessment challenges, professionals must expand their development of norm-referenced measures, standards-model instruments, dynamic assessment, and other innovations, and use the methods for the purposes for which they were intended. The following chapters present discussions of innovative assessments including curriculum-based assessment (Notari-Syverson & Losardo, Chapter 11), phonological evaluation (Stoel-Gammon, Chapter 4), dynamic assessment (Peña, Chapter 12), morphosyntactic evaluation (Leonard & Eyer, Chapter 5), prelinguistic development (McCathren, Warren, & Yoder, Chapter 3), measures derived from language samples (Evans, Chapter 10), and discourse assessment (McCabe, Chapter 6). Each of these chapters discusses innovative methods of identifying children's performance for skill areas and ideas for translating this knowledge into intervention practices.

Norm-referenced assessment practices also are addressed in several chapters. Rice and Watkins (Chapter 9) discuss vocabulary assessment practices and validate the use of norm-referenced tools such as the Peabody Picture Vocabulary Test for several purposes including diagnosis and research applications. In his chapter on parent report methods, Dale (Chapter 8) describes an innovative method of gathering normative data that allows accurate and early diagnosis of language delay.

Important limitations of some measurements in meeting assessment challenges also are addressed. Gutierrez-Clellen (Chapter 2) considers the limitations of some tools for use with children from nonmainstream cultures, and Cole and Fey (Chapter 7) challenge the widespread use of profiles of norm-referenced tests in determining eligibility for language intervention services.

Thal and Katich, in their chapter on early assessment (Chapter 1), point out an additional challenge in assessment and one that is central to accurate assessment: Single measures often are not adequate for describing and predicting an individual child's development; the younger the child, the more difficult it is to predict future performance. Even with an increased knowledge of prelinguistic milestones and assessment techniques, for example, as described by McCathren, Warren, and Yoder (Chapter 3), it still is necessary to look at the overall pattern of skills in order to be able to predict individual performance with confidence. Accurate assessment of communication skills requires multiple samples of ability, knowledge of a variety of techniques, and consideration of many approaches. The following chapters provide new ideas to help in meeting this challenge.

REFERENCES

Huang, R., Hopkins, J., & Nippold, M. (in press). Satisfaction with standardized language testing: A survey of speech-language pathologists. *Language, Speech, and Hearing Services in Schools.*

Taylor, C. (1994). Assessment for measurement or standards: The peril and promise of large-scale assessment reform. *American Educational Research Journal, 31,* 231–262.

Contributors

The Editors

Kevin N. Cole, Ph.D., Research Faculty, Department of Speech and Hearing Sciences, University of Washington, Box 357925, Seattle, WA 98195; and Research Associate, Washington Research Institute, 150 Nickerson Street, Suite 305, Seattle, WA 98109. Dr. Cole's research interests include efficacy of language intervention models, individual differences in response to intervention, and language intervention services to children from diverse cultural and linguistic backgrounds.

Philip S. Dale, Ph.D., Professor, Departments of Psychology, Linguistics, and Speech and Hearing Sciences, University of Washington, Box 351525, Seattle, WA 98195. Dr. Dale's research interests include assessment of young children's language, language development in exceptional populations including linguistically precocious children, early language and cognition, and the effects of various models of intervention for young children with disabilities.

Donna J. Thal, Ph.D., Professor, Department of Communicative Disorders, Director, Developmental Psycholinguistic Laboratory, San Diego State University, San Diego, CA 92182; Associate Research Psychologist, Center for Research in Language, University of California, San Diego, CA 92182. Dr. Thal's research has focused on early prediction of language impairment, relationships between language and nonlinguistic cognition, and cross-population studies of brain–behavior relationships in at-risk infants and toddlers.

The Chapter Authors

Julia L. Evans, Ph.D., Research Scientist, Department of Psychology, Carnegie Mellon University, Pittsburgh, PA 15213, with joint affiliation at Waisman Research Center, University of Wisconsin, Madison, WI 53705. Dr. Evans's research focuses primarily on characterizing language processing deficits of children with language impairments during spontaneous discourse. Her most recent work focuses on a dynamical systems approach to the study of variability in children's language performance.

Julia A. Eyer, Ph.D., Assistant Professor, Speech-Language Pathology, University of Texas at El Paso, Post Office Box 639, El Paso, TX 79968. Dr. Eyer's research interests concern the morphosyntactic development of children with specific language impairment.

Marc E. Fey, Ph.D., Associate Professor, School of Allied Health, Department of Hearing and Speech, University of Kansas Medical Center, 3901 Rainbow Boulevard, Kansas City, KS 66160. Dr. Fey's research and clinical work includes typically developing children as well as children with speech and language impairments. He has special interest in the experimental evaluation of the efficacy of intervention with children with language and literacy problems.

Vera F. Gutierrez-Clellen, Ph.D., Associate Professor and Bilingual Multicultural Professional Services Certificate Coordinator, Department of Communicative Disorders, San Diego State University, San Diego, CA 92182. Dr. Gutierrez-Clellen's research interests focus on language development and literacy in school-age children from Spanish-speaking backgrounds. In addition to her work on children's narratives, she has studied individual differences in mother–child interactions during early language stages.

Jeanette Katich, Graduate student, Department of Communicative Disorders, San Diego State University, San Diego, CA 92182.

Laurence B. Leonard, Ph.D., Distinguished Professor, Department of Audiology and Speech Sciences, Purdue University, West Lafayette, IN 47907. Dr. Leonard has published widely in the areas of language and phonological disorders. In addition to his work on word-finding problems, he has studied the early lexical and phonological characteristics of children with language impairments, as well as the factors affecting the morphosyntactic abilities of these children.

Angela Losardo, Ph.D., Associate Professor, Department of Communication Disorders, Appalachian State University, Boone, NC 28608. Dr. Losardo also teaches in the Birth to Kindergarten Program at Appalachian State University. Her principal research interests focus on language and communication of young children, alternative assessment/evaluation procedures, curricular approaches to early intervention, and preparation of personnel to work in early intervention.

Allyssa McCabe, Ph.D., Associate Professor, Department of Psychology, University of Massachusetts–Lowell, Lowell, MA 01854. Dr. McCabe's research has addressed age changes and parental effects on developing narrative structure, as well as cultural differences in narrative form and traditions, prior to focusing on narrative impairments in children and adults.

Rebecca B. McCathren, Ph.D., Assistant Professor, Department of Special Education, University of Missouri, Columbia, MO 65211. Dr. McCathren's research interests are in early communication and language development.

Jon F. Miller, Ph.D., Professor and Chair, Department of Communicative Disorders, University of Wisconsin–Madison, Madison, WI 53706. Dr. Miller has published widely in the areas of language disorder and language assessment. He is investigating the early language and communication development of children with Down syndrome.

Angela Notari-Syverson, Ph.D., Research Associate, Washington Research Institute, 150 Nickerson Street, Suite 305, Seattle, WA 98109. Dr. Notari-Syverson's work focuses on assessment and intervention in the areas of early language and literacy.

Elizabeth D. Peña, Ph.D., Assistant Professor, Department of Communication Sciences and Disorders, University of Texas at Austin, Austin, TX 78712-1089. Dr. Peña's research explores the role of dynamic assessment and mediated learning in identifying and treating culturally and linguistically diverse children with language disorders.

Mabel L. Rice, Ph.D., University Distinguished Professor, Department of Speech-Language-Hearing, and Director, Child Language Doctoral Program and the Merrill Advanced Studies Center, University of Kansas, Lawrence, KS 66045. Dr. Rice has held Visiting Scientist appointments at MIT and Harvard Graduate School of Education. She has extensive research and clinical experience with children with specific language impairment. Her research addresses several aspects of the condition of specific language impairment: morphosyntax, etiology, social and academic consequences, lexical learning, and preschool language intervention. Her publications include the edited volumes *Teachability of Language* and *Specific Language Impairments in Children* (with Ruth V. Watkins) as well as numerous journal articles and invited chapters.

Carol Stoel-Gammon, Ph.D., Professor, Department of Speech and Hearing Sciences, University of Washington, 1417 N.E. 42nd Street, Seattle, WA 98105-6246. Dr. Stoel-Gammon's research focuses on phonological acquisition in infants and toddlers with particular emphasis on the relationship between prelinguistic and early linguistic development and on early identification of phonological disorders.

Steven F. Warren, Ph.D., Professor, Department of Special Education and Department of Psychology and Human Development, Box 328, Peabody College, Vanderbilt University, Nashville, TN 37203. Dr. Warren also is Deputy Director of the John F. Kennedy Center for Research on Human Development at Vanderbilt University and Co-director of the center's Mental Retardation Research Training Program. He has conducted extensive research on communication and language intervention approaches.

Ruth V. Watkins, Ph.D., Assistant Professor, Department of Speech and Hearing Science, University of Illinois, 901 S. Sixth Street, Champaign, IL 61820. Dr. Watkins's research has focused on characterizing the linguistic impairments of children with specific language impairment and on approaches to intervention with young children with language impairments.

Paul J. Yoder, Ph.D., Associate Professor, Department of Special Education, Box 328, Peabody College, Vanderbilt University, Nashville, TN 37203. Dr. Yoder also is an investigator at the John F. Kennedy Center for Research on Human Development at Vanderbilt University. His research has focused on the social influences of language use and development in children both with and without disabilities. He is developing and testing the efficacy of language and prelinguistic communication interventions on toddlers with mental retardation.

Series Editors:
Steven F. Warren, Ph.D.
Joe Reichle, Ph.D.

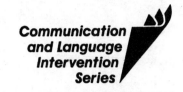

**Communication
and Language
Intervention
Series**

Volume 6

Assessment of
Communication and Language

1

Predicaments in Early Identification of Specific Language Impairment

Does the Early Bird Always Catch the Worm?

Donna J. Thal and Jeanette Katich

CONSIDER THE FOLLOWING SCENARIO: The mother of 2-year-old Kim is concerned because Kim produces only a few words, although he appears to understand as well as other 2-year-olds do and appears to be developing typically in all other respects. Her cousin, a speech-language pathologist, has told her that specific language impairment (SLI) can be a very serious problem and that she should take Kim for a complete language evaluation and be prepared to enroll him in therapy. These recommendations were accompanied by convincing examples of school children who have serious academic problems secondary to language impairment that was first manifested in the preschool years. Kim's pediatrician has told Kim's mother that it is too early to worry, that his level of language is in the typical range for a 2-year-old, and that Kim will catch up without any costly intervention. The pediatrician provided equally convincing examples of children who were late in starting to talk but caught up before starting school and were having no serious problems in school. Who is right? How is this mother to resolve this dilemma, one that parents of toddlers frequently face?

The recommendation of the speech-language pathologist is based on two premises. The first is that language delays identified in 2- to 3-year-old children are likely to persist into the school years and obstruct success in school. The second is that early intervention can correct those delays and prevent, or at least reduce the severity of, later language-learning problems. This chapter considers the first premise by examining the state of the art in early identification of risk for language impairment and attempts to determine whether language delay in 2- to 3-year-olds is a good predictor of SLI at school age.

This work was partially funded by National Institutes of Health Grant #DC00089, Grant #DC00482, and Grant #DC01289.

As a first step in evaluating the ability to identify SLI in the earliest stages, it is necessary to review the characteristics that define the disorder. Next, discussion of predictors of language development in typically developing children introduces the topic of long-term prediction of language development, and studies of outcome for children described as having SLI are presented. Finally, studies of infants and toddlers with language delays are discussed. The chapter concludes with an evaluation of the robustness[1] of proposed predictors of language impairment and recommendations for an appropriate course of action for concerned parents of infants and toddlers.

CHARACTERISTICS OF SPECIFIC LANGUAGE IMPAIRMENT

As the name implies, SLI generally is characterized as a delay in acquisition or as an atypical use of language skills in the presence of typical functioning in other areas, including auditory, neurological, socioemotional, and intellectual domains (Johnson, 1988; Leonard, 1994; Stark & Tallal, 1981). Children characterized as having SLI may have problems with any of the subsystems of language, which include semantics, grammar (syntax and morphology), pragmatics, and phonology. The disorder may manifest with different degrees of severity overall, and there may be distinct problems with comprehension and production. (See Watkins & Rice, 1994, for detailed discussions of SLI.) As this definition suggests, SLI may take many forms; and there are many questions concerning specific characteristics, long-term consequences, and etiology that continue to elude clear answers. Some of these questions make predicting risk for SLI more difficult. Two broadly stated issues are of particular interest: 1) whether SLI is really specific to language or is a result of some other underlying cognitive or perceptual ability and 2) whether SLI is a unitary phenomenon or is a label applied to a number of distinct phenomena. A third issue, heritability of SLI, may make prediction easier in some cases.

Is Specific Language Impairment Specific to Language?

Language impairment accompanies a number of other disorders. By definition, however, *specific* language impairment denotes the absence of other disorders. Ruling out SLI in the early stages of development is not too difficult when disorders such as mental retardation, autism, neurological disease, or serious hearing impairment also are present. As suggested by Whitehurst and Fischel (1994), the term *secondary language delay* is more appropriate here, and such delays should be considered significant risks for language disorders in the school years. However, the distinction between SLI and other language disorders, especially if the other disorders are not severe, is not always easy to determine. Autism, for example, often presents with symptoms very similar to SLI in the early years and

---

[1]Robust in the sense of being consistently reliable and valid; that is, if the particular factor is present, then there is a very high likelihood of a particular outcome.

is difficult to firmly diagnose before 4 years of age (Frith, Soares, & Wing, 1993; Siegel, Pliner, Eschler, & Elliott, 1988).

Differentiating between SLI and disorders in the intellectual domain can be particularly difficult. Many studies have reported relationships between language delay and symbolic play (Lovell, Hoyle, & Siddall, 1968; Lowe & Costello, 1976; Morehead, 1972; Rescorla & Goossens, 1992; Roth & Clark, 1987; Skarakis & Prutting, 1988; Terrell & Schwartz, 1988; Terrell, Schwartz, Prelock, & Messick, 1984; Thal & Bates, 1988; Udwin & Yule, 1983), suggesting a close relationship between language and other cognitive domains in the earliest developmental period. Other researchers have found intellectual delays in nonverbal tasks in older children who have been classified as having SLI (Cromer, 1983; Johnston & Ellis Weismer, 1983; Johnston & Ramstadt, 1983; Nelson, Kamhi, & Apel, 1987; Tallal, Stark, & Mellitis, 1985; see Johnston, 1994, for a review of these studies). Furthermore, studies that have focused on methods for identifying children with SLI for both research and clinical purposes have concluded that there is a serious lack of agreement across different methods.

Cole, Schwartz, Notari, Dale, and Mills (1995) examined the stability of classifying children as having SLI versus those with a more general developmental lag (GDL) (i.e., delayed in both cognitive and linguistic abilities). The children were between 3 and 7 years of age at the first assessment and were examined three times over a 2-year period. Cole and his colleagues reported that the classification of the children changed across assessments over time and varied according to the instrument used. Specifically, only 23% of 22 children originally diagnosed as having SLI and 27% of 26 children originally identified as having a GDL remained in the original category over all three test points. Because only 18% of the children scored within the typical range for both language and cognition at any of the test points (11% at the last test point), the changes in category for children originally identified as having SLI or GDL cannot be explained as recovery; that is, a number of children who were originally classified as having SLI fell into the GDL category at a later date, and vice versa. In fact, some of them switched more than once. It appears, then, that differentiating between SLI and GDL is not a straightforward task, a finding that is compatible with those of Aram, Morris, and Hall (1993) and with arguments posed by Lahey (1990).

Along related lines, Fey, Long, and Cleave (1994) argued that excluding children within the borderline range of intelligence (i.e., with performance IQs between 70 and 85) from being classified as having SLI creates an artificial group. They pointed out that the standard error of measurement rarely is considered when making such categorical assignments, so children who actually are within the typical range of intelligence may be excluded. In addition, because children at the upper end of the IQ score range usually are included, excluding children at the lower end artificially skews the sample of children described as having SLI. In their study, Fey et al. found that the language scores of children with language impairment and IQ scores between 70 and 85 did not differ significantly from those of children with SLI and IQ scores above 85, suggesting that this is not a useful inclusionary/exclusionary criterion for SLI.

Is Specific Language Impairment Unitary or Multifactorial?

Predicting which 2-year-olds are at serious risk for language or learning disabilities may be much more complicated if there are many different routes to language impairment. Determining whether SLI has a single underlying cause or is the result of many different factors is a difficult problem. As noted previously, SLI has a wide range of behavioral profiles, including problems with any of the subcomponents of language, in varying combinations. Although delays in vocabulary are common at the younger ages, the most prevalent symptoms of SLI in the school years are impairments in morphology (Dromi, Leonard, & Shteiman, 1993; Leonard, 1991; Leonard, Bortolini, Caselli, McGregor, & Sabbadini, 1993; Leonard, McGregor, & Allen, 1992; Oetting & Rice, 1993; Rice & Oetting, 1993; Watkins & Rice, 1991; Watkins, Rice, & Moltz, 1993). However, children with SLI may continue to have problems with semantics, pragmatics, and discourse (Bishop & Adams, 1991, 1992; Craig & Evans, 1989, 1993; Grove, Conti-Ramsden, & Donlan, 1993; Mentis, 1991; Vance & Wells, 1994). Arguments concerning the contribution of nonlinguistic cognitive factors also have been noted previously. Given these data, how could a unitary source of language impairment be possible?

If each of these linguistic domains were independent of the other, then children should have impairments in any one of them and typical development in the others. However, Bishop and Edmundson (1987a) pointed out that such patterns rarely occur, and those that occur do not support independence. Bishop and Edmundson described a hierarchy of vulnerability in language functions and argued that the patterns of impairment observed in SLI depend on the severity of the disorder. Disorders of comprehension reflect the most severe form of language impairment, followed by (in order of decreasing severity) disorders of expressive semantics, disorders of morphology and syntax, and disorders of phonology. Thus, children with disorders of language comprehension usually also have disorders of semantics, syntax and morphology, and phonology. Children with disorders of expressive semantics may have typical language comprehension, but they will have disorders of syntax and morphology and phonology. Other children may have disorders of phonology and typical abilities in all of the other areas of language. A maturational lag hypothesis has been proposed as an account for the possible unitary source of this behavioral pattern (Bishop & Edmundson, 1987b; Curtiss & Tallal, 1991). In a more detailed discussion of the research in this area, Bishop (1992) argued that the extant data support an information-processing capacity impairment source for SLI, a proposal that is compatible with the maturational lag hypothesis. Although much work must be done to clearly determine what the process or processes are, a unitary model such as this offers hope that some single measure might be developed to reliably predict SLI in very young children.

In contrast, other investigators (Aram, 1991; Aram & Nation, 1975; Rapin & Allen, 1983; Wilson & Risucci, 1986) have argued that there are distinct subtypes of SLI that may have different etiologies. From this perspective, each different causal mechanism may produce a disorder that is different and that requires a different approach to assessment and remediation. If this is the case, then attempting to identify a single entity will be nonproductive and confusing. In support of this position, Aram, Morris, and Hall (1992, 1993) described a number of studies in which criteria for identifying SLI were compared, and significant mismatches were found. In one study, identification with discrepancy criteria (like those studied by Cole et al., 1995, and Fey et al., 1994) were compared with identification using clinical criteria by "expert clinicians in the field of language disorders" (Aram et al., 1992, p. 551). The authors reported that discrepancy criteria identified only 40%–60% of the preschoolers identified by clinical criteria, depending on the restrictiveness of the discrepancy formula used. In another study, more than 45% of 8-year-olds, selected randomly from typical public school populations around Cleveland, Ohio, were identified as having a language disorder using a discrepancy criterion of 1 standard deviation (SD) difference between performance IQ and language score. When the criterion was changed to a difference of 2 SDs, only 19% were identified as having a language disorder. However, even this is much higher than the 3%–5% reported to occur in the typical population (Leske, 1981). In a third study, wide differences were found between children who were identified as having SLI using clinical versus research criteria (discrepancy formulas). Aram et al. (1993) reported that, depending on the particular formula used, 20%–71% of the children with SLI identified by clinical criteria were classified using the psychometrically defined research criteria. They suggested that using single measures of language and . nonverbal cognitive abilities will always be inadequate and recommended using at least two criteria. Finally, Aram et al. (1993) argued that the lack of cohesion in identifying SLI via the various methods they explored, along with other descriptions in the literature that document wide variation in children with SLI, suggests that SLI is a category that is too broad and nonspecific to be useful. As a result, "it may be necessary to abandon the term as clinically and academically illusive and spurious" (p. 589) and to focus on subtypes of SLI.

The broad disagreement represented by the two perspectives just described makes it clear that much more work must be done to characterize language disorders before truly robust predictors in infants and toddlers can be developed. However, this does not mean that the effort should be abandoned until the nature of language disorders is clearly and accurately defined. On the contrary, if subgroups of children with language impairment occur because of different underlying causes, then studies focused on early predictors may help identify some of the causes and sort out the SLI classification issues.

Familial Inheritance

Researchers have suspected heritability as a factor in SLI for many years. A number of studies in the 1970s and 1980s reported an incidence of family history of similar problems ranging from 20% to 63% (Byrne, Willerman, & Ashmorem, 1974; Heir & Rosenberger, 1980; Luchinger, 1970). These studies primarily were descriptive in nature and did not differentiate between speech and language disorders. In addition, because they did not include typical controls, they cannot reveal whether the incidence of language disorders is atypically high in families of children with language impairment. Fortunately, many studies that included typical controls and used more precisely delineated criteria for identifying subjects have followed.

Virtually all of the ensuing studies have reported a significantly higher proportion of first-degree relatives with histories of language impairment or learning disability in the families of children with SLI than in the families of typical control children. These include Bishop and Edmundson (1986), who reported 32% affected primary relatives; and Tallal, Ross, and Curtiss (1989b), who reported 36% affected mothers, 43% affected fathers, and 37% affected siblings compared with 18%, 24%, and 19%, respectively, for controls. Together, about 40% of the affected parents in the Tallal et al. study had children with SLI (compared with about 20% of the control parents), and children with SLI were significantly more likely than were controls to have at least one affected parent (77% versus 46%). Similar findings have been reported by Lahey and Edwards (1995); Tomblin (1989); and Tomblin, Hardy, and Hein (1991), and further support has been provided by twin studies (Bishop, North, & Donlan, 1995; Lewis & Thompson, 1992).

Some additional studies have attempted to go beyond measuring simple family incidence, and results have been somewhat conflicting. For example, Tallal, Townsend, Curtiss, and Wulfeck (1991) have suggested that children with inherited SLI may be more severely affected and have more problems with attention, activity, and auditory processing than those with no family history. Most of the children in this study had impairments in both comprehension and production, a result that is compatible with the claim by Bishop and Edmundson (1987a) that disorders of comprehension represent the most severe form of SLI. Bishop et al. (1995) and Lahey and Edwards (1995), however, have suggested that specific expressive language impairment may be more likely to be inherited than other forms of the disorder. In a related study, Tallal, Ross, and Curtiss (1989a) suggested that maternal history may be a more powerful factor than a history of language impairment in other relatives.

Two studies have examined family history in younger children. Paul (1991) found that the incidence of family history of language, speech, or learning problems was three to four times more frequent in 2-year-olds with specific language delay than in typical children. In contrast, Whitehurst et al. (1991) found no differences in family history of speech, language, and school problems in 2-year-olds with specific expressive language delay. Whitehurst et al. argued that the difference between their findings and Paul's are due to differences in the children studied. Whitehurst et al. restricted their sample to children with specific expressive language delay, whereas Paul's group contained some children with comprehension impairments. However, Bishop et al. (1995) and Lahey and Edwards (1995) argued that children with specific expressive language delay are more likely to have family histories of language disorders and learning disabilities. In addition, most of Paul's subjects no longer were classified as having SLI by the time they reached second grade (Paul, Hernandez, Herron, & Johnson, 1995), and those studied by Whitehurst had language within the typical range when retested at the age of 5½ (Whitehurst, Fischel, Arnold, & Lonigan, 1992).

Studies of family history of related language disorders have produced conflicting findings. The issue pursued in this chapter is whether 2- to 3-year-olds with a family history of language disorders are at greater risk for SLI than are those without that history. It is clear that there are more questions to be answered before the contribution of family history of language disorders to language assessment can be determined. Family history is known from birth, however, and, with further research, it could serve as a powerful early predictor of SLI.

Although precisely defining SLI (or even agreeing that such a syndrome exists) may not be possible, it is clear that some children have difficulty learning language, which, in turn, may affect the quality of their adult life. Research focused on clarifying the factors that characterize language impairment is moving forward and is likely to provide a clearer picture in the future. The next set of questions to consider, then, is related to outcome for people who have been identified during childhood as having language impairment. A substantial amount of work has been focused directly on determining long-term predictors of outcome for typically developing children and children with language delays. The remainder of the chapter focuses on these studies.

PREDICTING OUTCOME

Can outcome for children such as those previously described be successfully predicted? To answer this question, it is necessary to examine the expected outcome for children who meet the criteria for SLI. However, as the goal is predicting serious language problems at an earlier age, the literature on younger children also should be examined. To that end, it is necessary to examine predicting later language development in typically developing infants and toddlers. Finally, studies that examined outcomes for infants and toddlers with communicative delays are discussed. Because younger children may be either prelinguistic or just beginning to use language, there is very little language behavior to sample. As a result, other factors must be examined as well as the earliest emerging language skills.

Children with Specific Language Impairment

In the late 1970s and throughout the 1980s, researchers in speech-language pathology began to ask about the long-term outcome for children with SLI. A major problem with these studies is that they often did not exclude children with lower-than-normal intellectual levels and, thus, did not differentiate SLI from secondary language impairment. (See Aram & Hall, 1989, for a detailed review of the literature on long-term outcome for children with speech or language disorders.) In addition, the measures used to classify the children when they were originally identified as having language impairment varied widely. These studies, however, provided the first solid information about the longitudinal nature of language impairment.

Three studies have reported outcome at adolescence and/or adulthood for children who had speech or language delays in the school years. In two of the studies (Hall & Tomblin, 1978; King, Jones, & Lasky, 1982), children were identified by reviewing records from childhood, and outcome was determined by informant interview or questionnaire. In both studies, 50%–60% of the children with language impairment continued to have communication problems as adults, and they consistently scored lower on educational tests than did children with only articulation problems. Despite this difference, however, standardized tests indicated that the academic and language abilities of these adolescents generally were well within the typical range. Using a direct-testing method in the follow-up, Aram, Ekelman, and Nation (1984) reported an even higher proportion (69%) of children with continuing educational and/or language problems. The best predictor of outcome in this study was IQ score on the Leiter International Performance Scale (Leiter, 1969), a nonverbal test of intellectual ability. Thus, although some speech and language problem persisted in all of these groups, good academic, social, and emotional outcomes occurred in many of the individuals. In addition, because children with low IQ scores were excluded from only one of the studies and because IQ was the best predictor of outcome in another, it is impossible to eliminate more general cognitive factors as the possible cause of continued language problems.

Silva (1980) and his colleagues (Silva, McGee, & Williams, 1983; Silva, Williams, & McGee, 1987) conducted a population survey in which a large cohort of children selected to represent the typical range of language abilities was followed from birth to 11 years of age. At 3 years of age, the children with language delays were identified and divided into three groups: comprehension delay only, expressive delay only, and general language delay (both comprehension and production). Forty percent of all children with language delay at 3 years still experienced delay at 5 years, and 31% of those with delay at 5 years still experienced delay at 7 years, percentages that are much higher than expected by chance. Fifty-three percent to 79% of the children with general language delay (i.e., comprehension and production) at 3 years had continued delay at 5 years or

7 years, suggesting that this pattern is one of greatest risk. In addition, stable language delays (i.e., those that were present at all three data points) were associated with a greater prevalence of later low IQ and reading difficulties. Unfortunately, because no measures of IQ were taken at 3 years, it is impossible to determine whether the results reflect an outcome of early language delay or of early general intellectual delay. Silva et al. (1983) also noted much variability in the population studied: "More children moved out of the category of language delay between the ages of three to five and five to seven than stayed in it. At the same time, many children who were not delayed at age 3 were delayed at age 5 or 7" (p. 791). In their follow-up at 9 and 11 years of age, Silva et al. (1987) reported that all three groups were significantly overrepresented in the low-IQ group and in the group with low reading scores. However, at age 11, these results held only for the children with impairments in both comprehension and production. Thus, the poorest long-term outcome was reported for children who had a more general language delay. Because no IQ measures were administered at the earlier ages, however, it is impossible to rule out intellectual problems as a contributing source to the continued language and educational problems.

A number of shorter follow-up studies also have been conducted (Bishop & Adams, 1990; Bishop & Edmundson, 1987a, 1987b; Stark et al., 1984). Stark et al. (1984) compared outcome in 29 children with SLI, first tested between 4½ and 8 years, with that of 14 typically developing children when both groups were between 8 and 12 years of age. They reported that younger children with SLI improved more rapidly than did older children with SLI and that 25% of the children with SLI (usually the younger ones) were reclassified as typical at follow-up. The rest of the children with SLI showed some continued delay in language, and the ones who scored in the typical range still showed a significant gap between performance IQ and linguistic abilities. Bishop and her colleagues studied outcomes for a group of children with language impairment who were first studied at 4 years of age and were examined at regular intervals until they were 8½. At 5½, about half of the children still experienced delay (Bishop & Edmundson, 1987b). The best predictor of this outcome was expressive semantics exhibited in a discourse assessment task. At 8½, approximately 70% of the children who continued to experience delay at 5½ had reading and oral language problems. Many of those children demonstrated poor comprehension of what they read despite reading accuracy, and this was accompanied by impaired oral language comprehension. However, 96% of the children who had typical language at 5½ continued to have typical language and literacy skills at 8½ (Bishop & Adams, 1990).

A number of useful generalizations can be gleaned from the studies just described, generalizations that add to the information that will be useful in the search for predictors of risk from younger ages. First, it is consistently reported that younger children have a better prognosis. If children who are functioning within the typical range by 5 years have no trouble in school and if many children move into and out of the category of having language impairment across the period from 3 to 5 years of age, then identifying younger children who will have continuing problems will be very difficult. Second, lower intellectual level appears to be a frequent accompaniment of continued language delay; disorders that include problems with comprehension as well as production also have a poorer prognosis. Finally, many children continue to have some problems with language-related abilities later in life, even after many years of intervention, although those problems are not always severely disabling.

Typically Developing Infants and Toddlers

Many studies of development in typical children have focused on the problem of predicting later language and cognitive abilities from measures obtained in infancy. They are divided here into three categories: 1) those that examine behavioral and environmental variables, 2) those that use habituation or operant-looking preference paradigms to test the children, and 3) those that have used newer auditory evoked-response measures.

Behavioral and Environmental Variables In 1969, Bayley concluded that standardized tests were of little value in long-term prediction of intellectual skills prior to 24 months of age. Subsequent studies have upheld this conclusion and have identified other, more specific, factors that predict language and cognitive skills from infancy to preschool and early school years.

Bee et al. (1982) explored the ability of a number of behavioral and environmental variables identified in infancy to predict language and intellectual development at 3 and 4 years of age in healthy middle- and working-class children. Although no single variable was sufficient to predict preschool outcome, a cluster of variables (termed family ecology) was. These included social support of the mother during pregnancy, birth, and the first year and the mother's level of education. Siegel (1981, 1982) reported similar findings for pre- and full-term infants. In those studies, socioeconomic status (SES); birth order; maternal smoking; and, for the preterm infants only, severity of illness in the perinatal period were the best predictors of scores on the Reynell Developmental Language Scales (Reynell, 1977) at 2 and 3 years of age, the Bayley Scales of Infant Development (Bayley, 1969) at 2, and the Stanford-Binet Intelligence Scale (Terman & Merrill, 1960) at 3 years of age. Walker, Greenwood, Hart, and Carta (1994) found that early differences in the number of words produced, IQ, and SES were related to language and scholastic abilities in the school years. They argued that the language and IQ variables were related to different parenting styles that were directly related to SES. Hart and Risley (1995) supported this perspective; they reported that 3-year-old children from very low–SES families had consistently lower word production, had slower vocabulary growth between 1 and 3 years of age, and used a smaller number and variety of grammatical devices than did those from professional families. In addition, language level at 3 years of age predicted language level in the third grade. Detailed analysis of the language input and interactional styles experienced by the children in their homes when they were between 1 and 3 years of age pointed to specific sources for these differences. Parents in lower-SES families talked significantly less to their children and provided a narrower range of exemplars than did the professional families. They also provided significantly more negative feedback to their children and used significantly more negative imperatives than did the higher-SES parents. Thus, SES appears to be a very strong predictor of later language ability in typically developing children as a function of different parent interactional styles.

Two researchers have focused on specific language variables as predictors of later language development. In a group of typical toddlers studied biweekly from 12 to 20 months of age and then retested at 2 and 3 years of age, comprehension was the only reliable predictor of language development at 2 and 3 years (Rescorla, 1984). Production was much less useful and seemed to be more affected by other factors, such as phonological skills or motivational factors, than was comprehension. Similarly, Bates, Bretherton, and Snyder (1988) reported that comprehension (but not production) at 13 months of age was highly correlated with production vocabulary at 20 months and that production vocabulary at 20 months of age was the best predictor of mean length of utterance (MLU) at 2½ years of age, suggesting that comprehension plays a major role in the earliest stages of language development.

Habituation and Operant-Looking Preference Paradigms   Habituation and operant-looking preference measures are the most widely used techniques for learning about what infants know. In habituation studies, a visual stimulus is presented to infants until they tire of it and stop looking (i.e., they are habituated). Then a new stimulus is presented. If the infants recognize the new stimulus as something different, then they will begin looking again (i.e., they will dishabituate); if they do not recognize it as different, then habituation will continue, and they will have no interest in looking at the stimulus. In operant-looking studies, a reinforcement is associated with one stimulus versus another. Once the child is trained to look at a particular object or place when the stimulus appears, other stimuli are introduced. If the infant recognizes a new stimulus, then she or he will look in the direction of the reinforcer. Habituation studies often are used to examine memory and attention, while operant-looking studies usually examine threshold phenomena. Studies have consistently shown that habituation and operant-looking responses predict aspects of language and intelligence at later dates (Benasich & Tallal, 1994; Bornstein & Tamis-LeMonda, 1995; Fagan & McGrath, 1981; Henderson & Trehub, 1995; Lewis & Brooks-Gunn, 1981; Tamis-LeMonda & Bornstein, 1989; Tamis-LeMonda & Dyssegaard, 1994; Thompson, Fagan, & Fulker, 1991).

Good prediction of vocabulary at 3–4 years of age from visual recognition memory measured by habituation between 4 and 7 months of age has been demonstrated (Fagan & McGrath, 1981; Thompson et al., 1991), with higher predictions for comprehension than for production. Other researchers have included environmental variables specific to maternal input along with measures of infant memory to predict later language and cognitive abilities. Tamis-LeMonda and Bornstein (1989) examined the relationship between memory (as measured by habituation) and maternal encouragement of attention at 5 months of age and language (comprehension and production) and play at 13 months. Both factors were found to predict language and play at 13 months of age. This result has been replicated in a study of children in four different countries: Argentina, France, Japan, and the United States. In a later study, these 13-month measures predicted language and play at 21 months of age (Tamis-LeMonda & Dyssegaard, 1994), results that are compatible with an earlier report by Olson, Bates, and Bayles (1984). In other studies (reported in Bornstein & Tamis-LeMonda, 1995), Bornstein's group found that mothers who referred to objects more at 13 months had children with larger productive vocabularies, longer utterances, and greater semantic diversity at 20 months. They also reported that maternal verbal responsiveness at 9 months predicted child language level at 13 months, while verbal directiveness did not. These studies suggest that a number of factors may play a role in child language development. Some of them, such as the child's ability to process information, reside in the child. Other factors, such as the infant's experience with responsive parenting styles, reside in the external environment. They also are compatible with the SES findings reported previously, which point to the impact of diminished input.

Research with older children with SLI demonstrated a selective impairment in the ability of these children to process rapidly changing auditory stimuli (auditory temporal processing); the auditory processing impairment was highly correlated with the degree of language comprehension impairment (Tallal & Piercy, 1974; Tallal et al., 1985). Techniques for measuring auditory temporal processing in infants and toddlers have been developed, and researchers have begun to explore whether later language development can be predicted by this nonlinguistic ability. Benasich and Tallal (1995) have developed an operant conditioning paradigm for testing auditory temporal processing in infants using speech and speech-like stimuli that have been used with older children with language impairment. They found that auditory temporal processing ability at 5–10 months of age successfully predicted language in the second year. Similar results were reported by Henderson and Trehub (1995), who used pure tone stimuli to study auditory temporal processing abilities in infants. These studies suggest that auditory temporal processing ability in the first year of life is related to language ability in the second year of life and that it may be useful for identifying children who have difficulty processing rapidly occurring auditory stimuli. As this problem is found in many children classified as having SLI (Tallal & Piercy, 1973a, 1973b, 1974, 1975), techniques for measuring auditory temporal processing may be developed into a good early prediction test for some children who have serious language impairment that will persist into and throughout the school years.

Evoked-Response Measures   Evoked-response-potential (ERP) studies use the electrical activity of the brain as their basic measure. The ERP is a portion of a standard electroencephalogram (EEG) that is time locked to the onset of some event in the person's environment. Electrodes are attached to a number of places on the scalp, and the electrical output of the brain in response to various stimuli is measured at each of the sites. A number of studies have shown changes in locus of brain activity with increasing language ability (Mills, Coffey, & Neville, 1993, 1994; Mills, Coffey-Corina, & Neville, submitted; Mills, Thal, Di Iulio, Castaneda, & Neville, 1995), suggesting that this technique may be developed into a useful assessment tool.

Molfese (1989, 1994) and his colleagues examined the relationship between language stimuli and ERPs in early childhood and infancy in order to predict later language skills (Molfese, Burger-Judisch, & Hans, 1991; Molfese, Gill, & Benshoff, 1994; Molfese & Molfese, 1985, 1988; Molfese, Morse, & Peters, 1990). Auditory evoked responses were recorded from infants within the first 36 hours after birth (Molfese, 1989, 1994). Electrodes were placed on the scalp on sites directly over the temporal lobe on both sides of the head, and infants heard either artificially synthesized b + vowel or g + vowel syllables or nonspeech control stimuli matched to the formants of the speech syllables. At 3 years of age, the same children were tested on the verbal subscale of the McCarthy Scales of Children's Abilities (McCarthy, 1972). In one study (Molfese & Molfese, 1988), the children were divided into two equal groups by a median split based on the McCarthy Scales scores. For the high-language group only, infant ERPs on the left side (reflecting activity in the left hemisphere of the brain) showed higher activity for the speech stimuli. The right side was more active for the nonspeech stimuli. In a larger study (Molfese, 1994), 3-year-old children were divided into three groups based on scores on the Stanford-Binet Intelligence Scale language subscales: 16 children scored at least 1 SD below the mean, 47 scored within 1 SD, and 16 scored at least 1 SD above the mean. Infant ERPs successfully classified all 16 low children, 50 of the average children, and 13 of the high children. Many of these children were tested again at 5 years of age (Molfese et al., 1994), and the infant ERPs continued to predict their language level.

The studies of typical children just described are very helpful in suggesting behaviors to examine in children who are slow to develop language and also are helpful in suggesting measures that may help identify children who are at risk for serious language impairment. A number of variables appear to be consistently related to later language level: socioeconomic status, comprehension, and memory. A number of factors, some within the child and others related to environmental input, are likely to provide more solid prediction of later language than is any single factor. New technologies, including measures of auditory temporal processing and localization of brain-wave activity while attending to speech, provide hope that some relatively simple, direct measures of cognitive skills in infancy and early childhood may provide useful predictive information about later language development in the not-too-distant future.

Late-Talking Infants and Toddlers

Because there has been little agreement as to the reliability of identifying SLI as a clinically significant disorder prior to 3 or 4 years of age, researchers studying younger children with language delays refer to them as late talkers. Three longitudinal cohorts have been described in numerous studies by research groups in Pennsylvania (Rescorla, 1993a, 1993b, 1994; Rescorla & Goossens, 1992; Rescorla, Hadicke-Wiley, & Escarce, 1993; Rescorla & Schwartz, 1990), Oregon (Paul, 1991; Paul & Alforde, 1993; Paul et al., 1995; Paul & Jennings, 1992; Paul, Laszio, McFarland, & Midford, 1993; Paul, Lynn, & Lohr-Flanders, 1993; Paul & Riback, 1993; Paul & Schiffer, 1991), and New York (Whitehurst et al., 1993; Whitehurst et al., 1991; Whitehurst & Fischel, 1994). In the longest study, Rescorla's group (1993a, 1993b, 1994) described the outcome for approximately 25 late talkers who were followed yearly from 24 to 30 months through 8 years of age. Children in this cohort had typical nonverbal ability as indicated by the Bayley Scales of Infant Development; age-adequate receptive language; and expressive language, which was at least 5 months below their chronological age. At the first few follow-ups, the late talkers continued to experience delay, although they began (as a group) to move into the typical range in selected areas of language. At 3 years of age, they were at age level in receptive language; single-word expressive vocabulary; and the ability to use language to define, explain, and describe. They were, however, below age level in MLU, used fewer syntactically complete sentences containing a subject and a verb, and produced fewer morphemes in obligatory contexts. At 4 years of age, they continued to experience delay in grammatical competence. Rescorla and Schwartz (1990) noted that greater age at identification and severity of the expressive language delay were the best predictors of continued delay. By 5 years of age, however, late talkers scored within the typical range on the Verbal Factor Score of the Stanford-Binet Intelligence Scale and in syntax. They also were within norms on various prereading and reading skills tests. At 6 years of age, late talkers had average scores on a wide range of language skills and on tests of reading mastery and phonological awareness. Typical scores on tests of language and other academic skills continued at 7 and 8 years of age. At every age, however, the scores of the late talkers were significantly lower than those of the age-matched controls (who had been identified and followed at the same ages) on some standardized tests.

Paul's group (Paul & Alforde, 1993; Paul et al., 1995; Paul, Laszio, et al., 1993; Paul & Riback, 1993) carried out similar yearly evaluations of 30 late talkers from 18 to 30 months of age through second grade. At each yearly follow-up, their spontaneous language was analyzed using Developmental Sentence Scoring (DSS) (Lee, 1974), and they were compared with typical age-matched controls. At 3 years of age, 42% of the children had moved into the typical range on the DSS and were categorized as children with a history of expressive language delay (HELD); 58% continued to experience expressive language delay (ELD). SES was the only significant predictor of outcome at age 3 (Paul, 1989). The group with HELD did not perform exactly like typical controls, however. When specific word-class categories were analyzed, the group with HELD used significantly fewer pronouns and verbs than did typical controls. At 4 years of age, 63% of the children were classified as having HELD, and they did not differ significantly from typical controls on any of the specific word classes (Paul & Riback, 1993). Their MLU also was no different from typical controls, but they used fewer grammatical morphemes in obligatory contexts (Paul & Alforde, 1993). When they entered kindergarten, the groups with HELD and ELD were combined and compared with typical controls on a number of standardized measures (Paul, Laszio, et al., 1993). The late talkers scored within the typical range on standardized tests of language production and reading readiness but significantly lower than typical controls, a result that is compatible with those reported by Rescorla (1993a, 1993b, 1994). Using the DSS, 37% of the children continued to experience ELD at the kindergarten data point. In first grade, 27% continued to experience ELD; by second grade, it was only 14% (4 of 28 children). That is, by second grade, 86% (24 out of 28) of the children who were identified as late talkers between 18 and 24 months of age were within the typical range on spontaneous language production as analyzed by the DSS. Paul et al. (1995) also examined narrative structure in order to explore higher-level language skills. At kindergarten, the group with HELD and the group with ELD were lower than typical controls on lexical diversity in narratives and stage of narrative development (following Applebee, 1978), and the group with ELD (but not with HELD) was lower than controls on cohesive adequacy (following Liles, 1985). At first grade, the group with HELD and the group with ELD were lower than typical controls only on narrative stage assignment. At second grade, both groups of late talkers performed within the typical range on all measures of narrative use.

Similar long-term outcomes have been reported by Whitehurst's group (Whitehurst & Fischel, 1994; Whitehurst et al., 1992). They identified thirty-seven 2-year-old late talkers with expressive delays that were more severe than those studied by Rescorla's and Paul's research groups (at least 2 SDs below the mean on the Expressive One-Word Picture Vocabulary Test [Gardner, 1979]). They then measured phonological and expressive vocabulary outcome at 3½ and 5½ years of age. At 3½, 88% of the children had typical vocabulary, and 65% had typical phonological skills. At 5½, 96% had typical vocabulary, and 78% had typical phonology. Although they did not use any measures of syntax, they obtained reading and math scores from the schools for 22 of the late talkers when they were 7 years old; these scores were well within the typical range. Whitehurst et al. (1992) found a higher incidence of drooling and of choking on food in the late talkers than in typical children when they were 2 years of age. In addition, at a follow-up 5 months after identification, children with a higher proportion of consonants in their babble at identification had more rapid vocabulary growth (Whitehurst et al., 1991), and vocabulary size at identification was the best predictor of vocabulary status at the follow-up (Fischel, Whitehurst, Caulfield, & DeBaryshe, 1989). Because the vast majority of these children were within the typical range at the later follow-up points, however, there is no support for the claim that any of these factors could be reliable predictors of SLI. The evidence from these three longitudinal studies strongly suggests that children in the 2-year-old range who have delays only in expressive language are not at serious risk for continuing language and learning problems.

In San Diego, another research group has focused on language and nonlinguistic cognition in late talkers (Thal & Bates, 1988; Thal, Bates, Goodman, & Jahn-Samilo, 1995; Thal & Tobias, 1992, 1994; Thal, Tobias, & Morrison, 1991). All of the studies carried out by this group followed children over a shorter period of time, and most used a smaller number of children than did those described previously. However, because the researchers used more focused experimental measures rather than standardized tests, the studies help extend clinicians' understanding of the nature and course of SLI.

In the first outcome study from this group, Thal et al. (1991) reported a 1-year follow-up for 10 children who were identified as late talkers when they were between 18 and 28 months of age. At the follow-up, 4 of the 10 children still experienced delay, and 6 had typical expressive vocabulary and MLU. These two groups were then compared using data from the original assessment. The children who still experienced delay 1 year later experienced delay in word comprehension and gesture production (on structured gesture imitation tasks) at the first visit, whereas those who caught up had demonstrated typical levels of behavior in both of those domains. Thus, the children who caught up were those who were similar to children with ELD described by Rescorla's and Whitehurst's groups. Thal and Tobias (1992) then compared the use of communicative gestures at the first visit from the same two subgroups. They found that the late talkers who continued to experience delay used significantly fewer communicative gestures than did typical age-matched controls. Those who caught up, however, used significantly more gestures for communicative purposes than did age-matched controls and used them for a wider range of communicative purposes. Based on these studies, comprehension and gesture production were proposed as potential reliable predictors of language outcome.

Similar results for late talkers with specific ELD were reported with another cohort of late talkers (Oroz, Thal, & Cleveland, 1993; Thal, Oroz, Evans, Katich, & Leasure, 1995; Thal & Tobias, 1994). At the first visit, the late talkers with ELD demonstrated typical vocabulary comprehension and typical use of gestures, as in the earlier studies by Thal's group. In addition, they showed patterns of development similar to those described by the other three research groups. Within 1 year, expressive vocabulary was within the typical range. Analysis of vocabulary composition, however, revealed that late talkers with ELD did not use some of the later-developing word classes (specifically auxiliary verbs and conjunctions) as often as did typically developing children, and their MLU was significantly lower. By the 2-year follow-up, when children were around 4 years old, they performed like typical controls in use of auxiliary verbs and conjunctions and on MLU.

Thal, Oroz, et al. (1995) took another approach, which focused specifically on predictors of early delayed language development, using the MacArthur Communicative Development Inventories (CDI) (Fenson et al., 1993). The CDI are parent-report instruments that sample aspects of communicative development from 8 to 30 months of age. The CDI: Words and Gestures (Infant form) samples word comprehension, word production, and gesture production. It is normed on children between 8 and 16 months of age. The CDI: Words and Sentences (Toddler form) samples word production, utterance length, and grammatical complexity. Norms for this version cover 16–30 months of age. In two studies, data from the original norming population were used; in a third, new data were collected.

The two studies that used data from the original norming sample focused on children whose parents had completed the CDI twice in order to establish test–retest reliability. Subjects included 217 children whose parents filled out the Infant form when they were a mean age of 13 months and the Toddler form when they were approximately 20 months of age (Infant-Toddler cohort) and 185 children whose parents filled out the Toddler form twice, once when they were about 20 months and again when they were about 26 months of age (Toddler-Toddler cohort). These were largely middle-class children with typical birth histories, no medical syndromes, and no extended illnesses or other serious medical problems. All children were from monolingual English-speaking homes, although some exposure to a second language was not an exclusionary criterion. For both groups of children, a number of environmental variables were examined as possible predictors of later language ability: birth order, socioeconomic status, maternal education, paternal education, maternal vocation, paternal vocation, gender, ethnicity, presence of mild medical problems, and second-language exposure.

In this strongly middle-class sample, none of the environmental variables were identified as predictors of language delay at the second data point for either group of children. For the Infant-Toddler cohort, 30 children were in the lowest 10% for word production at the second data point, thus qualifying as late talkers. Word production, gesture production, and the percentage of receptive vocabulary produced (i.e., number of words produced divided by the number of words understood) at the first data point significantly differentiated between the children with delays and the children without delays. In addition, a regression analysis indicated that two of those factors—the number of gestures produced and the percentage of receptive vocabulary actually produced at 13 months of age—were the best predictors of language status at 20 months. For the Toddler-Toddler cohort, 24 children qualified as late talkers at the second data point. As a group, those children had been significantly behind the rest of the group on number of words produced, utterance length, and grammatical complexity at the first data point. Thus, for both groups of children, communicative status at the first data point, based on either language or gesture, predicted outcome 6–7 months later.

Because clinicians must make decisions about individual children, discriminate analysis was used to estimate the ability to predict continuity for individuals in the groups described. In the Infant-Toddler cohort, using the same factors that differentiated between children with and without delays in the group analysis just described (vocabulary production, gesture production, and the proportion of receptive vocabulary produced as predictors), 10% of the children who were late talkers at the second data point and 24% of the children who were typical at the second data point were misassigned. In the Toddler-Toddler cohort (using vocabulary production, utterance length, and grammatical complexity), 27% of the children who were late talkers at the second data point and 20% of the children who were typical were misassigned. Thus, although continuity clearly was present at a group level, the ability to predict outcome for individuals was much more limited.

In the third study reported by Thal, Bates, et al. (1995), 28 children were followed monthly with the CDI from 8 to 30 months of age. The Infant form was given from 8 to 16 months and the Toddler form from 17 to 30 months. Between 18 and 24 months (the age at which most studies of late talkers have identified their cohorts), 5 of the 28 children scored in the lowest 10% (qualifying as late talkers). Of those five, only one was in the lowest 10% at 30 months. The others scored at the 12th, 24th, 26th, and 73rd percentiles. Even if the child at the 12th percentile were classified as a late talker, only 40% of the children retained their late-talker status. Thus, the predictive value of late-talker status at 18–24 months was not useful for determining the status of these five individuals at 30 months of age.

Two other studies have examined individual outcome in a small number of subjects. Weismer, Murray-Branch, and Miller (1994) examined development of four late talkers over a 21-month period. Expressive vocabulary was within the typical range for three of the four children at 34–35 months of age and below it for one. The child who continued to experience delay and two of the children who caught up had received therapy, while the other child caught up without therapy. The child who did not receive therapy also was within the typical range for MLU. The child with continued vocabulary delay also experienced substantial delay in MLU. The other two children were below expectations for their age but did not experience serious delay on MLU. Weismer et al. (1994) reported that expressive language level (vocabulary and MLU) did not predict outcome for any of these children. Comprehension was not delayed enough in any of the children to attempt to use as a predictor. However, at least one of the children did not have typical vocabulary by 34–35 months, an outcome that might be expected from group studies of children with ELD. Finally, symbolic play (as measured by the Symbolic Play Test [Lowe & Costello, 1976]) did not predict outcome for the individual children. The subject with the best outcome had the poorest score on the Symbolic Play Test.

Tobias (1995) examined the development of three late talkers with expressive and receptive language delays over a period of 2 years. Two of the children were within the typical range for expressive vocabulary and MLU at the 2-year follow-up, although their trajectory of development was flatter (i.e., they developed more slowly) than for a comparable group of late talkers with typical comprehension. The third continued to experience delay in all aspects of language. Neither use of gestures in experimental gesture imitation tasks nor comprehension delay predicted that status of these late talkers 2 years later when they were about 4½ years old.

These late-talker studies converge on a number of important findings. As a group, children with early ELD but typical comprehension may be expected to function within the typical range in most areas of language by kindergarten, and they are not at risk for problems in later grades. In addition, a number of factors—language comprehension and production, gesture production, and SES—predict language outcome for late talkers *at the group level;* however, none of the variables that appear to be reliable predictors at the group level are adequate predictors of outcome for individual children, at least over the approximately 2-year period examined in studies that focused on individual children.

CONCLUSION

Returning to the scenario described at the beginning of this chapter, are there robust predictors that Kim's mother, the speech-language pathologist, and the pediatrician can use to determine whether Kim should be enrolled in therapy? The answer to that question must be no. No *single* known factor can reliably predict later language status even for well-defined groups of children and certainly not for an individual child. Yet decisions must be made about individual children. The problems arise from a number of different factors:

1. There still is no agreement as to the nature of this phenomenon. Separating SLI from more general mild intellectual impairment continues to be an obstacle, and it is not known whether SLI is a unitary phenomenon with a single cause or a number of different syndromes that each have a unique cause.

2. Outcome and symptomatology vary widely depending on the age of the child, and children move into and out of the SLI category at many different

ages, with and without therapy. As Whitehurst and Fischel (1994) pointed out, "The frequency and patterning of language delays vary so greatly with age that data taken from one age group ... may have little relevance to other age groups" (p. 639).

3.   Single measures of language are consistently inadequate for determining whether a child is developing typically or is experiencing delay at any age, and they become less and less reliable for younger and younger children.

Does this mean that there is nothing to be done, no valid advice to give parents of children like Kim? Again, the answer is no. Much has been learned about the nature of early language development, all of which is useful in a risk-factor model such as that used by physicians (and recommended by Whitehurst & Fischel, 1994, for use with late talkers). If a patient has a high cholesterol level, then there is an elevated risk of heart attack, but no physician can reliably predict that a heart attack will or will not occur. If the patient also has a family history of heart disease and does not exercise, then the risk is higher. However, physicians still cannot say if or when a heart attack will occur. Identifying serious language impairment in the earliest stages is a similar proposition.

The longitudinal studies of late talkers all suggest that the majority of children who have specific *expressive* language delay prior to 3 years of age are not at serious risk for language or language-learning disorders in the school years, even without intervention. After 3, and certainly by 5 years of age, however, specific expressive language delay is much more likely to continue into the school years and affect reading as well as other language-related learning. In addition, the literature on typically developing children and children with language delays strongly suggests that delays in addition to expressive language delay may add up to substantial risk, depending on the nature, severity, number, and duration of those delays. Some of the factors that have been consistently correlated with language outcome, across a number of studies and ages, include language comprehension, size of comprehension–production gap, use of communicative gestures, intellectual ability, presence of symbolic play, use of true consonants in babble, memory, information processing capacity, SES, family history, and parental interaction style. Furthermore, although studies on the effects of otitis media have been highly contradictory (e.g., Bishop & Edmundson, 1986; Lonigan, Fischel, Whitehurst, Arnold, & Valdez-Menchaca, 1992; Paul, 1991; Teele, Klein, & Rosner, 1980), a possible connection between otitis media and temporal processing impairments in children with SLI has been suggested (Tallal et al., 1996). These are some of the risk factors that must be evaluated in careful, accurate assessments of infants and toddlers who are at risk for language impairment. Depending on the number of factors present and how the child and family are handling any communication breakdowns, a number of interventions are possible. These include a variety of approaches across the whole spectrum of intensiveness and directness from the very indirect "watch and see" recommended by Paul (in press), to home programs administered by parents under the guidance of a speech-language pathologist, to more intensive intervention based on individual needs.

REFERENCES

Applebee, N. (1978). *The child's concept of story*. Chicago: University of Chicago Press.

Aram, D. (1991). Comments on specific language impairment as a clinical category. *Language, Speech, and Hearing Services in Schools, 22*, 84–87.

Aram, D., Ekelman, B., & Nation, J. (1984). Preschoolers with language disorders: 10 years later. *Journal of Speech and Hearing Research, 27*, 232–244.

Aram, D., & Hall, N. (1989). Longitudinal follow-up of children with preschool communication disorders: Treatment implications. *School Psychology Review, 18*, 487–501.

Aram, D., Morris, R., & Hall, N. (1992). The validity of discrepancy criteria for identifying children with developmental language disorders. *Journal of Learning Disabilities, 25*, 549–554.

Aram, D., Morris, R., & Hall, N. (1993). Clinical and research congruence in identifying children with specific language impairment. *Journal of Speech and Hearing Research, 36*, 580–591.

Aram, D., & Nation, J. (1975). Patterns of language behavior in children with developmental language disorders. *Journal of Speech and Hearing Research, 18*, 229–241.

Bates, E., Bretherton, I., & Snyder, L. (1988). *From first words to grammar.* New York: Academic Press.

Bayley, N. (1969). *Bayley Scales of Infant Development*. New York: The Psychological Corporation.

Bee, H., Barnard, K., Eyres, S., Gray, C., Hammond, M., Spietz, A., Snyder, C., & Clark, B. (1982). Prediction of IQ and language skill from perinatal status, child performance, family characteristics, and mother–infant interaction. *Child Development, 53*, 1134–1156.

Benasich, A., & Tallal, P. (1994, June). *Relationships among infant auditory temporal processing thresholds, perceptual-cognitive abilities and language development in the first two years.* Poster presented at the biennial meeting of the International Conference on Infant Studies, Paris, France.

Benasich, A., & Tallal, P. (1995). *Auditory temporal processing thresholds, habituation, and recognition memory in the first year of life.* Manuscript submitted for publication.

Bishop, D. (1992). The underlying nature of specific language impairment. *Journal of Child Psychology and Psychiatry, 33*, 3–66.

Bishop, D., & Adams, C. (1990). A prospective study of the relationship between SLI, phonological disorders, and reading retardation. *Journal of Child Psychology and Psychiatry, 31*, 1027–1050.

Bishop, D., & Adams, C. (1991). What do referential communication tasks measure? A study of children with specific language impairment. *Applied Psycholinguistics, 12*, 199–215.

Bishop, D., & Adams, C. (1992). Comprehension problems in children with specific language impairment: Literal and inferential meaning. *Journal of Speech and Hearing Research, 35*, 119–129.

Bishop, D., & Edmundson, A. (1986). Is otitis media a major cause of specific developmental language disorders? *British Journal of Communication Disorders, 21*, 321–338.

Bishop, D., & Edmundson, A. (1987a). Language-impaired 4-year-olds: Distinguishing transient from persistent impairment. *Journal of Speech and Hearing Research, 52,* 156–173.

Bishop, D., & Edmundson, A. (1987b). Specific language impairment as a maturational lag: Evidence from longitudinal data on language and motor development. *Developmental Medicine and Child Neurology, 29,* 442–459.

Bishop, D., North, T., & Donlan, C. (1995). Genetic basis of specific language impairment: Evidence from a twin study. *Developmental Medicine and Child Neurology, 37,* 56–71.

Bornstein, M., & Tamis-LeMonda, C. (1995). Language and nonlanguage factors in child development from prelinguistic vocalization to linguistic communication. In G. Konopczynski (Ed.), *Is early language performance predictive of later language development* (pp. 31–67). Calais, France: Ortho-Editions.

Byrne, B., Willerman, L., & Ashmorem, L. (1974). Severe and moderate language impairment: Evidence for distinctive etiologies. *Behavior Genetics, 4,* 331–345.

Cole, K., Schwartz, I., Notari, A., Dale, P., & Mills, P. (1995). Examination of the stability of two methods of defining specific language impairment. *Applied Psycholinguistics, 16,* 103–123.

Craig, H., & Evans, J. (1989). Turn exchange characteristics of SLI children's simultaneous and nonsimultaneous speech. *Journal of Speech and Hearing Disorders, 54,* 334–347.

Craig, H., & Evans, J. (1993). Pragmatics and SLI: Within-group variations in discourse behaviors. *Journal of Speech and Hearing Research, 36,* 777–789.

Cromer, R. (1983). Hierarchical planning disability in the drawings and constructions of a special group of severely aphasic children. *Brain and Cognition, 2,* 144–164.

Curtiss, S., & Tallal, P. (1991). On the nature of the impairment in language-impaired children. In J. Miller (Ed.), *Research on child language disorders: A decade of progress* (pp. 189–210). Austin, TX: PRO-ED.

Dromi, E., Leonard, L., & Shteiman, S. (1993). The grammatical morphology of Hebrew-speaking children with SLI: Some competing hypotheses. *Journal of Speech and Hearing Research, 36,* 760–771.

Fagan, J., & McGrath, S. (1981). Infant recognition memory and later intelligence. *Intelligence, 5,* 121–130.

Fenson, L., Dale, P., Reznick, J.S., Thal, D., Bates, E., Reilly, J., & Hartung, J. (1993). *The MacArthur Communicative Development Inventories: Manual and norms.* San Diego: Singular.

Fey, M., Long, S., & Cleave, P. (1994). Reconsideration of IQ criteria in the definition of specific language impairment. In R.V. Watkins & M.L. Rice (Eds.), *Communication and language intervention series: Vol. 4. Specific language impairments in children* (pp. 161–178). Baltimore: Paul H. Brookes Publishing Co.

Fischel, J.E., Whitehurst, G.J., Caulfield, M.B., & DeBaryshe, B.D. (1989). Language growth in children with expressive language delay. *Pediatrics, 82,* 218–222.

Frith, U., Soares, I., & Wing, L. (1993). Research into earliest detectable signs of autism: What the parents say. *Communication, 27,* 17–18.

Gardner, M.F. (1979). *Expressive One-Word Picture Vocabulary Test.* Novato, CA: Academic Therapy Publications.

Grove, J., Conti-Ramsden, G., & Donlan, C. (1993). Conversational interaction and decision making in children with specific language impairment. *European Journal of Disorders of Communication, 28,* 141–152.

Hall, P., & Tomblin, B. (1978). A follow-up study of children with articulation and language disorders. *Journal of Speech and Hearing Disorders, 43,* 227–241.

Hart, B., & Risley, T. (1995). *Meaningful differences in the everyday experience of young American children.* Baltimore: Paul H. Brookes Publishing Co.

Heir, D., & Rosenberger, P. (1980). Focal left temporal lobe lesions and delayed speech acquisition. *Developmental and Behavioral Pediatrics, 1*, 54–57.

Henderson, J., & Trehub, S. (1995, April). *Infant temporal processing: Subsequent language*. Poster presented at the biennial meeting of the Society for Research on Child Development, Indianapolis, IN.

Johnston, J. (1988). Specific language disorders in the child. In N. Lass, J. Northern, L. McReynolds, & D. Yoder (Eds.), *Handbook of speech-language pathology and audiology* (pp. 685–715). Philadelphia: B.C. Decker.

Johnston, J. (1994). Cognitive abilities of children with language impairment. In R.V. Watkins & M.L. Rice (Eds.), *Communication and language intervention series: Vol. 4. Specific language impairments in children* (pp. 107–121). Baltimore: Paul H. Brookes Publishing Co.

Johnston, J., & Ellis Weismer, S. (1983). Mental rotation abilities in language-disordered children. *Journal of Speech and Hearing Research, 26*, 397–403.

Johnston, J., & Ramstadt, V. (1983). Cognitive development in preadolescent language-impaired children. *British Journal of Disorders of Communication, 18*, 49–55.

King, R., Jones, C., & Lasky, E. (1982). In retrospect: A fifteen-year follow-up report of speech-language–disordered children. *Language, Speech, and Hearing Services in Schools, 13*, 24–32.

Lahey, M. (1990). Who shall be called language disordered? Some reflections and one perspective. *Journal of Speech and Hearing Disorders, 55*, 612–620.

Lahey, M., & Edwards, J. (1995). Specific language impairment: Preliminary investigation of factors associated with family history and with patterns of language performance. *Journal of Speech and Hearing Research, 38*, 643–657.

Lee, L. (1974). *Developmental Sentence Scoring*. Evanston, IL: Northwestern University Press.

Leiter, R.G. (1969). *The Leiter International Performance Scale*. Chicago: Stoetling.

Leonard, L. (1991). Specific language impairment as a clinical category. *Language, Speech, and Hearing Services in Schools, 22*, 66–68.

Leonard, L. (1994). Some problems facing accounts of morphological deficits in children with specific language impairments. In R.V. Watkins & M.L. Rice (Eds.), *Communication and language intervention series: Vol. 4. Specific language impairments in children* (pp. 91–105). Baltimore: Paul H. Brookes Publishing Co.

Leonard, L., Bortolini, U., Caselli, M.C., McGregor, K., & Sabbadini, L. (1993). Morphological deficits in children with specific language impairment: The status of features in the underlying grammar. *Language Acquisition, 2*, 151–179.

Leonard, L., McGregor, K., & Allen, G. (1992). Grammatical morphology and speech perception in children with specific language impairment. *Journal of Speech and Hearing Research, 35*, 1076–1085.

Leske, M. (1981). Prevalence estimates of communicative disorders in the U.S.: Speech disorders. *Asha, 23*, 217–225.

Lewis, B., & Thompson, L. (1992). A study of developmental speech and language disorders in twins. *Journal of Speech and Hearing Research, 35*, 1086–1094.

Lewis, M., & Brooks-Gunn, J. (1981). Visual attention at three months as a predictor of cognitive functioning at two years of age. *Intelligence, 5*, 131–140.

Liles, B. (1985). Narrative abilities in normal and language disordered children. *Journal of Speech and Hearing Research, 28*, 123–133.

Lonigan, C., Fischel, J., Whitehurst, G., Arnold, D., & Valdez-Menchaca, M. (1992). The role of otitis-media in the development of expressive language disorder. *Developmental Psychology, 28*, 430–440.

Lovell, K., Hoyle, H., & Siddall, M. (1968). A study of some aspects of the play and language of young children with delayed speech. *Journal of Child Psychology, Psychiatry & Allied Disciplines, 3*, 41–50.

Lowe, M., & Costello, A. (1976). *The Symbolic Play Test.* Windsor, England: NFER-Nelson.

Luchinger, R. (1970). Inheritance of speech deficits. *Folia Phoniatrica, 22,* 216–230.

McCarthy, D. (1972). *McCarthy Scales of Children's Abilities.* San Antonio, TX: The Psychological Corporation.

Mentis, M. (1991). Topic management in the discourse of normal and language-impaired children. *Journal of Childhood Communication Disorders, 14,* 45–66.

Mills, D., Coffey, S., & Neville, H. (1993). Language acquisition and cerebral specialization in 20-month-old infants. *Journal of Cognitive Neuroscience, 5,* 317–334.

Mills, D., Coffey, S., & Neville, H. (1994). Variability in cerebral organization during primary language acquisition. In G. Dawson & K. Fischer (Eds.), *Human behavior and the developing brain* (pp. 427–455). New York: Guilford Press.

Mills, D., Coffey-Corina, S., & Neville, H. (submitted). Language comprehension and cerebral specialization in 13–17-month-old-infants. In D. Thal & J. Reilly (Eds.), *Special issue on origins of language disorders: Developmental neuropsychology.*

Mills, D., Thal, D., Di Iulio, L., Castaneda, C., & Neville, H. (1995). *Auditory sensory processing and language abilities in late talkers: An ERP study* (Tech. Rep. #CND-9508). La Jolla: University of California, San Diego, Center for Research in Language, Project in Cognitive & Neural Development.

Molfese, D. (1989). Electrophysiological correlates of word meanings in 14-month-old human infants. *Developmental Neuropsychology, 5,* 79–103.

Molfese, D. (1994). *Electrophysiological responses obtained during infancy and their relation to later language development: Further findings.* Unpublished manuscript.

Molfese, D., Burger-Judisch, L., & Hans, L. (1991). Consonant discrimination by newborn infants: Electrophysiological differences. *Developmental Neuropsychology, 7,* 177–195.

Molfese, D., Gill, L., & Benshoff, S. (1994). Predicting language performance at 5 years from evoked potentials recorded at birth. *Infant Behavior and Development, 17,* 830.

Molfese, D., & Molfese, V. (1985). Electrophysiological indices of auditory discrimination in newborn infants: The bases for predicting later language development? *Infant Behavior and Development, 8,* 197–211.

Molfese, D., & Molfese, V. (1988). Right-hemisphere responses from preschool children to temporal cues to speech and nonspeech materials: Electrophysiological correlates. *Brain and Language, 33,* 245–259.

Molfese, D., Morse, P., & Peters, C. (1990). Auditory evoked responses to names for different objects: Cross-modal processing as a basis for infant language acquisition. *Developmental Psychology, 26,* 780–795.

Morehead, D. (1972). Early grammatical and semantic relations: Some implications for a general representational deficit. *Papers and Reports on Child Language Development, 4,* 1–12.

Nelson, L., Kamhi, A., & Apel, K. (1987). Cognitive strengths and weaknesses in language-impaired children: One more look. *Journal of Speech and Hearing Disorders, 52,* 36–43.

Oetting, J., & Rice, M. (1993). Plural acquisition in children with specific language impairments. *Journal of Speech and Hearing Research, 36,* 1236–1248.

Olson, S., Bates, J., & Bayles, K. (1984). Mother–infant interaction and the development of individual differences in children's cognitive competence. *Developmental Psychology, 20,* 166–179.

Oroz, M., Thal, D., & Cleveland, S. (1993, November). *Lexical and grammatical development in normal and late-talking toddlers.* Poster presented at the annual convention of the American Speech-Language-Hearing Association, Anaheim, CA.

Paul, R. (1989, April). *Profiles of toddlers with delayed expressive language development*. Paper presented at the biennial meeting of the Society for Research in Child Development, Kansas City, MO.

Paul, R. (1991). Profiles of toddlers with slow expressive language development. *Topics in Language Disorders, 11*, 1–13.

Paul, R. (in press). Clinical implications of the natural history of slow expressive language development. *American Journal of Speech Language Pathology.*

Paul, R., & Alforde, S. (1993). Grammatical morpheme acquisition in 4-year-olds with normal, impaired, and late-developing language. *Journal of Speech and Hearing Research, 36*, 1271–1275.

Paul, R., Hernandez, R., Herron, L., & Johnson, K. (1995, June). *Narrative development in children with normal, impaired, and late developing language: Early school age.* Poster presented at the annual Symposium on Research in Child Language Disorders, Madison, WI.

Paul, R., & Jennings, P. (1992). Phonological behavior in toddlers with slow expressive language development. *Journal of Speech and Hearing Research, 35*, 99–107.

Paul, R., Laszio, C., McFarland, L., & Midford, N. (1993). Language outcomes in late-talkers: Kindergarten. *Society for Research in Child Development Abstracts, 9*, 534.

Paul, R., Lynn, T., & Lohr-Flanders, M. (1993). History of middle ear involvement and speech-language development in late talkers. *Journal of Speech and Hearing Research, 36*, 1055–1062.

Paul, R., & Riback, M. (1993, November). *Sentence structure development in late talkers.* Poster presented at the annual meeting of the American Speech-Language-Hearing Association, Anaheim, CA.

Paul, R., & Schiffer, M. (1991). Expression of communicative intentions in normal and 'late talking' young children. *Applied Psycholinguistics, 12*, 419–431.

Rapin, I., & Allen, D. (1983). Developmental language disorders: Nosologic considerations. In V. Kirk (Ed.), *Neuropsychology of language, reading and spelling* (pp. 155–184). New York: Academic Press.

Rescorla, L. (1984). Individual differences in early language development and their predictive significance. *Acta Pediologica, 1*, 97–115.

Rescorla, L. (1993a). Outcome for toddlers with specific expressive language delay (SELD) at ages 3, 4, 5, 6, 7, & 8. *Society for Research in Child Development Abstracts, 9*, 566.

Rescorla, L. (1993b, July). *Toddlers with specific expressive language delay (SELD): Outcome at age 8.* Poster presented at the Sixth International Congress for the Study of Child Language, Trieste, Italy.

Rescorla, L. (1994, June). *Identification and outcome of early expressive language delay.* Paper presented at the XVIII Congreso Nacional de AELFA, Mexico City, Mexico.

Rescorla, L., & Goossens, M. (1992). Symbolic play development in toddlers with specific expressive language impairment. *Journal of Speech and Hearing Research, 35*, 1290–1302.

Rescorla, L., Hadicke-Wiley, M., & Escarce, E. (1993). Epidemiological investigation of expressive language delay at age two. *First Language, 13*, 5–22.

Rescorla, L., & Schwartz, E. (1990). Outcome of toddlers with specific expressive language delay. *Applied Psycholinguistics, 11*, 393–407.

Reynell, J. (1977). *Reynell Developmental Language Scales.* Los Angeles: Webster Psychological Services.

Rice, M., & Oetting, J. (1993). Morphological deficits of children with SLI: Evaluation of number marking and agreement. *Journal of Speech and Hearing Research, 36*, 1249–1257.

Roth, F., & Clark, D. (1987). Symbolic play and social participation abilities of language-impaired and normally developing children. *Journal of Speech and Hearing Disorders, 52*, 17–29.

Siegel, B., Pliner, C., Eschler, J., & Elliott, G. (1988). How children with autism are diagnosed: Difficulties in identification of children with multiple developmental delays. *Developmental and Behavioral Pediatrics, 9*, 199–204.

Siegel, L. (1981). Infant tests as predictors of cognitive and language development at two years. *Child Development, 52*, 545–557.

Siegel, L. (1982). Reproductive, perinatal, and environmental factors as predictors of the cognitive and language development of preterm and full-term infants. *Child Development, 53*, 963–973.

Silva, P. (1980). The prevalence, stability and significance of developmental language delay in preschool children. *Developmental Medicine and Child Neurology, 22*, 768–777.

Silva, P., McGee, R., & Williams, S. (1983). Developmental language delay from three to seven years and its significance for low intelligence and reading difficulties at seven. *Developmental Medicine and Child Neurology, 25*, 783–793.

Silva, P., Williams, S., & McGee, R. (1987). A longitudinal study of children with developmental language delay at age three: Later intelligence, reading, and behavior problems. *Developmental Medicine and Child Neurology, 29*, 630–640.

Skarakis, E., & Prutting, C. (1988). Characteristics of symbolic play in language-disordered children. *Human Communication, 12*, 7–18.

Stark, R., Bernstein, L., Condino, R., Bender, M., Tallal, P., & Catts, H. (1984). Four-year follow-up study of language-impaired children. *Annals of Dyslexia, 34*, 49–68.

Stark, R., & Tallal, P. (1981). Selection of children with specific language deficits. *Journal of Speech and Hearing Disorders, 46*, 114–122.

Tallal, P., Miller, S., Bedi, G., Byma, G., Wang, X., Nagarijan, S., Schreiner, C., Jenkins, W., & Merzenich, M. (1996). Language comprehension in language-learning impaired children improved with acoustically modified speech. *Science, 271*, 81–84.

Tallal, P., & Piercy, M. (1973a). Defects of non-verbal auditory perception in children with developmental aphasia. *Nature, 241*, 468–469.

Tallal, P., & Piercy, M. (1973b). Developmental aphasia: Impaired rate of nonverbal processing as a function of sensory modality. *Neuropsychologia, 11*, 389–398.

Tallal, P., & Piercy, M. (1974). Developmental aphasia: Rate of auditory processing and selective impairment of consonant perception. *Neuropsychologia, 12*, 83–94.

Tallal, P., & Piercy, M. (1975). Perceptual and linguistic factors in the language impairment of developmental dysphasics: An experimental investigation with the Token test. *Cortex, 11*, 196–205.

Tallal, P., Ross, R., & Curtiss, S. (1989a). Familial aggregation in specific language impairment. *Journal of Speech and Hearing Disorders, 54*, 167–173.

Tallal, P., Ross, R., & Curtiss, S. (1989b). Unexpected sex-ratios in families of language/learning-impaired children. *Neuropsychologia, 27*, 987–998.

Tallal, P., Stark, R., & Mellitis, E. (1985). Identification of language-impaired children on the basis of rapid perception and production skills. *Brain and Language, 25*, 314–322.

Tallal, P., Townsend, J., Curtiss, S., & Wulfeck, B. (1991). Phenotypic profiles of language-impaired children based on genetic/family history. *Brain and Language, 41*, 81–95.

Tamis-LeMonda, C., & Bornstein, M. (1989). Habituation and maternal encouragement of attention in infancy as predictors of toddler language, play, and representational competence. *Child Development, 60*, 738–751.

Tamis-LeMonda, C., & Dyssegaard, B. (1994, June). *Children's language-play associations in the second year: Describing individual profiles.* Poster presented at the International Conference on Infant Studies, Paris, France.

Teele, D., Klein, J., & Rosner, B. (1980). Epidemiology of otitis media in children. *Annals of Otology, Rhinology and Laryngology, 89,* 5–6.

Terman, L., & Merrill, M. (1960). *Stanford-Binet Intelligence Scale.* Newton, MA: Houghton Mifflin.

Terrell, B., & Schwartz, R. (1988). Object transformations in the play of language-impaired children. *Journal of Speech and Hearing Disorders, 53,* 459–466.

Terrell, B., Schwartz, R., Prelock, P., & Messick, C. (1984). Symbolic play in normal and disordered children. *Journal of Speech and Hearing Research, 27,* 424–429.

Thal, D., & Bates, E. (1988). Language and gesture in late talkers. *Journal of Speech and Hearing Research, 31,* 115–123.

Thal, D., Bates, E., Goodman, J., & Jahn-Samilo, J. (1995). *Continuity of language-learning abilities in late- and early-talking toddlers.* Project in Cognitive Neurodevelopment, Technical Report # CND9505 and under review *Developmental Neuropsychology.*

Thal, D., Oroz, M., Evans, D., Katich, J., & Leasure, K. (1995, June). *From first words to grammar in late-talking toddlers.* Paper presented at the annual Symposium on Research in Child Language Disorders, Madison, WI.

Thal, D., & Tobias, S. (1992). Communicative gestures in children with delayed onset of oral expressive vocabulary. *Journal of Speech and Hearing Research, 35,* 1281–1289.

Thal, D., & Tobias, S. (1994). Relationships between language and gesture in normal developing and late-talking toddlers. *Journal of Speech and Hearing Research, 37,* 157–170.

Thal, D., Tobias, S., & Morrison, D. (1991). Language and gesture in late talkers: A 1-year follow-up. *Journal of Speech and Hearing Research, 34,* 604–612.

Thompson, L., Fagan, J., & Fulker, D. (1991). Longitudinal prediction of specific cognitive abilities from infant novelty preference. *Child Development, 62,* 530–538.

Tobias, S. (1995). *Language and gesture in 3 toddlers with expressive and receptive language delay.* Unpublished master's thesis, San Diego State University, San Diego.

Tomblin, B. (1989). Familial concentration of developmental language impairment. *Journal of Speech and Hearing Disorders, 54,* 287–295.

Tomblin, B., Hardy, J., & Hein, H. (1991). Predicting poor-communication status in preschool children using risk factors present at birth. *Journal of Speech and Hearing Research, 34,* 1096–1105.

Udwin, O., & Yule, W. (1983). Imaginative play in language-disordered children. *British Journal of Disorders of Communication, 18,* 197–205.

Vance, M., & Wells, B. (1994). The wrong end of the stick: Language-impaired children's understanding of non-literal language. *Child Language Teaching and Therapy, 10,* 23–46.

Walker, D., Greenwood, C., Hart, B., & Carta, J. (1994). Prediction of school outcomes based on early language productions and socioeconomic factors. *Child Development, 65,* 606–621.

Watkins, R., & Rice, M. (1991). Verb particle and preposition acquisition in language-impaired preschoolers. *Journal of Speech and Hearing Research, 34,* 1130–1141.

Watkins, R.V., & Rice, M.L. (Eds.). (1994). *Communication and language intervention series: Vol. 4. Specific language impairments in children.* Baltimore: Paul H. Brookes Publishing Co.

Watkins, R., Rice, M., & Moltz, C. (1993). Verb use by language-impaired and normally developing children. *First Language, 13,* 133–143.

Weismer, S., Murray-Branch, J., & Miller, J. (1994). A prospective longitudinal study of language development in late talkers. *Journal of Speech and Hearing Research, 37*, 852–867.

Whitehurst, G., Arnold, D., Epstein, J., Angell, A., Smith, M., & Fischel, J. (1993). A picture book intervention in daycare and home for children from low-income families. *Society for Research in Child Development Abstracts, 9*, 219.

Whitehurst, G., Arnold, D., Smith, M., Fischel, J., Lonigan, C., & Valdez-Menchaca, M. (1991). Family history in developmental language delay. *Journal of Speech and Hearing Research, 34*, 150–157.

Whitehurst, G., & Fischel, J. (1994). Early developmental language delay: What, if anything, should the clinician do about it? *Journal of Child Psychology and Psychiatry, 35*, 613–648.

Whitehurst, G., Fischel, J., Arnold, D., & Lonigan, C. (1992). Evaluating outcomes with children with expressive language delay. In S.F. Warren & J. Reichle (Eds.), *Communication and language intervention series: Vol. 1. Causes and effects in communication and language intervention* (pp. 277–313). Baltimore: Paul H. Brookes Publishing Co.

Wilson, B., & Risucci, D. (1986). A model for clinical quantification classification. Generation I: Application to language-disordered preschool children. *Brain and Language, 27*, 281–309.

2

Language Diversity

Implications for Assessment

Vera F. Gutierrez-Clellen

THE NUMBER OF CHILDREN FROM ethnic groups who were classified as having mental retardation decreased during the 1970s, perhaps as a result of civil rights litigation; since then, however, there has been a parallel increase in the number of children from ethnic groups classified as having learning disabilities and with special needs receiving no services. Reports concerning the overrepresentation of children from ethnic groups in special education classes for those with mental retardation have noted that despite the shift in disability designation, a disproportionate number of children from ethnic groups continue to be categorized as having learning disabilities (Ortiz & Yates, 1983, 1984; Tucker, 1980). Increasingly, there has been an awareness that the language measures and methods commonly used to identify children who need special services and the underlying model driving assessments can have adverse consequences for linguistically or culturally diverse groups of children. Historically, the primary reason that children for whom English is not their first language have been referred to special education services is their lack of communicative proficiency in English (Damico, 1991; Ortiz & Wilkinson, 1987). Children with limited English proficiency (LEP) who need language services are less likely to be referred to special education programs when placed in bilingual classrooms. The underreferral of these children for services has been considered a reaction to the inadequacies of the system in meeting children's needs (García & Ortiz, 1988; Mehan, Hertweck, & Meihls, 1986). Furthermore, language assessment of children learning English as a second language (ESL) often results in placing children with LEP in classes in which academic instruction is in English, a language that they do not fully comprehend (Collier, 1987; Faltis, 1993; Snow, 1990). Such placement may hinder children's learning and diminish children's academic potential. These practices suggest that language assessment and, consequently, inappropriate educational placement of children for whom English is not their first language may be based, in part, on misunderstood principles of language proficiency and second-language acquisition.

Low test scores of some children on psychometric measures used to make placement decisions have prompted various attempts to remediate the problem. For example, the ruling in *Larry P. v. Riles* (1979) nullified in California the use of standardized IQ tests for the educational placement of African American children based on its finding that these tests resulted in an overrepresentation of these children in special education. The court's ruling and subsequent litigation challenging the ban as discriminatory (e.g., *Crawford v. Honig,* 1994) have raised questions about the use of standardized language tests that rely on correlations with IQ tests or that convert raw scores to IQ or mental age–equivalent scores (Larry P. Task Force, 1989). Examples of language tests that may incorporate such characteristics include the Expressive One-Word Picture Vocabulary Test (EOWPVT) (Gardner, 1981) and the Peabody Picture Vocabulary Test–Revised (PPVT–R) (Dunn & Dunn, 1981), both widely used in language assessments (Wyatt, 1993). However, as will be evidenced later, the use of alternative language tests may not necessarily result in less-biased outcomes. Limiting representation of children from ethnic groups in certain programs, changing the designation or the categories of disorder, reducing the number of referrals, or abolishing the use of certain tests does not eliminate the inadequacies of the current assessment process or the legal and ethical ramifications. These issues underscore the need for a shift in the model or principles underlying assessment in order to meet the needs of all children. The following sections illustrate the complexities of the process by discussing the limitations of available language measures, the underlying presumptions of assessment approaches, traditional concepts of language proficiency and bilingualism, and the available options for reducing bias in assessment.

LIMITATIONS OF TRADITIONAL LANGUAGE TESTS

Standardized tests play an important role in traditional language assessment. Their widespread use may be related to their relative cost efficiency in administration and reporting (Miller-Jones, 1989) as well as the "privileging of easily quantifiable, rather than messy and complex, displays of skill and knowledge" (Wolf, Bixby, Glenn, & Gardner, 1991, p. 43) in clinical assessments. Arguments in support of testing emphasize the role of tests in assessing the effectiveness of clinicians and treatments (i.e., accountability), selecting and sorting children for educational placement (i.e., classification), and making decisions about treatment. In spite of these institutionalized functions, the premises of language tests are largely questionable. Standardized tests presumably are impervious to extraneous contextual or sociolinguistic factors and only test what is intended. They also presumably identify the presence of a language disorder in the test taker or predict later performance (Plante & Vance, 1994). That standardized tests are objective, neutral, or somewhat independent of contextual influences that may affect the measurement of language behavior is incompatible with a perspective that recognizes language variation and sociocultural diversity within and across speech communities. Because language tests assume a high degree of homogeneity of exposure to the content of test items (Figueroa & García, 1994) and to the sociolinguistic aspects of testing situations within groups of test takers (Mehan et al., 1986; Miller-Jones, 1989), it is uncertain whether they can accurately measure the language competence of children from diverse backgrounds.

Although correlations between language tests may suggest that the tests are assessing the same thing (i.e., concurrent validity), deviations in children's test performance may indicate cultural differences in interpretation of the test items, the test's format, or the testing situation. Miller-Jones (1989) offered a good example of how the performance of a 5-year-old African American child could be affected by the constraints of a standardized language test context. The child was expected to explain the similarities between two elements (e.g., "How are wood and coal alike? How are they the same?"). Instead, the child provided simple associations ("They're hard") and used these associations for other hard objects (e.g., a ship, an automobile). The child's verbal attempts to define the testing situation indicated that the responses to the test reflected the child's interpretation of the task, not the child's language ability in the targeted area. For example, when the examiner explained, "Yeah, I'm writing down what you say so I can remember it later," the child asked incredulously, "Cause you don't know what it's for?" (Miller-Jones, 1989, p. 362). Because standard formats do not permit probes, alternative answers, or feedback, the child's misinterpretation of the task may permeate most test responses and significantly affect overall scores. Thus, scores on a given language test may reflect knowledge of the culture of testing rather than language ability. Moreover, there is evidence that the examiner's directions, feedback, and cues in testing situations are not consistent across test takers because testing occurs in socially situated interactions or as part of a social/institutional activity (Mehan et al., 1986). Thus, the characteristics of tests and testing situations may never be free of contextual influences on children's test scores.

If tests were capable of isolating specific language skills, then they would accurately identify children with language disabilities. Such is not the case; the limitations or inadequacies of language tests in accurately discriminating typical and impaired language are widely known (e.g., McCauley & Swisher, 1984a, 1984b; Plante & Vance, 1994). One of these limitations concerns the tests' predictive validity, or how well the instrument will predict future performance on a criterion measure. A review of tests used to assess language and school readiness indicates the limited capability of tests in this area. For example, Figueroa and García (1994) examined the predictive coefficients of school-readiness tests and noted that few tests use real-life achievements (e.g., grades) as criteria. When school-based criteria were used, the test scores predicted only between 4% and 9% of the variance in achievement. Evidence also indicates that standardized tests do not predict a student's response to instruction (Camp, Drummond, Carter, & Parker, 1988; Mercer, 1988). Measures of predictive validity may not accurately predict the future performance of individual children because correlations between pretest and posttest performance are based on group data, not on individual children (Haywood, Brown, & Wingenfeld, 1990).

Using standardized tests has serious implications for children from certain groups. The risk of misdiagnosing children when standardized tests are used in assessment is alarming. A study designed to obtain normative data for the Test for Auditory Comprehension of Language (TACL, Spanish version) (Carrow, 1973) with 60 monolingual and bilingual native Mexican children found that the children's language age–equivalent scores fell below language norms derived from English-speaking children (Wilcox & McGuinn Aasby, 1988). Discrepancies also have been reported within groups of English-speaking children using the English TACL. Primarily African American preschool children enrolled in a Head Start program ($N = 299$) received scores more than 1 standard deviation (SD) below the mean of the normative sample (Ramsey Musselwhite, 1983). Specifically, 56% of these children scored below 1 SD below the mean of children from middle–socioeconomic status (SES) backgrounds. Discrepancies still remained when scores were compared with the means of children from low-SES backgrounds. Using this criterion, about 15% of the children scored below 1 SD below the mean.

The Hannah-Gardner Test of Verbal and Nonverbal Language Functioning (Hannah & Gardner, 1978) was administered to 540 English-speaking preschool children participating in a Head Start program, including 376 African American children, 82 Hispanic children, and 82 Anglo children. The items on the expressive subtest were adapted to address the dialectal differences of speakers of African American and Hispanic English. Even with this adaptation, more than 68% of the children tested scored at least 1 SD below the mean of the normative sample (Norris, Juarez, & Perkins, 1989). The comparisons continued to reveal significant differences using different cutoff scores. About 32% of the Head Start children scored below 2 SDs from the mean. The chance of underestimating the language skills of these children was significant for all ethnic groups. When standardized tests are used, there also is the risk of underreferral—of missing children who may have language disorders. Peña, Quinn, and Iglesias (1992) found no significant differences in the performance of Hispanic and African American children with typical language skills and with language disorders on the EOWPVT. Rather, children from *both* groups scored more than 1 SD from the mean. Thus, standardized tests may not accurately differentiate groups with different language abilities.

The finding that standardized tests may not discriminate differences from disorders within groups also has been confirmed by research focused on the effects of dialects such as African American English (AAE) on the scoring of tests. For example, Cole and Taylor (1990) administered three standardized tests to African American children from low-income homes who attended a Mississippi public school and compared their performance according to the phonological rules of AAE and standard English. Results indicated differences across tests in the number of children identified as having disorders. Performance differences when the AAE scoring criteria were used suggested that dialect-specific test adaptations could reduce the likelihood of confusing dialectal differences with disorders. However, there is some indication that the AAE scoring procedure may not be effective for assessing other groups of AAE speakers. Washington and Craig (1992a) compared the responses of 28 African American, low-income preschool children from a metropolitan Detroit area using both standard English and AAE scoring procedures. Contrary to Cole and Taylor's results, there were no significant differences in the scores generated by the two procedures. The findings illustrate the difficulties of assuming language homogeneity among members of speech communities. Not only do speakers of AAE differ from speakers of standard English, but there also may be differences among groups of AAE speakers. Attempts to adjust test scores according to the idealized ways of speaking of a given speech community may not neutralize differences among groups.

Similar difficulties occur when translated tests are used. Figueroa (1989) reported differences in the rank ordering of vocabulary test items of the Wechsler Intelligence Scale for Children–Revised (WISC–R) (Wechsler, 1974) when they were translated from English to Spanish. The first half of the vocabulary subtest was easier in Spanish than in English, whereas the opposite occurred for the remaining half; thus, direct translations may not result in equivalent tests or comparable psychometric properties.

Notwithstanding the limitations and presumptions of standardized tests, researchers and clinicians have continued to attempt technical modifications. Efforts have been devoted to developing local norms for popular English language tests, translating English tests to other languages, using dialect-specific scoring procedures, and including various ethnic groups in normative samples. The failure of these test adaptations in reducing test bias was illustrated in a study with low-income, African American preschool and kindergarten children. Washington and Craig (1992b) examined the performance of 105 children on the PPVT–R. The test norms were based on a sample that included African Americans in similar percentages as in the general population (10% of the sample). The results of the study indicated that the mean standard score for the 105 children placed them at about the 10th percentile of the normative sample. About 65% of the children were identified as having receptive vocabulary impairments based on a cutoff score of 1 SD below the mean. Clearly, using a representative sample as a referent does not reduce test bias. Moreover, the results showed that even when children were given credit for items missed by 50% of the sample, most children scored below the mean of the normative sample (86%), and 51% scored more than 1 SD below the mean. Contrary to common wisdom, using multiple tests to increase the accuracy of language assessments can, in fact, increase the likelihood of misidentification. Plante and Vance (1994) examined the accuracy of preschool language tests in discriminating between children with typical language development and children with impaired language development. They found that when the scores of their best test discriminator were combined with those of tests with weaker discriminant ability, the results had less discriminant capacity. Using multiple tests did not increase the accuracy of the tests in identifying children with specific language impairment as having language impairment. On the contrary, it actually increased misclassification.

Standardized tests are not appropriate for all children, even if developed locally. Differences related to educational background, income, geographic variables, cultural experience, and/or acculturation may be difficult to adequately represent in the normative sample. In addition, the development of local norms may generate lower standards and lower expectations for certain groups with concurrent negative social and educational consequences.

LIMITATIONS OF AVAILABLE
MEASURES OF SPONTANEOUS LANGUAGE

One way of reducing bias in language assessment is to critically evaluate the construct validity of available language measures. Evidence of variability in children's performance on specific language measures may not be indicative of a disorder if the language measures are not appropriate for a given language or speech community. For example, English language assessments often include questions about a child's morphological development because the analysis of the child's learning processes may inform the identification of language disorder. Language samples typically are obtained to determine the mean length of utterance (MLU) in morphemes and the use of grammatical morphemes and to assign the child to a developmental level (Nelson, 1993). Although these practices have been criticized because of the lack of normative morphological data (Lahey, 1994), similar procedures have been proposed for the language assessment of Spanish-speaking children in the United States who are learning ESL (e.g., Linares, 1981; Merino, 1992). Yet differences across the two languages preclude comparing MLU scores based on developmental data from English-monolingual children with MLU scores obtained from Spanish language samples or from the English samples of bilingual children. Such comparisons are likely to overestimate the language development of Spanish-monolingual children and may not provide an appropriate assessment of the English proficiency of bilingual children. For example, in English, articles are represented by only two items (a, the) indicating indefiniteness and definiteness, whereas the Spanish language marks gender, number, and indefiniteness versus definiteness using nine different articles (un, una, unos, unas; el, la, los, las; lo). The inflections of Spanish verbs differentiate tense, mood, person, and number in 46 distinct forms; whereas English has few inflections for tense, person, and number (Merino, 1992) and relies more heavily on free morphemes to code this information. Given the nature of Spanish morphology, attempts to calculate MLU in Spanish are likely to generate large scores even at the very early stages of language development (see Linares, 1981, for a description of such procedure). Clinicians also have proposed to reduce the number of inflections to be computed in an effort to neutralize differences between English and Spanish MLU scores, to match subjects by MLU, and to obtain developmental data (García, Maez, & Gonzalez, 1981; Kvaal, Shipstead-Cox, Nevitt, Hodson, & Launer, 1988). Yet the meaning and, ultimately, the clinical relevance of MLU scores with this language group remain uncertain.

The difficulties in applying morphological measures to the assessment of children learning languages other than English also are apparent in the case of dual language acquisition. Merino (1992) reported variability in the rate and order of acquisition of Spanish morphemes between bilingual (Spanish-English) children in the United States and monolingual, Spanish-speaking children in Mexico. Individual differences in the use of Spanish morphemes by the bilingual children may be attributed to first-language attrition (i.e., subtractive bilingualism) in children who had more exposure to English than to Spanish in the early school years, or to transfer processes from the second language. Thus, morphological use or morphological complexity may not be a stable language measure for comparison even within speakers of the language.

The acquisition of grammatical morphemes may require different learning processes across different languages that, in turn, may explain differences in performance on these measures. For example, there is some evidence that articles are learned earlier in Spanish than in English, perhaps because they are semantically more salient as they carry gender and number information (Kvaal et al., 1988). Thus, although both languages use articles, cross-linguistic differences in the "informational load" of these morphemes may pose different language-learning demands on the child and may have an effect on rate of acquisition. Discrepancies between English and Spanish also occur for the order of acquisition of verb forms and prepositions. For example, there is some indication that Spanish regular verb forms are learned before irregular forms, in contrast to English expectations, and *en* [in, on] prepositions may appear later in Spanish than in English (Kvaal et al., 1988). Differences in the acquisition and use of prepositions may be related to differences in the ways these languages mark directionality. Whereas English uses prepositions and particles to indicate location and directionality, as in "go up" or "go down," Spanish frequently conveys directionality in the verb, as in *subir* (to go up) and *bajar* (to come down) (Slobin & Bocaz, 1988). Similarly, the preposition *en* may be less salient to the Spanish learner because it may be incorporated into verbs like *meter* (put *in*) or *poner* (put *on*).

The previous analysis illustrates the complexities of applying measures used in the language assessment of children learning ESL to the assessment of children learning other languages. Cross-linguistic or cross-dialectal differences, as just exemplified, may influence the types of processes required to learn a given grammatical structure and, eventually, the way a language disorder is expressed in a given language or speech community.

Child language disorders may not be manifested in universal ways across language groups. For example, the morphological difficulties exhibited by English-speaking children with language disorders may be related to the lack of phonetic or semantic substance of bound morphemes and function words in English (Leonard, 1991a, 1991b). Because grammatical morphemes in English are unstressed syllables or consonant affixes, children may need to pay increased attention to phonetic cues in order to perceive and produce these morphemes (Bedore & Leonard, 1995). Thus, English-speaking children with limited processing abilities may have difficulty perceiving and using English morphemes. Similarly, the limited morphological skills of English-speaking children with language disorders also may be related to the frequency of inflections in the language and the somewhat secondary role of these morphological markers in determining relations among parts of a sentence (Dromi, Leonard, & Shteiman, 1993). Thus, children with limited language-processing skills may prefer and, consequently, rely on word order cues because of their centrality to English learning and, as a result, may pay less attention to morphology. These issues suggest that a language disorder in children learning a more heavily inflected language with a relatively more perceptually and semantically salient morphological system may not manifest itself in morphological limitations (Dromi et al., 1993). Thus, applying morphological measures to the language assessment of children learning languages such as Spanish, German, or Hebrew may not be clinically useful.

Research examining the relevance of available language measures with different languages or dialects is needed to develop clinical measures appropriate to a child's first language. A first step in that direction may include the analysis of language-specific phenomena such as the use of ellipsis in pro-drop languages in which subject information is carried redundantly by the verb. For example, in the Spanish sentence "Me *llamaron* del banco"("[*They*] *called* me from the bank"), the verb inflections provide information about the identity of the subject. Thus, children may take longer to learn how to use appropriate subjects and other referents. There is some indication that preschool Spanish-speaking children performing at the low end of the language continuum may omit referent information in their oral narratives by using ellipsis to introduce people or referents for the first time (Gutierrez-Clellen & Heinrichs-Ramos, 1993). For example, one of these children indicated the actions and consequences in a narrative without mentioning the characters or protagonists of the story. Although the verb inflections indicated that there was one or more characters at a time, they were insufficient to clearly identify the protagonist.

These cross-linguistic variations underscore the need for a reexamination of the measures used in language assessment. The lack of equivalency of measures across languages has important implications in clinical assessment of children from different language backgrounds. First, it illustrates some of the problems involved in the translation of language tests. Certain tests may identify the language-learning difficulties of English-speaking children, but their translations into other languages may not indicate whether language disorder exists for children learning those languages. Second, the development of norms for different language groups in the United States may require the development of alternative language measures. If available measures of language development do not assess equivalent language-learning processes across children, then they may not be clinically sensitive for the differential diagnosis of language-learning ability.

ISSUES IN ASSESSING CHILDREN'S BILINGUAL COMPETENCE

Language Dominance Revisited

Assessments and interventions in the least restrictive environment require that children be tested in their primary language to avoid underestimating competence based on proficiency in their second language. Accordingly, one of the strategies proposed for the language assessment of children learning ESL is to establish the child's dominant language (Caterino, 1990; Westby, 1994). The results of language-dominance testing typically are used to decide which language to use for assessment and/or to determine the language of instruction (Chamberlain & Medinos-Landurand, 1991; Kayser, 1989). The assumption underlying these decisions, however, is that language dominance involves superior performance that is uniform across language areas. The following examples show that the patterns of language development evidenced by bilingual children may not be uniform between or within languages.

Figure 1 represents the Spanish and English language skills relative to average expected performance of Child A, age 4;9 years old, with severe to profound language delays. The child has been exposed to both languages at home. The child evidences weaknesses in phonology, vocabulary, and syntax in both languages yet exhibits strengths in the use of speech acts in both languages. Based on these language levels, there is no clear language dominance. Although both languages appear to achieve similar levels of development overall, specific language processes within a given area may have different patterns of development across the two languages. For example, for this child, consonant clusters in English appear more advanced than those in Spanish, a phenomenon perhaps related to their low frequency of occurrence and their low complexity in Spanish. In other words, the relatively higher frequency and complexity of English consonant clusters compared with Spanish may provide more opportunities and cues for perceiving and producing them.

Figure 2 displays the language profile of Child B, an 8;5-year-old with mild to severe language delays. For this child, patterns of phonological development

Child A

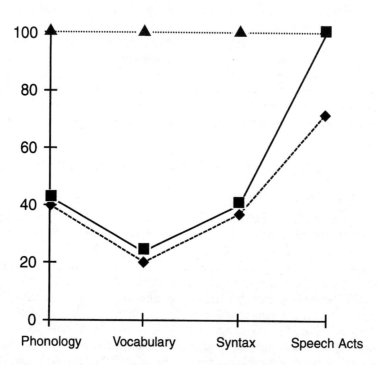

Figure 1. Spanish and English language skills of Child A. (◆ = Spanish; ■ = English; ▲ = expected achievement.)

appear slightly more advanced in English than in Spanish. Spanish vocabulary and syntax show a higher level of achievement than in English, and narrative performance appears similarly low in both languages. As with Child A, assessment in only one language would provide an inadequate appraisal of this child's language skills.

For many bilingual children, with and without language delays, there is no dominant language. Their developmental levels in each language may be lower than age expectations, or areas of strength in one language may correspond to areas of weakness in the other language. The risks of underestimating children's language skills when assessments are conducted in the presumably dominant language also are significant for children who are tested only in English by virtue of their exit from a transitional bilingual program and placement in an English-only class (Chamberlain & Medinos-Landurand, 1991). These children's English skills may be lower than those of monolingual English-speaking peers because of limited ESL instruction, not because of language-learning difficulties. Furthermore, a review of available tests of language dominance indi-

Child B

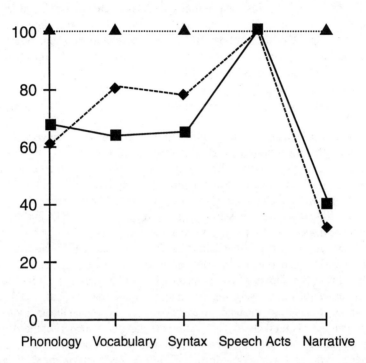

Figure 2. Spanish and English language skills of Child B. (◆ = Spanish; ■ = English; ▲ = expected achievement.)

cates that the tests focus on only one or two language areas (e.g., vocabulary, syntax) (Caterino, 1990), an insufficient assessment of the children's skills in any language.

The variability in the language development of bilingual children refutes the plausibility of viewing the language status of a bilingual child from a monolingual, or single-language, perspective. Grosjean (1989) argued that a monolingual view of bilingualism presumes an idealized concept of perfectly balanced bilingualism in which the bilingual person is equally and fully fluent in two languages, "like two monolinguals in one person" (p. 3). In contrast, he proposed a bilingual (or holistic) view of bilingualism in which the bilingual person's two languages may differ from the corresponding monolingual languages. Because the prevailing concept of bilingualism is the monolingual view, instances of code switching, or language borrowing, are regarded as anomalous cases of interference rather than as signs of bilingual competence. As a result, the language standards and assessment methods applied to bilingual people are those of monolingual rather than bilingual speakers (i.e., Spanish and English monolinguals as frames of reference for the assessment of a bilingual Spanish-English speaker). These presumptions also are prevalent in the bilingual research literature. For example, in Spanish acquisition studies conducted in the United States, it is common to treat children's exposure to English as a confounding variable that contaminates the study of Spanish-language development when, in fact, the development of Spanish in a bilingual environment should be the focus of research with these children. This shift in focus would be consistent with the linguistic characteristics of Spanish-speaking groups in the United States and would allow developmental and comparative studies based on authentic speech communities.

The competencies of bilingual children in each language may vary according to the type of bilingualism. Bialystok and Cummins (1991) argued that bilingual language skills should be described in terms of simultaneous and successive bilingualism rather than in bilingual/monolingual distinctions. Children who acquire two languages simultaneously are more likely to achieve a more balanced bilingualism (and possibly greater proficiency in each language) than children who successfully acquire a second language after the first has developed. There also is evidence that children who develop language in a subtractive bilingual environment (i.e., when academic and cognitive development mediated by input in the first language is replaced by input in a weak second language) may not attain the same levels of performance in either language as would children who learn language in an additive environment (i.e., when the addition of a second language is unlikely to displace the first language such as in the Anglophone community of Quebec, Canada). Children in a subtractive bilingual environment performed worse on a formal definition task and on the California Achievement Test than did children raised in a bilingual additive environment (Snow, 1990). When the first language does not develop beyond when the second language is introduced, children may experience arrested development of the first language (Shiff-Myers, 1992). In subtractive situations, learners may lose Spanish for academic language functions and maintain it for conversational uses (Hakuta, Ferdman, & Díaz, 1987). In addition, language loss in subtractive environments may have long-term negative consequences for communication between children and adult family members with limited or no English proficiency (Wong Fillmore, 1991). Furthermore, it is important to note that there is almost no evidence of perfectly balanced bilingualism in the bilingual research literature (Watson, 1991). A review of studies examining the phonological processing and production of simultaneous bilinguals judged as fully native in both languages indicates that bilinguals may not be equally capable of performing the same speech tasks in the two languages (Sharwood Smith, 1991; Watson, 1991).

Bilingualism: Two Separate Systems or One?

An alternative strategy to assessments in the assumed dominant language is to conduct assessments in both languages (Chamberlain & Medinos-Landurand,

1991). Because areas of strength in one language may correspond to areas of weakness in the other language, it is reasonable to combine test scores in each language to derive a holistic bilingual competence score. For example, combining expressive vocabulary scores from the first and second languages would yield a total vocabulary score that may be higher than the scores for each separate language and closer to the child's true language abilities. In fact, a study using this procedure for assessing the vocabulary production of infants and toddlers found no significant differences in scores between Spanish-English bilingual and English monolingual children (Pearson, Fernández, & Oller, 1993). Yet in traditional assessments, the bilingual child's performance in each language typically is compared with the corresponding monolingual language referent as if the languages formed two separate systems, not one. The use of English and Spanish in Table 1 from spontaneous language samples of 4;10-year-old twins demonstrates that the two languages of bilinguals contribute to a unitary language system.

The data from these children's language samples appear to indicate that the children code switch between languages at word, phrase, and utterance boundaries. Within-utterance code switches, as illustrated in Table 2, suggest that when speakers use a "bilingual speech mode," the two languages may not be separated or treated as autonomous language systems (Grosjean, 1989). The language performance of many bilingual children, as presented in the examples in Table 2, may not reflect two distinct language referents (Grosjean, 1989). Contrary to the monolingual model of bilingualism, there is evidence that, at least for production, bilinguals may develop two language systems that differ from those of monolinguals (Watson, 1991) and may use them simultaneously (Cook, 1992). A bilingual perspective in assessment would, therefore, address the typical variation described in the language performance of bilinguals and include a careful analysis of the communicative functions of code-switching behavior within linguistic and nonlinguistic constraints (Grosjean, 1982, 1989).

The previous examples illustrate the various grammatical functions of code switching described for Southwestern English and Spanish dialects as well as for bilingual communities in New York (Amastae & Elías-Olivares, 1982; Eastman, 1992). These grammatical functions range from the use of alternate morphemes to words, phrases, and sentences. In addition to filling a linguistic need (for a lex-

Table 1.   English and Spanish utterances from spontaneous language samples of 4;10-year-old twins

Utterances	Adán	Abel
Total number of utterances	71	62
English	16	11
Spanish	39	38
Utterances with midsentence code switches	16	13

Table 2. Examples of within-utterance code switches for English and Spanish

Code switch[a]	English translation
Otro *piece* aquí	Another piece here
Aquí *amma* pónlo	Here I'm gonna put it
I wash it éso	I wash it that
Ya cayó oso *here*	Bear just fell down here
Go yo *to donkey*	I go to the donkey
Me no *see* nada	Me don't see anything
My mojo todo	My wet everything

[a]The italicized words in these examples represent the code switch.

ical item, phrase, or sentence), code switching may be used for various communicative purposes within bilingual and bidialectal communities (Grosjean, 1982). Examples of these functions include expressing group identity and status, conveying confidentiality, changing the role of the speaker, and crossing social or ethnic boundaries.

In spite of the common use of code switching by proficient bilinguals, research in bilingual language development has suggested that code switching represents a developmental stage in the early acquisition of a second language, which is followed by a gradual separation of the two languages (Fantini, 1985). For example, switches between the stem of a word and its affix, such as *washear* (to wash) or *taipear* (to type), traditionally are viewed as characteristic of code switching in a language learner or as language borrowing (Langdon & Merino, 1992). These concepts appear to be consistent with the monolingual model of bilingualism, discussed previously, which views the alternation and integration of two languages by bilinguals as a transitory stage that is overcome with age or development. However, these language mechanisms are common examples of typical language use in bilingual settings (Eastman, 1992) and may indeed be what differentiates the language system(s) of bilinguals from that of monolinguals.

While the debate awaits further research, assessments should attempt to differentiate typical language differences from disorders by including an analysis of code-switching behavior. One may determine whether the switches operate under linguistic and nonlinguistic constraints (Grosjean, 1982); that is, switches may be expected to preserve word meanings as judged by bilingual listeners and be grammatically constrained by the structure of the languages of the bilingual speaker. For example, "My mojo todo" ("My wet everything") may be an inappropriate switch. A bilingual listener would expect "/Me/ mojo todo" ("Me wet everything"), which contains an appropriate English personal pronoun rather than the possessive (which cannot precede a verb unless it is nominalized). Dialectal differences may be validated by comparing the child's language patterns with those of members of the family or speech community (Terrell, Arensberg, & Rosa, 1992). Performance under nonlinguistic constraints may be assessed by observing the child interacting in naturalistic monolingual and bilingual contexts. The purpose of this approach would be to examine the child's ability to use code switching as an appropriate communicative strategy. It is expected that under true monolingual conditions (unlike those in which the examiner switches languages or asks the child to speak in the "other" language), more competent children will avoid communication breakdowns (i.e., speaking a language that the listener does not understand).

Language Proficiency Revisited

The previous sections in this chapter have outlined some of the issues concerning language dominance and bilingualism and have presented several options for assessing bilingual children. The complexity of these issues requires a clear understanding of language proficiency and how it may best be described in assessment. As discussed previously, the language systems of bilingual children differ from the language systems of monolingual children, and the interrelationships between the two languages indicate a unique structure and organization of their language competencies. Thus, if the languages learned by bilingual children reflect, in part, a general language-learning ability, then the challenge is to determine what achievements may be used to predict these children's language development or what model of language proficiency would best describe their language abilities.

A domain model of language proficiency would evaluate the child's knowledge of phonology, morphology, syntax, lexicon, and pragmatics. Alternatively, a componential model of language proficiency that distinguishes between modalities of processing may examine the child's listening, speaking, signing, interpreting, reading, writing, or thinking skills (Oller & Damico, 1991). A domain model of language proficiency applied to children with language delays, such as Child A and Child B (see Figures 1 and 2), appears to indicate that second-language development parallels first-language development. Low performance in a first language in these cases also is replicated in the second language. In effect, the bilingual research literature provides strong support for the concept of linguistic interdependence for certain language activities (for a review, see Cummins, 1991). For example, studies with various language groups have indicated correlations between aspects of language proficiency such as verbal analogies (Malakoff, 1988) or discourse cohesion (Cummins, Lopes, & King, 1988) across the languages of bilingual learners. Even for children who have experienced language loss, first-language proficiency in conversational or context-supported interactions may predict similar achievements in the second language. There is evidence, however, that these models may not capture differences in the demands of various language activities and, therefore, may be insufficient to describe the language proficiencies of bilingual children. For example, children learning English in a subtractive environment may not achieve second-language development for decontextualized or academic language skills, based on conversational skills in the first language (Hakuta et al., 1987). There appears to be a low correlation between measures of basic interpersonal communicative skills (BICS) and measures of cognitive academic language proficiency (CALP) (Cummins, 1983) and no correlation between conversational skills and school language achievement (Snow, Cancino, Gonzalez, & Shriberg, 1989) within or between languages.

Alternatively, an integrated approach to language proficiency, focusing on the demands of different language tasks, may provide more accurate information regarding language development and directions for intervention. A language-task model applied to assessment would define the demands of language tasks in terms of contextualized/decontextualized dimensions (Snow, 1987) and would consider the degree of audience participation, presumption of shared background knowledge, and message complexity as parameters (Snow, 1991). The model should define the type of task used to assess language performance, as well as the type of competence invoked by the task (Bialystok & Cummins, 1991). Although the application of this model to bilingual assessments remains to be tested, its principles are promising. They are based on the prediction that aspects of first- and second-language proficiency, which appear unrelated (e.g., conversational versus definitional skills), may not be related to differences within the child but to the quality and quantity of the second-language instruction (Cummins, 1991). Thus, the model is consistent with the concept that assessments should examine children's language experiences as well as the ways families and teachers mediate school language and cultural knowledge.

ISSUES IN ASSESSING LINGUISTICALLY DIVERSE SCHOOL-AGE CHILDREN

Cross-Cultural Interpretation of Children's Language Behavior

Before determining what is typical or deviant language, it is important to note that language ability standards are based on a socially constructed set of rules that dictate appropriate or idealized ways of speaking for a given group (Erickson, 1984; Gumperz, 1982). Sociolinguistic research in interpersonal communication suggests that language assessments should be socially situated, not simply a matter of conforming to norms of linguistic appropriateness (Gumperz, 1982). In assessment situations, both examiner and examinee infer what is intended based on the values, beliefs, and attitudes of their speech communities. For example, the interpretive processes underlying the assessment of "nonstandard" language behavior may be ruled by the consensus that certain forms, dialects, or accents are associated with upward social mobility. Thus, English dialects such as Standard American English, African American English, or Chicano English may become more or less prestigious because their users are attributed different socioeconomic status or levels of assimilation to the dominant cultural group. Ideally, knowledge of the grammatical rules, lexicon, and use of these diverse dialects applied to assessment would facilitate the recognition of a typical language difference and prevent misdiagnosing a disorder. Yet, given that the standard language behavior in assessment reflects the social parameters and ways of speaking of the dominant culture or group, performance differences in the form or content of a language still may penalize children from diverse backgrounds.

The inherent cultural and linguistic biases of language assessment are best exemplified in the assessment of children's discourse competence. Research in language and education has shown that the examiner's cultural values and presumptions about language competence are inseparable components of language assessment. One study used two groups of informants, African American and Caucasian graduate students at Harvard University, to judge the well-formedness of the oral narrative of an African American child (Michaels, 1991). The narrative text was a mimicked version of the original, edited to maintain the child's rhythm and intonation, but with the grammatical and phonological features of standard English. Listener evaluations revealed differences in the judgments of narrative development across the two groups. Whereas the Caucasian informants unanimously found the story incoherent and suggestive of language-learning problems, the African American informants found it easy to understand and indicative of academic achievement.

Although a number of scholars have advocated for the assessment of language use or discourse to optimize the performance of children from diverse backgrounds (e.g., Damico, 1991; Ripich & Spinelli, 1985), such assessments are *not* necessarily less biased. Assessments that apply naturalistic methods to determine language competence (e.g., criterion-referenced measures of conversational discourse) may be more appropriate for diverse cultural groups than would traditional testing methods that rely on discrete point measures (e.g., vocabulary, syntax). Yet integrative assessments of language use are not culturally different from assessments of vocabulary or grammar because they also assess what the child presumably has learned within a given speech community. Thus, they incorporate assumptions about past learning experiences or opportunities, which may be difficult to verify or validate.

Expectations based on sociocultural knowledge play a critical role in interpreting children's discourse in language assessments. One way of addressing this issue in assessment is to acknowledge that children's language strategies may be ruled by different culture-specific values and beliefs. There is a vast body of literature describing the communication styles of different groups, which may inform assessments (for reviews, see Battle, 1993; Cheng, 1987; Langdon, 1992; Lynch & Hanson, 1992). However, the characterization of different groups as an explanatory strategy to interpret seemingly deviant communicative behavior also may reinforce cultural stereotypes. This approach obscures the concept that traditional language assessments are inherently based on the social and communicative rules of the dominant group (i.e., those individuals who presumably make educational decisions for the child and the family). Furthermore, the practice of "matching" by cultural membership (either by comparing the child to a cultural referent or by using bicultural assessors) is based on the questionable assumption that speech communities are homogeneous and stable. Thus, any attempt to isolate a set of communication features as the referent criteria for a given group may not neutralize cultural bias.

Individual and Cultural Differences

Assessments should distinguish performance differences that are related to differences in language-learning ability from those that reflect differences in language-learning experience. There is some evidence that the pragmatic behaviors selected for assessing school-age children represent the communication rules and cultural expectations of American classroom settings. Thus, for many children, performance differences in these areas may simply reflect nonfamiliarity with school discourse, not necessarily language ability.

An early study of Hispanic children learning ESL found that the use of certain pragmatic behaviors could predict children's later language-based academic performance in English-only classrooms (Damico, Oller, & Storey, 1983). The pragmatic criteria included discourse measures such as children's use of revisions, delayed responses, nonspecific vocabulary (i.e., use of deictic referents), inappropriate responses (i.e., unexpected topic shifts), poor topic maintenance, and other "on-line" processes (e.g., linguistic nonfluencies, need for repetition). Children who demonstrated these communicative behaviors at the outset made smaller gains in academic achievement after 7 months of exposure to a general English-language classroom than did children categorized as not having language disorders on the basis of the pragmatic criteria. However, there is evidence that children who appear to use inappropriate communicative behavior based on school culture expectations may be demonstrating characteristics typical of second-language learners (e.g., revisions, dysfluencies, delayed responses) and/or previously learned communication styles, *not* disorders. For example, children who are not talkative may be exhibiting their language socialization experiences (Gutierrez-Clellen, 1995; Gutierrez-Clellen, Peña, & Quinn, 1995). Similarly, children who do not respond directly may be using topic-associating discourse or other styles (Gutierrez-Clellen & Quinn, 1993; Kay-Raining Bird & Kluppel Vetter, 1994; Michaels, 1986).

A major focus in assessing school-age children has been to examine oral language tasks that are presumed to facilitate the achievement of literacy because they tend to be associated with academically successful groups in American schools (Michaels, 1991). For example, children's performance on decontextualized language tasks that treat language as an object may be related to variations in literacy achievement or school-related experiences, and experience with formal definitions and story understanding have been associated with pre-reading skills (e.g., print production, decoding) (Velasco, 1989). However, children's language performance during these assessments may not reflect innate language ability but rather the byproduct of cultural mediation in specific school and home settings (Gutierrez-Clellen et al., 1995). There is some indication that the skills assessed for school-age children largely are learned in school or are promoted through formal classroom interactions (Scribner & Cole, 1981; Snow, 1991). Studies have shown important differences in children's experiences with these tasks. Anderson-Yockel and Haynes (1994) found significant differences in the frequency of maternal questions during book readings between African American and European American adult–toddler dyads. Kindergarten children from middle-class backgrounds have been found to exhibit greater proficiency in their ability to provide formal definitions and to indicate story understanding than have working-class children (Dickinson & Snow, 1987). Similar group differences also have been reported for story comprehension and production (Feagans, 1982). Results of a study with children learning French as a second language suggest that school experience has a stronger influence on children's performance of decontextualized language tasks than does home exposure to these tasks (Snow, 1991). In fact, a seminal study conducted in Liberia with nonliterates, English-schooled literates, nonschooled Vai script literates, and nonschooled Arabic literates demonstrated that formal schooling promotes both familiarity with the tasks used in assessment and experience with verbal exposition (Scribner & Cole, 1981). In this study, schooled individuals outperformed nonliterates and nonschooled literates in language tasks, including explanation of sorting stimuli, syllogisms in which the responses ran counter to life experience, grammatical rules, game instructions, and answers to hypothetical questions about name switching. In contrast, assessment tasks that most closely resembled the linguistic practices of nonschooled Vai script literates revealed their specialized training in metalinguistic tasks. For example, blending syllables (rather than word units) in the construction of sentences is an activity required by the complexity of the Vai script. These findings suggest that nonschooled literacies (e.g., Vai script, Arabic) may not involve the same language processes used for acquiring literacy in school contexts. Moreover, the study describes the extent to which the language skills targeted in assessment are mediated within actual literacy and school practices. The research underscores that children's poor performance in assessment may reflect differences in learning experiences or educational opportunity in school-culture settings rather than reflect intrinsic disability.

That the language behaviors selected for the language assessment of school-age children tend to reflect the communication rules and practices of American school settings also has been supported by ethnographic research in education. This research has repeatedly demonstrated that when children do not use expected academic discourse rules or behaviors, language differences are perceived as disorders, and assessments are used to *confirm* a disability (e.g., Mehan et al., 1986).

These issues have important implications for assessment for two reasons. If certain oral language skills can develop without cultural mediation, then it will be possible to design objective assessments that presumably isolate targeted language behavior from its social context. Alternatively, if language performance in a given context reflects cultural mediation, then the challenge is to determine what the goal of language mediation within a given culture is and what its social purposes are. The answers to this challenge may be key to conducting nondiscriminatory assessments.

An Ecological Perspective on Language-Learning Disability

Children with mild language-learning disabilities are most often identified in school. Cultural differences across groups regarding appropriate or typical communicative behavior may lead to a mismatch between the family's and the clinician's views and assumptions. An ethnographic study of Puerto Rican parents' views of disability found that their parameters of "normalcy" were much wider than those used by the educational system (Harry, 1992). They objected to using academic learning as a criterion for disability, noting, for example, that their children had achieved a level of bilingualism that exceeded that of most adult family members. In addition, parents of children labeled as having learning disabilities attributed the problem to a weakness of the school system in properly teaching their children rather than to an intrinsic, child-specific impairment.

These views on disability are revealing. Together with the research reviewed previously, they justify a paradigm shift in assessment from a traditional focus on what the child does (or does not do) to an assessment of the ways families and teachers mediate school language and school cultural knowledge (Gutierrez-Clellen et al., 1995). Furthermore, the assessment of language in its social context requires further research examining the effects of children's exposure to different language experiences and tasks on performance during assessment. For instance, there is evidence that using a film versus a book to elicit children's narratives may generate different types of complex language. A study comparing the syntactic complexity in oral narratives of Mexican American typical and low achievers (from kindergarten to fifth grade) indicated that, regardless of achievement, children exhibited a greater use of subordinate clauses and phrases under the movie condition than when a book was used to elicit stories (Gutierrez-Clellen & de García, 1994). Future studies also should examine the teaching strategies used in instructional settings, their language demands, and the extent to which language learning is promoted in classrooms. This type of empirical research will lead to language assessments that evaluate children's language-learning ability based on their actual learning experiences and *not* on hypothetical mental constructs or culturally specific assumptions about language performance.

ALTERNATIVE ASSESSMENT APPROACHES

In an attempt to reduce bias in assessment, researchers have proposed several strategies to modify the testing situation. Examples include rewording instructions, providing additional time or practice, asking the child to provide an explanation for incorrect responses, having a parent or another trusted adult administer the test, and using repeated presentations of test stimuli (Erickson & Iglesias, 1986; Kayser, 1989; Weddington, 1987).

Taken together, these modifications may reduce assessment bias, but they may not provide sufficient explanatory information about the child's language difficulties or language-learning ability. Damico (1991) proposed using "explanatory analysis" in the interpretation of a child's school language performance. An initial concern based on the child's language difficulties in classroom settings would be followed by a series of questions about whether the observed communication difficulties could be attributed to test anxiety, second-language acquisition, dialectal phenomena, cross-cultural "interference," a subtractive bilingual environment, or test bias. Descriptive observations designed to answer these questions would determine whether there were extrinsic variables affecting the child's language performance in the observed contexts. The evaluator assumes that the reported problematic language behaviors are attributable to extrinsic factors until all such possibilities have been reasonably eliminated. Only then would the problem be associated with an intrinsic language disability. These strategies may reduce the probability of misdiagnosis. However, an exclusive focus on the child as a learner may shift attention away from the language-mediation skills of teachers and other adults. If assessments are intended to test language knowledge, then a crucial component should include an assessment of the skills of those adults who mediate such knowledge.

The issues discussed thus far suggest that it may be unproductive, if not impossible, to neutralize technical or situational bias in language assessments. There is a paucity of data on the language development of different cultural linguistic groups in the United States and the means by which language learning is mediated across different sociocultural environments. Criterion-referenced measures also require culturally and linguistically valid criteria (Kriger Wilen & van Maanen Sweeting, 1986; Terrell et al., 1992).

Ethnographic interviewing, language sampling in culturally relevant contexts, and observing in settings in which actual communicative competence is revealed may help the clinician determine the type of mediated learning experiences teachers and family have provided for the child and the extent to which children's language performance reflects those experiences. For the assessment of young children, ethnographic interviews employing techniques such as those described by Westby (1990) may be significant during data collection. Parental reports also may be used as a valid tool to gather information about a child's language status. A study designed to assess lexical acquisition in infants and toddlers learning Spanish as a first language administered the Inventario del Desarrollo de las Habilidades Comunicativas MacArthur (MacArthur Communicative Development Inventories) (Jackson-Maldonado, Thal, Marchman, Bates, & Gutierrez-Clellen, 1993) toddler form and found that parents from low-income/educational backgrounds can provide reliable information if the examiner uses culturally and linguistically appropriate interview questions and language inventories (Jackson-Maldonado et al., 1993).

Furthermore, ethnographic methods can inform the development of language-sampling procedures that will be relevant to a given group or family. Mastergeorge (1994), over a period of 2 years, interviewed and observed 30 families of children with typical and delayed development in their homes using ethnographic methods. Her research demonstrated that everyday problem-solving contexts, such as pairing shoes and sorting laundry, provided valuable information about the tutorial strategies families used with their children and their beliefs about their children's learning. Thus, rather than assuming universal contexts for language sampling (e.g., asking parents to play as they would at home), ethnographic procedures may be applied to elicit language samples that reflect the actual language-learning experiences of children.

Ethnographic methods also can help diverse language uses gain recognition as skilled forms of language. Wyatt (1995) described the use of "baby rap," verbal disputes, and "playing the dozens" in a group of African American preschoolers as clear demonstrations of their emerging sociolinguistic knowledge within their speech communities. Thus, knowledge of these group-specific speech events also may be used to assess children with different levels of language experience or ability within these communities. The analysis of peer–peer language interactions may serve as a basis by which to identify children who may be less skilled at these "language contests" and who may benefit from increased mediated socialization within their speech communities.

CONCLUSION

Assessments should be able to integrate performance data and contextual effects to explain and maximize performance (i.e., test the limits). Accordingly, clinicians should use language measures and tasks that address the experiences and social expectations of children. Given the diversity of these experiences, even these assessments may not reveal the child's true language-learning ability. Such information will be obtained only through analyses of both the child's responsiveness to adult mediations and the quality of those mediated language-learning experiences (see Chapter 12).

This chapter addressed some of the issues involved in the assessment of children's language from an interactionist and constructivist perspective that considers language ability and disability in its sociocultural context. This perspective contrasts with prevailing medical models that view language disability as a trait and state residing in the individual. If language assessments are to recognize cultural and linguistic diversity, a redefinition of language disability (and ability) will be necessary:

> Disability... exists neither in the head of educators nor in the behavior of students. It is, instead, a function of the interaction between educators' categories, institutional machinery, and students' conduct. That is, designations like "disability" and "handicap" do not exist apart from the institutional practices and cultural-meaning systems that generate and nurture them. (Mehan et al., 1986, p. 164)

REFERENCES

Amastae, J., & Elías-Olivares, L. (1982). *Spanish in the United States: Sociolinguistic aspects.* New York: Cambridge University Press.

Anderson-Yockel, J., & Haynes, W.O. (1994). Joint book-reading strategies in working-class African American and White mother–toddler dyads. *Journal of Speech and Hearing Research, 37*(3), 583–593.

Battle, D.E. (1993). *Communication disorders in multicultural populations.* Stoneham, MA: Butterworth-Heinemann.

Bedore, L.M., & Leonard, L.B. (1995). Prosodic and syntactic bootstrapping and their clinical applications: A tutorial. *American Journal of Speech-Language Pathology, 4,* 66–72.

Bialystok, E., & Cummins, J. (1991). Language, cognition, and education of bilingual children. In E. Bialystok (Ed.), *Language processing in bilingual children* (pp. 222–232). New York: Cambridge University Press.

Camp, J., Drummond, R., Carter, T., & Parker, W. (1988). The predictive validity of the Florida College Level Academic Skills Test (CLAST) for predicting grade point average with university seniors and recent graduates. *Educational and Psychological Measurement, 48,* 963–967.

Carrow, E. (1973). *Test for Auditory Comprehension of Language.* Austin, TX: Urban Research Group.

Caterino, L.C. (1990). Step-by-step procedure for the assessment of language minority children. In A. Barona & E. García (Eds.), *Children at risk: Poverty, minority status, and other issues in educational equity* (pp. 269–282). Washington, DC: National Association of School Psychologists.

Chamberlain, P., & Medinos-Landurand, P. (1991). Practical considerations for the assessment of LEP students with special needs. In E.V. Hamayan & J.S. Damico (Eds.), *Limiting bias in the assessment of bilingual students* (pp. 111–156). Austin, TX: PRO-ED.

Cheng, L.L. (1987). *Assessing Asian language performance.* Gaithersburg, MD: Aspen Publishers, Inc.

Cole, P.A., & Taylor, O.L. (1990). Performance of working class African-American children on three tests of articulation. *Language, Speech, and Hearing Services in Schools, 21,* 171–176.

Collier, V. (1987). Age and rate of acquisition of second language for academic purposes. *Teaching English to Speakers of Other Languages Quarterly, 21,* 617–641.

Cook, V.J. (1992). Evidence for multicompetence. *Language Learning, 42*(4), 557–591.

Crawford v. Honig, 21 IDELR 799 (9th Ca. Cir. 1994).

Cummins, J. (1983). Language proficiency and academic achievement. In J. Oller (Ed.), *Current issues in language testing research* (pp. 121–153). Rowley, MA: Newbury House.

Cummins, J. (1991). Interdependence of first- and second-language proficiency in bilingual children. In E. Bialystok (Ed.), *Language processing in bilingual children* (pp. 70–89). New York: Cambridge University Press.

Cummins, J., Lopes, J., & King, M.L. (1988). The language use patterns, language attitudes, and bilingual proficiency of Portuguese-Canadian children in Toronto. In B. Harley, P. Allen, J. Cummins, & M. Swain (Eds.), *The development of bilingual proficiency. Vol. III: Social context and age.* (Final report submitted to the Social Sciences and Humanities Research Council.) Toronto, Canada: Ontario Institute for Studies in Education.

Damico, J.S. (1991). Descriptive assessment of communicative ability in limited English proficient students. In E.V. Hamayan & J.S. Damico (Eds.), *Limiting bias in the assessment of bilingual students* (pp. 157–217). Austin, TX: PRO-ED.

Damico, J.S., Oller, J.W., & Storey, M.E. (1983). The diagnosis of language disorders in bilingual children: Surface-oriented and pragmatic criteria. *Journal of Speech and Hearing Disorders, 48,* 385–393.

Dickinson, D.K., & Snow, C.E. (1987). Interrelationships among prereading and oral language skills in kindergartners from two social classes. *Early Childhood Research Quarterly, 2,* 1–26.

Dromi, E., Leonard, L.B., & Shteiman, M. (1993). The grammatical morphology of Hebrew-speaking children with specific language impairment: Some competing hypotheses. *Journal of Speech and Hearing Research, 36,* 760–771.

Dunn, L., & Dunn, L. (1981). *Peabody Picture Vocabulary Test–Revised.* Circle Pines, MN: American Guidance Service.

Eastman, C.M. (1992). Codeswitching as an urban language, contact phenomenon. *Journal of Multilingual and Multicultural Development, 13,* 1–17.

Erickson, F. (1984). Rhetoric, anecdote, and rhapsody: Coherence strategies in a conversation among Black American adolescents. In D. Tannen (Ed.), *Coherence in spoken and written discourse* (pp. 81–154). Norwood, NJ: Ablex.

Erickson, J.G., & Iglesias, A. (1986). Assessment of communication disorders in non-English proficient children. In O. Taylor (Ed.), *Nature of communication disorders in culturally and linguistically diverse populations* (pp. 181–218). San Diego: College-Hill Press.

Faltis, C. (1993, December/January). Programmatic and curricular options for secondary schools serving limited English proficient students. *High School Journal,* 171–181.

Fantini, A. (1985). *Language acquisition of a bilingual child: A sociolinguistic perspective.* San Diego: College-Hill Press.

Feagans, L. (1982). The development and importance of narratives for school adaptation. In L. Feagans & D.C. Farran (Eds.), *The language of children reared in poverty* (pp. 95–116). New York: Academic Press.

Figueroa, R.A. (1989). Psychological testing of linguistic-minority students: Knowledge gaps and regulations. *Exceptional Children, 56,* 145–152.

Figueroa, R.A., & García, E. (1994, Fall). Issues in testing students from culturally and linguistically diverse backgrounds. *Multicultural Education,* 10–19.

García, E., Maez, L., & Gonzalez, G. (1981). A national study of Spanish-English bilingualism in young Hispanic children of the U.S. *Bilingual Education Paper Series, 4*(12).

García, S.B., & Ortiz, A.A. (1988). Preventing inappropriate referrals of language minority students to special education. *New Focus: Occasional Papers in Bilingual Education, 5,* 1–12. Wheaton, MD: The National Clearinghouse for Bilingual Education.

Gardner, M. (1981). *Expressive One-Word Picture Vocabulary Test.* Novato, CA: Academic Therapy Publications.

Grosjean, F. (1982). *Life with two languages: An introduction to bilingualism.* Cambridge, MA: Harvard University Press.

Grosjean, F. (1989). Neurolinguists, beware! The bilingual is not two monolinguals in one person. *Brain and Language, 36,* 3–15.

Gumperz, J.J. (1982). *Discourse strategies.* New York: Cambridge University Press.

Gutierrez-Clellen, V.F. (1995). Narrative development and disorders in Spanish-speaking children: Implications for the bilingual interventionist. In H. Kayser (Ed.), *Bilingual speech-language pathology: An Hispanic focus* (pp. 97–128). San Diego: Singular.

Gutierrez-Clellen, V.F., & de García, L. (1994, November). *Syntactic complexity of Latino children with low and normal achievement.* Paper presented at the national convention of the American Speech-Language-Hearing Association, New Orleans.

Gutierrez-Clellen, V.F., & Heinrichs-Ramos, L. (1993). Referential cohesion in the narratives of Spanish-speaking children: A developmental study. *Journal of Speech and Hearing Research, 36,* 559–567.

Gutierrez-Clellen, V.F., Peña, E., & Quinn, R. (1995). Accommodating cultural differences in narrative style: A bilingual perspective. *Topics in Language Disorders, 15*(4), 54–67.

Gutierrez-Clellen, V.F., & Quinn, R. (1993). Assessing narratives in diverse cultural/ linguistic populations: Clinical implications. *Language, Speech, and Hearing Services in Schools, 24*(1), 2–9.

Hakuta, K., Ferdman, B.M., & Díaz, R.M. (1987). Bilingualism and cognitive development: Three perspectives. In S. Rosenberg (Ed.), *Advances in applied psycholinguistics. Vol. II: Reading, writing, and language learning* (pp. 284–319). Cambridge, MA: Cambridge University Press.

Hannah, E.P., & Gardner, J.O. (1978). *Hannah-Gardner Test of Verbal and Nonverbal Language Functioning.* Northridge, CA: Lingua Press.

Harry, B. (1992). Making sense of disability: Low-income, Puerto Rican parents' theories of the problem. *Exceptional Children, 59*(1), 27–40.

Haywood, H.C., Brown, A.L., & Wingenfeld, S. (1990). Dynamic approaches to psychoeducational assessment. *School Psychology Review, 19,* 411–422.

Jackson-Maldonado, D., Thal, D., Marchman, V., Bates, E., & Gutierrez-Clellen, V.F. (1993). Early lexical development in Spanish-speaking infants and toddlers. *Journal of Child Language, 20*(3), 523–549.

Kay-Raining Bird, E., & Kluppel Vetter, D. (1994). Storytelling in Chippewa-Cree children. *Journal of Speech and Hearing Research, 37*(6), 1354–1368.

Kayser, H. (1989). Speech and language assessment of Spanish-English speaking children. *Language, Speech, and Hearing Services in Schools, 20*(3), 226–241.

Krigcr Wilcn, D., & van Maanen Sweeting, C. (1986). Assessment of limited English proficient Hispanic students. *School Psychology Review, 15,* 59–75.

Kvaal, J.T., Shipstead-Cox, N., Nevitt, S.G., Hodson, B.W., & Launer, P.B. (1988). The acquisition of 10 Spanish morphemes by Spanish-speaking children. *Language, Speech, and Hearing Services in Schools, 19*(4), 384–394.

Lahey, M. (1994). Grammatical morpheme acquisition: Do norms exist? *Journal of Speech and Hearing Research, 37*(5), 1192–1194.

Langdon, H.W. (1992). Language communication and sociocultural patterns in Hispanic families. In H.W. Langdon (Ed.), *Hispanic children and adults with communication disorders* (pp. 99–131). Gaithersburg, MD: Aspen Publishers, Inc.
Langdon, H.W., & Merino, B.J. (1992). Acquisition and development of a second language in the Spanish speaker. In H.W. Langdon (Ed.), *Hispanic children and adults with communication disorders* (pp. 132–168). Gaithersburg, MD: Aspen Publishers, Inc.
Larry P. v. Riles, 495 F. Supp. 926, (N.D. Ca. 1979); 83–84 EHLR DEC. 555:304, California.
Larry P. Task Force. (1989). *Larry P. Task Force Report: Policy and alternative assessment guideline recommendations.* Sacramento, CA: Resources in Special Education.
Leonard, L.B.(1991a). Specific language impairment as a clinical category. *Language, Speech, and Hearing Services in Schools, 22,* 66–68.
Leonard, L.B.(1991b). The cross-linguistic study of language impaired children. In J.F. Miller (Ed.), *Research on child language disorders: A decade of progress* (pp. 379–386). Austin, TX: PRO-ED.
Linares, N. (1981). Rules for calculating mean length of utterance in morphemes for Spanish. In J.G. Erickson & D.R. Omark (Eds.), *Communication assessment of the bilingual bicultural child* (pp. 291–295). Baltimore: University Park Press.
Lynch, E.W., & Hanson, M.J. (Eds.). (1992). *Developing cross-cultural competence: A guide for working with young children and their families.* Baltimore: Paul H. Brookes Publishing Co.
Malakoff, M.E. (1988). The effect of language of instruction on reasoning in bilingual children. *Applied Psycholinguistics, 9*(1), 17–38.
Mastergeorge, A.M. (1994, November). *The role of ethnography: Understanding everyday contexts, cognition, and language.* Paper presented at the national convention of the American Speech-Language-Hearing Association, New Orleans.
McCauley, R.J., & Swisher, L. (1984a). Psychometric review of language and articulation tests for preschool children. *Journal of Speech and Hearing Disorders, 49,* 34–42.
McCauley, R.J., & Swisher, L. (1984b). Use and misuse of norm-referenced tests in clinical assessment: A hypothetical case. *Journal of Speech and Hearing Disorders, 49,* 338–348.
Mehan, H., Hertweck, A., & Meihls, J.L. (1986). *Handicapping the handicapped: Decision making in students' educational careers.* Stanford, CA: Stanford University Press.
Mercer, J. (1988). Ethnic differences in IQ scores: What do they mean? (A response to Lloyd Dunn). *Hispanic Journal of Behavioral Sciences, 10*(3), 199–218.
Merino, B.J. (1992). Acquisition of syntactic and phonological features in Spanish. In H.W. Langdon (Ed.), *Hispanic children and adults with communication disorders* (pp. 57–98). Gaithersburg, MD: Aspen Publishers, Inc.
Michaels, S. (1986). Narrative presentations: An oral preparation for literacy with first graders. In J. Cook-Gumperz (Ed.), *The social construction of literacy* (pp. 94–116). Cambridge, England: Cambridge University Press.
Michaels, S. (1991). The dismantling of narrative. In A. McCabe & C. Peterson (Eds.), *Developing narrative structure* (pp. 303–351). Hillsdale, NJ: Lawrence Erlbaum Associates.
Miller-Jones, D. (1989). Culture and testing. *American Psychologist, 44*(2), 360–366.
Nelson, N.W. (1993). *Childhood language disorders in context: Infancy through adolescence.* New York: Macmillan.

Norris, M.K., Juarez, M.J., & Perkins, M.N. (1989). Adaptation of a screening test for bilingual and bidialectal populations. *Language, Speech, and Hearing Services in Schools, 20,* 372–380.

Oller, J.W., & Damico, J.S. (1991). Theoretical considerations in the assessment of LEP students. In E.V. Hamayan & J.S. Damico (Eds.), *Limiting bias in the assessment of bilingual students* (pp. 77–110). Austin, TX: PRO-ED.

Ortiz, A.A., & Wilkinson, C.Y. (1987). *Limited English proficient and English proficient Hispanic students with communication disorders: Characteristics at initial assessment and at reevaluation.* Austin: The University of Texas, Handicapped Minority Research Institute on Language Proficiency.

Ortiz, A.A., & Yates, J.R. (1983). Incidence of exceptionality among Hispanics: Implications for manpower planning. *National Association for Bilingual Education Journal, 7*(3), 41–53.

Ortiz, A.A., & Yates, J.R. (1984). Linguistically and culturally diverse handicapped students. In R. Podemski, B. Price, T. Smith, & G. Marsh, II (Eds.), *Comprehensive administration of special education* (pp. 114–141). Rockville, MD: Aspen Systems Corp.

Pearson, B.Z., Fernández, S.C., & Oller, D.K. (1993). Lexical development in bilingual infants and toddlers: Comparison to monolingual norms. *Language Learning, 43*(1), 93–120.

Peña, E., Quinn, R., & Iglesias, A. (1992). The application of dynamic methods to language assessment: A nonbiased procedure. *The Journal of Special Education, 26*(3), 269–280.

Plante, E., & Vance, R. (1994). Selection of preschool language tests: A data-based approach. *Language, Speech, and Hearing Services in Schools, 25,* 15–24.

Ramsey Musselwhite, C. (1983). Pluralistic assessment in speech-language pathology: Use of dual norms in the placement process. *Language, Speech, and Hearing Services in Schools, 14,* 29–37.

Ripich, D.N., & Spinelli, F.M. (1985). *School discourse problems.* San Diego: College-Hill Press.

Scribner, S., & Cole, M. (1981). *The psychology of literacy.* Cambridge, MA: Harvard University Press.

Sharwood Smith, M. (1991). Language modules and bilingual processing. In E. Bialystok (Ed.), *Language processing in bilingual children* (pp. 10–24). New York: Cambridge University Press.

Shiff-Myers, N.B. (1992). Considering arrested language development and language loss in the assessment of second language learners. *Language, Speech, and Hearing Services in Schools, 23,* 28–33.

Slobin, D.I., & Bocaz, A. (1988). Learning to talk about movement through time and space: The development of narrative abilities in Spanish and English. *Lenguas Modernas* (Universidad de Chile), *15,* 5–24.

Snow, C.E. (1987). Beyond conversation: Second language learners' acquisition of description and explanation. In J. Lantolf & A. Labarca (Eds.), *Research in second language learning: Focus on the classroom* (pp. 3–16). Norwood, NJ: Ablex.

Snow, C.E. (1990). Rationales for native language instruction: Evidence from research. In A.M. Padilla, H.H. Fairchild, & C. Valadez (Eds.), *Bilingual education: Issues and strategies* (pp. 60–74). Beverly Hills: Sage Publications.

Snow, C.E. (1991). Diverse conversational contexts for the acquisition of various language skills. In J.F. Miller (Ed.), *Research on child language disorders: A decade of progress* (pp. 105–124). Austin, TX: PRO-ED.

Snow, C.E., Cancino, H., Gonzalez, P., & Shriberg, E. (1989). Giving formal definitions: An oral language correlate of school literacy. In D. Bloome (Ed.), *Classroom and literacy*. Norwood, NJ: Ablex.

Terrell, S.L., Arensberg, K., & Rosa, M. (1992). Parent–child comparative analysis: A criterion-referenced method for the nondiscriminatory assessment of a child who spoke a relatively uncommon dialect of English. *Language, Speech, and Hearing Services in Schools, 23*, 34–42.

Tucker, J.A. (1980). Ethnic proportions in classes for the learning disabled: Issues in nonbiased assessment. *The Journal of Special Education, 14*(1), 93–105.

Velasco, P. (1989). *The relationship of oral decontextualized language and reading comprehension in bilingual children*. Unpublished doctoral dissertation, Harvard Graduate School of Education, Boston.

Washington, J.A., & Craig, H.K. (1992a). Articulation test performances of low-income, African-American preschoolers with communication impairments. *Language, Speech, and Hearing Services in Schools, 23*, 203–207.

Washington, J.A., & Craig, H.K. (1992b). Performances of low-income preschool and kindergarten children on the Peabody Picture Vocabulary Test–Revised. *Language, Speech, and Hearing Services in Schools, 23*, 329–333.

Watson, I. (1991). Phonological processing in two languages. In E. Bialystok (Ed.), *Language processing in bilingual children* (pp. 25–48). New York: Cambridge University Press.

Wechsler, D. (1974). *Wechsler Intelligence Scale for Children–Revised*. New York: The Psychological Corporation.

Weddington, G.T. (1987). *The assessment and treatment of communication disorders in culturally diverse populations*. Unpublished manuscript.

Westby, C.E. (1990). Ethnographic interviewing: Asking the right questions to the right people in the right ways. *Journal of Childhood Communication Disorders, 13*, 101–111.

Westby, C.E. (1994). Multicultural issues. In J.B. Tomblin, H.L. Morris, & D.C Spriestersbach (Eds.), *Diagnosis in speech-language pathology* (pp. 29–51). San Diego: Singular.

Wilcox, K.A., & McGuinn Aasby, S. (1988). The performance of monolingual and bilingual Mexican children on the TACL. *Language, Speech, and Hearing Services in Schools, 19*, 34–40.

Wolf, D., Bixby, J., Glenn, J., III, & Gardner, H. (1991). To use their minds well: Investigating new forms of student assessment. *Review of Research in Education, 17*, 31–74.

Wong Fillmore, L. (1991). Language and cultural issues in early education. In S.L. Kagan (Ed.), *The care and education of America's young children: Obstacles and opportunities* (pp. 30–49). Chicago: University of Chicago Press.

Wyatt, T.A. (1993, May). Standardized language assessment and Larry P.: A review. *California Speech-Hearing Association*, 17–18.

Wyatt, T.A. (1995). Language development in African-American English child speech. *Linguistics and Education, 7*, 7–22.

3

Prelinguistic Predictors
of Later Language Development

Rebecca B. McCathren,
Steven F. Warren, and Paul J. Yoder

IDENTIFYING COMMUNICATION AND LANGUAGE DELAYS and disabilities as early as possible is of vital importance. The cumulative, often pervasive, effects of such delays and disorders on peer relationships, emotional and behavioral development (Baker & Cantwell, 1982), and later school achievement (Silva, Williams, & McGee, 1987) are well documented. Yet language delays often are not identified until children are 3 or 4 years of age or older (Wetherby & Prizant, 1992). The availability of reliable, valid prelinguistic assessments could lead to much earlier identification of children with communication delays and disorders, thus allowing intervention efforts to be implemented earlier in the developmental process.

Two hurdles must be cleared to develop valid prelinguistic assessments. First, good predictors of later language development must be identified. Second, assessment situations that reliably elicit infants' and young children's most sophisticated communication skills must be created. Researchers are making substantial progress on clearing both of these hurdles.

This chapter identifies four proven prelinguistic predictors of later language development and critiques relevant available assessments that measure these predictors. A brief overview of research needs and recommendations for practitioners concludes the chapter. Issues related to the selection of nonspeech systems for young children are beyond the scope of this chapter (see Reichle, 1991).

PRELINGUISTIC COMMUNICATION DEVELOPMENT

The prelinguistic communication period of development begins at birth and fades as children begin to use words as their primary means of communicating

Preparation of this chapter was supported by the National Institute of Child Health and Human Development Grant #T32HD07226 and Grant #RO1HD27594 and U.S. Department of Education Grant #HO23C20152.

thoughts, feelings, and needs. This period is divided into preintentional and intentional communication stages. The preintentional communication stage is characterized by behaviors that have no intended outcome and are not directed toward a partner. The infant's behavior is communicative only because another person assigns communicative meaning to it. For example, an infant reaches for a distant toy. Her father observes this and gets the toy for the baby. Acts like this are termed *perlocutionary*, which Bates (1976) defined as acts that are not intentional but have communicative effects.

At about 8–9 months of age, infants begin to act in ways that clearly are intended to have an effect on the listener (Bates, 1979a; McLean, 1990). Bates (1976) termed these *intentional communication acts*. McLean (1990) divided this stage into two substages—illocutionary and locutionary—to distinguish between intentional unconventional communication and the development of conventional gestures. The illocutionary substage is distinguished by the emergence of coordinated attention. Infants include (i.e., coordinate between) both their communicative partner and an object, event, or other person in the communication act by alternating gazes between them.

The conventional illocutionary substage typically begins at about 12 months and is marked by the addition of conventional gestures that clarify the infant's communication. These gestures include pointing to objects that are out of reach or using an open palm to request an object. During this stage, the infant also uses ritualized vocalizations to label objects (e.g., ba-ba for baby). Babbling during this stage is characterized by prosody and syllabic differentiation that is language-like, but the sounds themselves are usually unintelligible (McLean, 1990).

The prelinguistic period begins to fade from 12 to 17 months as the infant moves into the locutionary substage. Increasingly, the infant uses words to express thoughts, feelings, and needs. These initial words often are accompanied by gestures and vocalizations (Iverson & Thal, in press).

PREDICTORS OF LATER LANGUAGE DEVELOPMENT

Numerous variables are predictive of overall language development. Many of these factors are related to developmental delay in general (e.g., Down syndrome, neurological impairments). The focus of this chapter is on four variables that appear to be closely related to language development and that independently predict language development irrespective of the presence or absence of other factors (e.g., Down syndrome, fragile X syndrome). This small set of predictors includes three communication components that emerge during the prelinguistic period: 1) babbling, 2) development of pragmatic functions, and 3) vocabulary comprehension. The fourth predictor is the development of combinatorial and symbolic play skills.

Babbling

One of the more frequently examined areas of prelinguistic development is babbling. The stages of typical vocal development have been described by a number of researchers (e.g., Oller & Lynch, 1992; Stark, 1980; Stoel-Gammon, 1992). Researchers also have investigated babbling in infants to determine continuities between babbling and later speech and to determine whether expressive language development can be predicted from babbling (Kagan, 1971; Locke, 1989; Stoel-Gammon, 1989).

Stages of Vocalization   The earliest stages of prelinguistic vocal development are marked by vocalizations that contain only vowels (Oller & Lynch, 1992). As the infant's vocal repertoire expands, the use of consonants increases. At about 5 months, infants enter the canonical syllable stage, which is characterized by consonant–vowel (CV) syllables with adult-like consonant-to-vowel transitions. These canonical syllables are divided into two types: *reduplicated* and *variegated*. In reduplicated babbling, the infant repeats the same syllable (e.g., ma-ma, ba-ba). In variegated babbling, the infant changes the consonant, the vowel, or both (e.g., da-ba, do-ga). In the final stage, the infant mixes babbling with meaningful speech.

Relationship Between Babbling and Spoken Language   Babbling may be predictive of later spoken language for two reasons. First, there appears to be a direct relationship based on the similarity of form (Locke, 1989). Second, babbling is one of the early behaviors typically responded to and labeled as communicative by adults. Harding (1983) reported that most of the mothers in her study consistently responded to all vocalizations as communicative.

Canonical babbling may be more strongly related to later spoken language than other kinds of vocalizations. There are two possible reasons for this. First, adults may be more apt to attribute meaning to canonical babbling because of its wordlike sounds than to other types of vocalizations and thus respond to canonical babbling as if the infant had spoken real words (McCune, 1992; Papousek, 1993). Second, infants who are good babblers may have better-developed oral-motor skills and neurological functioning than might infants with less-developed babbling (Locke, 1989).

The empirical research showing a correlation between early babbling and later spoken language has used two measures of babbling: amount of vocalization and consonant use in vocalizations.

Amount of Vocalization   Researchers have found the amount of vocalization in the prelinguistic period to be predictive of later speech for typically developing children (Camp, Burgess, Morgan, & Zerbe, 1987; Kagan, 1971; Roe, 1977). High vocalization rates are predictive of 1) higher vocabulary development for girls but not for boys (Kagan, 1971); 2) amount of talking at 3 years, as well as vocabulary development and performance on a reading task at 5 years for boys (Roe, 1977); and 3) word use at 1 year for both boys and girls (Camp et al., 1987).

Consonant Use in Vocalizations   Locke (1983) examined the similarity between babbling and early speech. He identified 12 consonants that account for 92%–95% of consonants used by infants 11–12 months old and found that this same set of consonants also is the most frequently used in early word production. He also found that the CV syllable type, which is characteristic of canonical babbling, typifies early speech.

Consonant use in the prelinguistic communication period also is predictive of some aspects of spoken language (Murphy, Menyuk, Liebergott, & Schultz, 1983; Stoel-Gammon, 1989; Whitehurst, Smith, Fischel, Arnold, & Lonigan, 1991). Studies have shown that complexity of babbling (as measured by consonant use) is positively correlated with 1) earlier entry into the stage of meaningful speech (Stoel-Gammon, 1989); 2) earlier attainment of a 50-word productive vocabulary (Murphy et al., 1983); 3) advanced phonological development at 3 years (Vihman & Greenlee, 1987); and 4) expressive language gains (Whitehurst et al., 1991).

In summary, research indicates that both the amount of vocalization and the use of consonants during the prelinguistic period are predictive of spoken language. Amount of vocalization predicts amount of speech and vocabulary development. Complexity of vocalization predicts language milestones and phonological and expressive language development.

Development of Pragmatic Functions

Bruner (1981) identified three categories of pragmatic functions that develop in the first year of life: 1) behavioral regulation—controlling another's behavior to get him or her to perform an action (e.g., giving a bottle, manipulating a toy); 2) social interaction—getting another's attention for social purposes (e.g., playing peekaboo, showing off); and 3) joint attention—directing another's attention to establish a shared focus on an activity, object, or person. The exact age and order of onset for these pragmatic skills vary across children (Carpenter, Mastergeorge, & Coggins, 1983).

Behavioral regulation occurs when the infant tries to get someone to do or cease doing something. The infant uses requests and protests to elicit the desired behavior from the adult. This includes behaviors like obtaining out-of-reach objects and manipulating objects. Mosier and Rogoff (1994) reported requesting behavior in infants as young as 6 months in situations that were designed to elicit these behaviors. In children with Down syndrome, frequency of prelinguistic requesting has been found to be positively associated with both expressive (Mundy, Sigman, Kasari, & Yirmiya, 1988; Smith & vonTetzchner, 1986) and receptive (Mundy et al., 1988) language.

Social interaction is used by infants to get adults to focus attention on them. Games like peekaboo and social routines like waving "hi" or "bye" are demonstrations of social interaction. Rates of social interaction predict expressive language for children with Down syndrome and both expressive and receptive language for typically developing children (Mundy, Kasari, Sigman, & Ruskin, 1995).

Joint attention entails the infant using behaviors to direct the adult's attention to an object or event that the infant is noticing. Loud noises, unexpected events, and interesting objects can serve as the topic of the infant's "comments." In studies of children with Down syndrome, the rate of commenting was significantly associated with receptive but not expressive language (Mundy et al., 1988; Smith & vonTetzchner, 1986). Mundy and colleagues (1988) found that the rate of commenting of typically developing infants was predictive of both receptive and expressive language. Joint attention also is predictive of language development for children with autism (Mundy, Sigman, & Kasari, 1990).

Behavioral regulation and joint attention often are expressed through the infant's use of coordinated attention. Examples of coordinated attention include giving or showing an object to an adult or pointing to an object while looking at the adult (Yoder & Munson, 1995). Coordinated attention is most important as an indicator of the infant's intention to communicate.

In the course of prelinguistic development, infants should use all three of these pragmatic functions (Wetherby, Cain, Yonclas, & Walker, 1988). Failure to do so indicates potential impairment (Wetherby & Prutting, 1984).

Vocabulary Comprehension

Vocabulary comprehension in typically developing prelinguistic infants is correlated with later word production (Bates, Benigni, Bretherton, Camaioni, & Volterra, 1979; Bates, Bretherton, & Snyder, 1988). Similarly, in a study of late talkers, Thal, Tobias, and Morrison (1991) found that the difference between late talkers whose productive language was within typical limits a year later and late talkers whose productive language was still delayed a year later was their vocabulary comprehension at the beginning of the study; the children with the smallest receptive vocabularies made the least gains in production.

Unfortunately, comprehension is very difficult to measure for children under the age of 2 (Bates, 1993). Receptive language typically has been measured by asking infants to touch objects or pictures or to demonstrate an action that has been named. Distinguishing noncompliance from not knowing is virtually impossible with infants.

One of the ways around this dilemma is to use parent reports instead of child performance to determine comprehension. Bates (1993) stated that valid parent report measures depend on following three guidelines: 1) ask about behaviors that are happening now, not that have happened in the past; 2) ask about what is new and changing; and 3) ask parents to recognize, not re-create (i.e., provide a checklist rather than a blank piece of paper). Bates and her colleagues (1979) reported that parent report measures were better predictors of later language than was laboratory or home observation.

Development of Combinatorial and Symbolic Play Skills

Although play usually is not considered a communicative skill, the complexity of a child's play has been found to be predictive of later language development (Bloom, 1993). Also, play is a primary intervention context for young children, and level of play skills has been shown to predict the success of prelinguistic communication intervention (Yoder, Warren, & Hull, 1995).

Piaget (1962) specified a developmental continuum that includes three types of play with objects. The first, exploratory play, is the banging, shaking, or mouthing of objects. The next type, combinatorial play, is demonstrated by the infant's relating objects to each other, such as building a tower, putting a toy person in a toy car, or pounding pegs with a hammer. The final, most sophisticated, type of play is symbolic. In symbolic play, one object stands for another (e.g., pretending a block is a car or a stick is a gun). Concurrent with prelinguistic development, infants engage in exploratory play, then move to combinatorial play, and later engage in symbolic play.

Combinatorial play skills predict language development for both typically (Bates et al., 1979; Bloom, 1993) and atypically developing infants (Mundy et al., 1988). For typically developing infants, higher levels of combinatorial play are predictive of higher levels of receptive language (Bates et al., 1979), and earlier onset of combinatorial play is predictive of earlier onset of speech (Bloom, 1993). For children with developmental delays (Casby & Ruder, 1983), hearing impairments (Casby & McCormack, 1985), Down syndrome (Mundy et al., 1988), or autism (Mundy et al., 1990), both level and rates of combinatorial and symbolic play are predictive of language development.

Play skills also may be useful for distinguishing between children in need of intervention and those who will "catch up" without intervention. Thal and colleagues (1991) compared the play scheme development of children who appeared to have language delays but later "caught up" with the play scheme development of children who continued to exhibit language delays a year later. Thal and colleagues found that the children who continued to have delays in play scheme development performed significantly worse on all play measures than did the children who later caught up.

Play also is important because object manipulation is a frequent focus of prelinguistic commenting and requesting. Object play is an excellent context for prelinguistic communication intervention (Yoder et al., 1995). Children who do not demonstrate interest or skill in object play are harder to engage in the types of interactions that facilitate communication development. Yoder and colleagues reported that lesser amounts of combinatorial and symbolic play are related to slower rates of increasing prelinguistic requesting during intervention with children with mental retardation.

In summary, rates and complexity of babbling, rates of pragmatic use, level of vocabulary comprehension, and complexity and rates of play all have been found to predict some aspects of later language development. Assessing and monitoring the development of infants in these four skill areas can allow identification of communication delays and disorders well before a child "fails" to talk. Subsequently, intervention efforts can begin months or years earlier than might otherwise be the case. At least in principle, this should lead to more successful outcomes. It is first necessary, however, to have valid, reliable assessments of these four predictors.

PRELINGUISTIC ASSESSMENTS

Without valid and reliable assessment, predictors of later language development that are generated through research cannot be used by clinicians to distinguish typically developing infants from those in need of intervention. The eight assessment instruments shown in Table 1 frequently are used to assess early communication development. Nonstandardized assessments of early communication development (e.g., Miller & Paul, 1995) are not included. Six of the assessments in Table 1 either do not measure the four predictors or are so limited in their measurement that they are of little use in early identification. The two instruments that do measure the four predictors are the Assessing Prelinguistic and Early Linguistic Behaviors in Developmentally Young Children (ALB) (Olswang,

Table 1. Assessments of prelinguistic communication skills

Assessment instrument	Babbling	Pragmatic functions	Vocabulary comprehension	Play skills
Bayley Scales of Infant Development–Second Edition (Bayley, 1993)	X		X	
Assessing Prelinguistic and Early Linguistic Behaviors in Developmentally Young Children (Olswang et al., 1987)	X	X	X	X
Communication and Symbolic Behavior Scales (Wetherby & Prizant, 1993)	X	X	X	X
MacArthur Communicative Development Inventory/ Infants (Fenson et al., 1993)			X	X
Preschool Language Scale–3 (Zimmerman, Steiner, & Pond, 1992)	X		X	
Receptive-Expressive Emergent Language Scale (Bzoch & League, 1971)	X		X	
Reynell Developmental Language Scales (Reynell & Huntley, 1985)	X		X	
Sequenced Inventory of Communication Development (Hedrick, Prather, & Tobin, 1975)		X	X	

Stoel-Gammon, Coggins, & Carpenter, 1987) and the Communication and Symbolic Behavior Scales (CSBS) (Wetherby & Prizant, 1993). Although the MacArthur Communicative Development Inventory/Infants (CDI/I) (Fenson et al., 1993) does not measure all four predictors, it has been shown to predict vocabulary comprehension and expressive vocabulary. Following is a description of how these assessments measure the four predictor skills and an examination of the issues related to reliability, validity, and test administration and scoring.

Babbling

Mean babbling level has been reported to predict the onset of speech (Stoel-Gammon, 1989). Both the ALB and the CSBS measure babbling. In the ALB, a mean babbling level is computed based on the complexity of the child's vocalizations. Vocalizations are divided into three levels. Level 1 vocalizations have a vowel and/or a consonant that is not a true consonant but a glide or a glottal. Level 2 vocalizations contain at least one CV or VC sequence with a true consonant. Level 3 vocalizations have at least two true consonants differing in placement or articulation. In a 50-utterance sample, the mean babbling level would be computed in the following manner:

$$
\begin{array}{lll}
\text{Level 1} & 20 \text{ vocalizations} \times 1 = & 20 \\
\text{Level 2} & 10 \text{ vocalizations} \times 2 = & 20 \\
\text{Level 3} & 20 \text{ vocalizations} \times 3 = & \underline{60} \\
& & 100
\end{array}
$$

100 vocalizations ÷ 50 utterances = mean babbling level of 2

The CSBS has two communicative clusters that measure aspects of babbling. The *Communicative Means–Vocal cluster* has four babbling scales: 1) vocal acts without gesture, 2) inventory of consonants, 3) frequency of syllables with consonants, and 4) frequency of acts containing multisyllables. The *Communicative Means–Gestural cluster* includes a fifth babbling scale: vocal acts with gesture. Although the constructs "syllables with consonants" and "acts containing multisyllables" have been found to predict later language (Camp et al., 1987; Stoel-Gammon, 1989; Vihman & Greenlee, 1987), proportions rather than frequency counts are predictive. The scores of the four scales, like all of the CSBS scales, are assigned a value of 1–5 on a Likert scale. The use of the Likert scale reduces the variation among children, which may make prediction more difficult. Therefore, it is unclear whether this cluster score measure can yield a reliable prediction of later language.

Development of Pragmatic Functions

Both the ALB and the CSBS measure pragmatic functions. The ALB provides a frequency tally for commenting, requesting, requesting information, acknowledging, and answering. The CSBS measures behavioral regulation, social interaction, and joint attention. The frequency of communicative acts that function as behavioral regulation and joint attention is counted. The third pragmatic function, social interaction, is included as a proportion with joint attention and behavioral regulation in the scale termed Sociability of Functions. The scores on each of the scales are then assigned a Likert score ranging from 1 to 5. Research is needed to determine the relative proportions of the three pragmatic functions that predict positive developmental outcomes and those that signal that there may be a problem. Also, the use of a Likert scale may reduce individual child variance to the point that it interferes with the predictive validity.

Vocabulary Comprehension

The CDI/I is the only assessment that measures vocabulary comprehension in a way that is supported in the research literature. The vocabulary comprehension section of the CDI/I is a parent report form for children 8–16 months old that asks parents to mark the words from a list that their child understands. The list consists of 368 words in 19 categories (e.g., animal names, vehicles, food and drink, people). The number of words that the child understands predicts later expressive language development.

Development of Combinatorial and Symbolic Play Skills

The CDI/I, the ALB, and the CSBS each measures some aspects of play. The CDI/I asks parents whether their child engages in specific functional and symbolic play schemes. Combinatorial play is not included in the assessment as a distinct category. The ALB has 12 discrete play behavior levels that are used to categorize children's play skills. The child's highest level of play is reported. The CSBS has three scales related to combinatorial and symbolic play. The first is an inventory of the number of different action schemes. The second uses a weighting system based on the complexity of the action schemes. The third rates combinatorial play skills. These scores are assigned values of 1–5 on a Likert scale.

Reliability

Reliability is the degree to which scores on a test are stable and consistently measured (Overton, 1992). Kamphaus, Dresden, and Kaufman (1993) recommended that reliability be reported using measures for test–retest and internal consistency. Because of the subjectivity implied in interpreting prelinguistic communication, interrater reliability also will be included. All three assessments report some reliability information.

Test–Retest Both the CDI/I and the CSBS report test–retest correlations. Test–retest scores measure the stability of a child's performance over time. Because communication changes so dramatically in the first 2 years of life, attention must be paid to the amount of time between testing. Changes in scores may reflect development, not error in measurement. For this reason, it is expected that test–retest measures for early communication development will be higher over shorter periods of time rather than over longer periods (e.g., 1 month versus 3 months). The CDI/I reports acceptable levels of test–retest reliability for 500 children tested 6 weeks apart. Although the CSBS reports test–retest reliability, the time period between testings (an average of 2.85 months) is too long to provide a good measure of reliability.

Internal Consistency   The CDI/I and the CSBS report measures of internal consistency. Internal consistency measures the extent to which different scales measure the same construct (Kamphaus et al., 1993). Internal consistency correlations for both the CDI/I and the CSBS are high. However, the Social-Affective Signaling cluster of the CSBS includes "gaze shift" and "negative affect," which are negatively correlated. These items should not be included in the same cluster because a negative correlation demonstrates that they do not measure the same construct.

Interrater Reliability   Interrater reliability is the extent to which two different people assign the same score or code to the behavior being assessed. The CDI/I uses parent reports to obtain information about a child; therefore, interrater reliability is not applicable. High rates of interrater reliability are reported for the ALB, although ongoing training and monitoring are needed to maintain reliability. Interrater reliability for the CSBS for two of the three pairs of coders is unacceptably low (below .8) on 16 of the 44 comparisons. Training clinicians and researchers to reliably code both the ALB and the CSBS is a difficult and time-consuming task.

The three tests do report reliability data. Both the CSBS and the CDI/I manuals include reliability data using measures of test–retest and internal consistency. The reported reliability for the CDI/I generally is good. Unfortunately, some of the correlations on the CSBS are low. Test–retest measures conducted over shorter periods of time may indicate that the CSBS is more stable than previously shown. Including negatively correlated items in the same cluster on the CSBS creates a problem with internal consistency. The ALB manual includes only interrater reliability.

Validity

Validity is the degree to which a test performs its designated task (Sattler, 1990). The question to ask about validity is not, "Is this test valid?" but rather, "Is this test valid for this use?" The objective of assessing prelinguistic communication is to predict which children will require further monitoring and/or intervention. The other important validity issue is the extent to which the norms provided in the manuals reflect typical development.

Predictive and Discriminate Validity   The CDI/I reports predictive validity. Discriminate validity is reported in the CSBS manual. The CDI/I manual reports that early productive vocabulary predicts later productive vocabulary, and early vocabulary comprehension predicts later vocabulary comprehension.

The discriminate validity of the CSBS is demonstrated by its ability to identify children who are at risk for potential delays and disorders. To establish this, the scores for children identified as having pervasive developmental disorder (PDD) or specific language impairment (SLI) are included with the scores from typically developing children. The CSBS is able to differentiate between these groups at levels greater than chance.

The available data on the predictive and discriminate validity of all three assessments is minimal, at best. To facilitate effective clinical practice, cutoff scores, or patterns of scores, are needed to distinguish between children with delayed development who will catch up on their own and children in need of intervention.

Norms Norms of a test represent the typical performance of a large group of people on that test (Sattler, 1990). For the norms to be deemed valid, the group of people tested must represent the gender, ethnicity, socioeconomic status (SES), and geographic variation of the instrument's target population. Sattler (1990) recommends a sample of at least 100 people for each age. The norming samples for the CDI/I, the ALB, and the CSBS are considerably smaller than this.

Of the three tests, the CDI/I provides the most complete normative data as well as the largest sample. The CDI/I was normed on 679 typically developing children, 86.9% of whom were Caucasian, 4% of whom were African American, 4.5% of whom were Hispanic, 2.9% of whom were Asian, and 1.7% of whom were assigned to a group known as "other." The norming sample of the CSBS raises several concerns. First, it includes a larger proportion of children with language disabilities than is representative of the population. Second, it provides limited demographic information. Third, the size of the standardization sample, 282 infants, is insufficient to identify accurately the parameters of typical communication development. The ALB provides limited demographic information and relies on a very limited sample size ($N = 20$).

The validity of the norms of all three assessments would be enhanced by substantially larger data sets that reflect the ethnic, geographic, and SES diversity that is representative of the current U.S. population. Until then, percentile ranking must be interpreted with caution, particularly for non-Caucasian, lower-SES children.

Test Administration and Scoring

Both the CSBS and the ALB take approximately 1 hour to administer. Both instruments utilize the child's parent and allow the parent to interact with the child during testing. The testing formats are standardized with some room for flexibility, and the manuals provide the protocols that are to be followed. Like most standardized tests, learning the test protocol takes time and training. Once learned, however, neither is particularly difficult to administer. The ALB designates 30 minutes for unstructured play and 30 minutes for more structured tasks.

With the CSBS, the majority of time is spent in relatively naturalistic but structured interaction. To allow later scoring, videotaping is required for the CSBS and for the unstructured play section of the ALB.

Scoring for both the CSBS and the ALB is a complicated, time-consuming, and therefore expensive task. Scoring the tests can take anywhere from 1 to 3 hours depending on how frequently the child communicated. Maintaining reliability in coding is another ongoing concern. Nevertheless, both the CSBS and the ALB provide information about the child's prelinguistic and early linguistic skills that would not be apparent from observation or parent reports alone. The difficulty and expense of scoring assessments, however, obviously affects whether a particular test will be used.

In contrast to the time and attention needed to administer and code the CSBS and the ALB, the CDI/I is relatively quick and easy. It takes parents from 15 to 45 minutes to complete, depending on the number of words the child understands. Scoring the assessment is done simply by counting responses. Because of its ease of administration, relatively representative norms, and the demonstrated usefulness in the empirical literature (Fenson et al., 1994), the CDI/I should be used as part of any communication assessment of prelinguistic children. Because of the time and expense needed to administer and score the tests, however, the CSBS and the ALB should be used primarily when a detailed description of a child's communication is needed to develop an effective intervention.

RESEARCH DIRECTIONS

Given the limited time and resources available, identifying potential developmental delays and intervening effectively is extremely important. To do this with any degree of certainty, several questions must be addressed: What are the parameters of typical prelinguistic communication development? Which children need intervention and which will "catch up" by themselves? Which prelinguistic skills are the best predictors of later language development? Do the assessment instruments have predictive validity? Can intervention enhance prelinguistic communication development? What effect do cultural differences have on the validity of the four predictor skills?

What Are the Parameters of Typical Prelinguistic Communication Development?

Identifying what is typical communication development for young children is the first step in identifying what is outside the typical developmental range. Without well-established parameters, deciding what is outside the typical range may be based more on intuition than on fact. The CSBS and the ALB, in conjunction with the CDI/I, measure all of the important predictors of later language development. The norming population (679 infants) for the CDI/I is large enough to represent the parameters for vocabulary comprehension. The CSBS and the ALB, however, must expand their norming populations using stratified sampling methods before the norms and rankings provided by these assessments can be credible.

A related need is establishing communicative profile norms. Some factors may be good predictors of continued delay only in combination with other factors (e.g., a large difference between comprehension and production, limited use of one pragmatic function when compared with others, high rates of coordinated attention with low rates of canonical babbling). Children with PDD, SLI, or other disabilities may have communicative profiles that are consistent with children with the same disability. Establishing communication profile norms on large groups of children may substantially aid in earlier identification and intervention.

Which Children Need Intervention and Which Will "Catch Up" by Themselves?

Distinguishing late talkers who will catch up by themselves from children who truly need intervention is a major research challenge (Fenson et al., 1994). The development of complex babbling and combinatorial and symbolic play skills is predictive of the onset of speech. However, the onset of speech can vary dramatically, even for children who are developing typically. Identifying those skills or communicative profiles that are specifically related to continued delays and not just to later onset is an important research goal. So far, vocabulary comprehension and symbolic and combinatorial play have been the most reliable markers when trying to distinguish so-called late bloomers from children in need of intervention (Thal et al., 1991). Late bloomers rarely show significant delays on these variables.

Which Prelinguistic Skills Are the Best Predictors of Later Language Development?

The ALB and the CSBS generate detailed information about early communication. All of this information may not be necessary, however, to identify children with delays or to develop appropriate interventions. Perhaps two or three variables can provide all of the information needed to intervene effectively. More information does not automatically mean more useful knowledge. Reducing the number of variables to be measured may make assessment instruments more "user friendly." Practitioners may be more apt to use these assessments if the amount of information to be collected were reduced and the scoring process were streamlined. Of course, it may be that simplifying measurement instruments will make them less accurate and valid, a common concern about many relatively simple screening instruments.

Do the Assessment Instruments Have Predictive Validity?

Typical communication development is extremely variable. This variability creates problems for valid assessment. Are children who score low on early communication assessments really at risk for language delays or disabilities? Is a high score a guarantee that language will develop without delay or impairment? Research on the predictive validity of specific assessments can help ensure that these tests reflect the actual developmental trajectory for a given child.

Can Intervention Enhance Prelinguistic Communication Development?

Little research has explored the effects of enhancing the development of the four predictor skills when development is delayed. Assuming intervention can enhance the development of one or more of the four predictor skills, will this trigger a corresponding change in later language or communication development? What are the best ways to enhance each of these skills? Are there developmental markers that would signal the child's readiness and ability to progress on each of these skills?

Most of the prelinguistic intervention research through 1996 has targeted pragmatic functions. Warren, Yoder, Gazdag, Kim, and Jones (1993); Wilcox (1992); and Yoder, Warren, Kim, and Gazdag (1994) have published research on teaching requesting and commenting functions to young children with developmental delays. Using a single-subject design, Warren and colleagues showed clear increases in prelinguistic requesting that generalized across setting and communication partner in four children. These effects were replicated by Yoder and colleagues. However, as of 1996, there have been no studies published on the long-term effects on language development of teaching pragmatic functions.

What Effect Do Cultural Differences Have on the Validity of the Four Predictor Skills?

Cultural differences provide a major challenge for accurately assessing prelinguistic communication skills, just as they complicate other types of assessment. Furthermore, most of the important questions about prelinguistic communication development have not yet been answered from a cross-cultural perspective. For example, if adults' responses to children's prelinguistic communications vary across cultures, how are children's emergent communication skills affected? Do the four predictors identified predict language development in cultures in which adults have a different set of beliefs and behaviors relative to language learning and infant development? Are these predictors universal and invariant across cultures, or does their power wax and wane from culture to culture? Behaviors such as sustained eye gaze or face-to-face vocal "conversations" between mother and infant, attributing communicative intent to prelinguistic infants, and the use of motherese are valued and expected in Caucasian, middle-class, American families. There are, however, cultures in which these same behaviors may be considered inappropriate and may not occur with any regularity (Schieffelin & Ochs, 1983).

The four prelinguistic predictors of later language development probably are universal and should have predictive validity across cultures. However, adults' responses to these behaviors surely are not universal. All typically developing infants babble. What seems to differ across cultures is not the specific features of babbling but the way in which adults respond to babbling. For example, according to Schieffelin and Ochs (1983), the Kaluli people in New Guinea believe that infants are not able to understand adults. Therefore, adults do not address infants as conversational partners, nor do they respond to infants' babbling as if it were meaningful. Researchers studying infants growing up in Caucasian, middle-class, American families have documented that mothers consistently respond to infants' vocalizations (Harding, 1983). Given the difference in responses to babbling, are the rates or syllabic shape of babbling still predictive of the onset of speech across cultures? Further research should have important implications for efforts to establish the overall validity of the four prelinguistic predictors. In the meantime, practitioners must continue making assessment and treatment decisions.

RECOMMENDATIONS FOR PRACTITIONERS

The two earliest predictors to emerge in infants are babbling and the onset of intentional communication demonstrated through the use of pragmatic functions. If an infant is babbling infrequently or the complexity of the babbling does not progress, then a comprehensive hearing assessment should be conducted. If the infant's hearing is normal, then the next step is to assess the motor abilities relevant to the physical aspects of babbling. Different intervention strategies may be called for depending on the apparent cause of the delay in the child's vocal development.

By the time infants are 12 months old, they should be requesting, commenting, greeting, and protesting (Wetherby et al., 1988). If an infant's communication is characterized by extensive use of only one or two of the basic pragmatic functions and little use of the other functions, then the ALB or the CSBS should be used to obtain a clear picture of the child's pragmatic functioning in preparation for intervention.

The last two predictive skills to emerge—vocabulary comprehension and play skills—are representational abilities. These skills are best assessed after the child is able to intentionally communicate. Both vocabulary comprehension and symbolic play indicate that the child is able to use one thing (e.g., a toy, a symbol) to represent another thing (e.g., another object, a meaning). The ease and efficiency of measurement with the CDI/I may make vocabulary comprehension and play skills the two prelinguistic skills that should be assessed first if the child does show some evidence of intentional communication. If the CDI/I indicates a delay, then the CSBS or the ALB will provide useful information to facilitate intervention planning.

Reliably assessing infants who come from backgrounds other than Caucasian, middle-class, American for delayed or atypical prelinguistic development may be difficult, at best. This problem may be eased somewhat by including in the assessment process an adult who shares the infant's culture and who is knowledgeable about early communicative development. This person may be able to respond to concerns about the infant's communication development while helping practitioners distinguish between behaviors that are problematic and those that are just culturally different.

CONCLUSION

The field of prelinguistic communication assessment is young and evolving. Researchers have identified four important predictors of later language development and are working to identify variables that can distinguish children who will catch up on their own from those in need of intervention. Prelinguistic communication assessments such as the CSBS and the ALB are dramatic improvements over what was available only a decade before them. It is hoped that these instruments will lead the way to a new generation of less complicated, reliable, valid, user-friendly assessments (e.g., the CDI/I) that will allow communication delays to be identified as early as possible in a young child's life.

REFERENCES

Baker, L., & Cantwell, D.P. (1982). Developmental, social, and behavioral characteristics of speech and language disordered children. *Child Psychiatry and Human Development, 12*, 195–206.
Bates, E. (1976). *Language and context: The acquisition of pragmatics*. New York: Academic Press.
Bates, E. (1979a). Intentions, conventions, and symbols. In E. Bates, L. Benigni, I. Bretherton, L. Camaioni, & V. Volterra (Eds.), *The emergence of symbols: Cognition and communication in infancy* (pp. 33–68). New York: Academic Press.
Bates, E. (1979b). On the evolution and development of symbols. In E. Bates, L. Benigni, I. Bretherton, L. Camaioni, & V. Volterra (Eds.), *The emergence of symbols: Cognition and communication in infancy* (pp. 1–32). New York: Academic Press.
Bates, E. (1993). Comprehension and production in early language development. *Monographs of the Society for Research in Child Development, 58*, 222–242.
Bates, E., Benigni, L., Bretherton, I., Camaioni, L., & Volterra, V. (1979). Cognition and communication from nine to thirteen months: Correlational findings. In E. Bates, L. Benigni, I. Bretherton, L. Camaioni, & V. Volterra (Eds.), *The emergence of symbols: Cognition and communication in infancy* (pp. 69–140). New York: Academic Press.
Bates, E., Bretherton, I., & Snyder, L. (1988). *From first words to grammar: Individual differences and dissociable mechanisms*. Cambridge, MA: Cambridge University Press.
Bayley, N. (1993). *Bayley Scales of Infant Development* (2nd ed.). San Antonio, TX: The Psychological Corporation.
Bloom, L. (1993). Developments in cognition. In L. Bloom, *The transition from infancy to language: Acquiring the power of expression* (pp. 214–242). New York: Cambridge University Press.
Bruner, J. (1981). The social context of language acquisition. *Language and Communication, 1*, 155–178.
Bzoch, K.R., & League, R. (1971). *Receptive-Expressive Emergent Language (REEL) Scale*. Austin, TX: PRO-ED.

Camp, B., Burgess, D., Morgan, L., & Zerbe, G. (1987). A longitudinal study of infant vocalizations in the first year. *Journal of Pediatric Psychology, 12,* 321–331.

Carpenter, R.L., Mastergeorge, A.M., & Coggins, T.E. (1983). The acquisition of communicative intentions in infants eight to fifteen months of age. *Language and Speech, 26*(2), 101–116.

Casby, M.W., & McCormack, S.M. (1985). Symbolic play and early communication development in hearing-impaired children. *Journal of Communication Disorders, 18,* 67–78.

Casby, M.W., & Ruder, K.F. (1983). Symbolic play and early language development in normal and mentally retarded children. *Journal of Speech and Hearing Research, 26,* 404–411.

Fenson, L., Dale, P.S., Reznick, J.S., Bates, E., Thal, D., & Pethick, S.J. (1994). Variability in early communicative development. *Monographs of the Society for Research in Child Development, 59*(5), 1–188.

Fenson, L., Dale, P.S., Reznick, J.S., Thal, D., Bates, E., Hartung, J.P., Pethick, S., & Reilly, J.S. (1993). *MacArthur Communicative Developmental Inventories.* San Diego: Singular.

Harding, C.G. (1983). Setting the stage for language acquisition: Communication development in the first year. In R.M. Golinkoff (Ed.), *The transition from prelinguistic to linguistic communication: Issues and implications* (pp. 93–113). Hillsdale, NJ: Lawrence Erlbaum Associates.

Hedrick, D.L., Prather, E.M., & Tobin, A.R. (1975). *Sequenced Inventory of Communication Development test manual* (Rev. ed.). Seattle: University of Washington Press.

Iverson, J.M., & Thal, D.J. (in press). Communicative transitions: There's more to the hand than meets the eye. In A.M. Wetherby, S.F. Warren, & J. Reichle (Eds.), *Communication and language intervention series: Vol. 7. Transitions in prelinguistic communication: Preintentional to intentional and presymbolic to symbolic.* Baltimore: Paul H. Brookes Publishing Co.

Kagan, J. (1971). *Change and continuity in infancy.* New York: John Wiley & Sons.

Kamphaus, R.W., Dresden, J., & Kaufman, A.S. (1993). Clinical and psychometric considerations in the cognitive assessment of preschool children. In J.L. Culbertson & D.J. Willis (Eds.), *Testing young children: A reference guide for developmental, psychoeducational, and psychological assessments* (pp. 55–72). Austin, TX: PRO-ED.

Locke, J.L. (1983). *Phonological acquisition and change.* New York: Academic Press.

Locke, J.L. (1989). Babbling and early speech: Continuity and individual differences. *First Language, 9,* 191–206.

McCune, L. (1992). First words: A dynamic systems view. In C.A. Ferguson, L. Menn, & C. Stoel-Gammon (Eds.), *Phonological development: Models, research, implications* (pp. 313–336). Parkton, MD: York Press.

McLean, L.K.S. (1990, September). Communication development in the first two years of life: A transactional process. *Zero to Three,* 13–19.

Miller, J.F., & Paul, R. (1995). *The clinical assessment of language comprehension.* Baltimore: Paul H. Brookes Publishing Co.

Mosier, C.E., & Rogoff, B. (1994). Infants' instrumental use of their mothers to achieve their goals. *Child Development, 65,* 70–79.

Mundy, P., Kasari, C., Sigman, M., & Ruskin, E. (1995). Nonverbal communication and early language acquisition in children with Down syndrome and in normally developing children. *Journal of Speech and Hearing Research, 38,* 157–167.

Mundy, P., Sigman, M., & Kasari, C. (1990). A longitudinal study of joint attention and language development in autistic children. *Journal of Autism and Developmental Disorders, 20*(1), 115–128.

Mundy, P., Sigman, M., Kasari, C., & Yirmiya, N. (1988). Nonverbal communication skills in Down syndrome children. *Child Development, 59,* 235–249.

Murphy, R., Menyuk, P., Liebergott, J., & Schultz, M. (1983). *Predicting rate of lexical acquisition.* Paper presented at the Biennial Meeting of the Society for Research in Child Development, Detroit, MI.

Oller, D.K., & Lynch, M.P. (1992). Infant vocalizations and innovations in infraphonology: Toward a broader theory of development and disorders. In C.A. Ferguson, L. Menn, & C. Stoel-Gammon (Eds.), *Phonological development: Models, research, implications* (pp. 509–536). Parkton, MD: York Press.

Olswang, L., Stoel-Gammon, C., Coggins, T., & Carpenter, R. (1987). *Assessing Prelinguistic and Early Linguistic Behaviors in Developmentally Young Children.* Seattle: University of Washington Press.

Overton, T. (1992). *Assessment in special education: An applied approach.* Columbus, OH: Charles E. Merrill.

Papousek, M. (1993, March). *Stages of infant-directed speech: Relation to stages in the infant's interactional vocal repertoire.* Paper presented at the meeting of the Society for Research in Child Development, New Orleans, LA.

Piaget, J. (1962). *Play, dreams, and imitation in childhood.* New York: Norton.

Reichle, J. (1991). Defining the decisions involved in designing and implementing augmentative and alternative communication systems. In J. Reichle, J. York, & J. Sigafoos (Eds.), *Implementing augmentative and alternative communication: Strategies for learners with severe disabilities* (pp. 39–60). Baltimore: Paul H. Brookes Publishing Co.

Reynell, J.K., & Huntley, M. (1985). *Reynell Developmental Language Scales manual* (2nd ed.). Windsor, England: NFER-NELSON.

Roe, K.V. (1977). *Relationship between infant vocalizations at three months and preschool cognitive functioning.* Paper presented at the Annual Meeting of the Washington Psychological Association, Seattle.

Sattler, J.M. (1990). *Assessment of children* (3rd ed.). San Diego: J.M. Sattler.

Schieffelin, B.B., & Ochs, E. (1983). A cultural perspective on the transition from prelinguistic to linguistic communication. In R.M. Golinkoff (Ed.), *The transition from prelinguistic to linguistic communication: Issues and implications.* (pp. 115–131). Hillsdale, NJ: Lawrence Erlbaum Associates.

Silva, P.A., Williams, S., & McGee, R. (1987). A longitudinal study of children with developmental language delay at age three: Later intelligence, reading and behavior problems. *Developmental Medicine and Child Neurology, 29,* 630–640.

Smith, L., & vonTetzchner, S. (1986). Communicative, sensorimotor, and language skills of young children with Down syndrome. *American Journal of Mental Deficiency, 91*(1), 57–66.

Stark, R.E. (1980). Stages of speech development in the first year of life. In G. Yeni-Komshian, J. Kavanagh, & C. Ferguson (Eds.), *Child phonology* (pp. 73–92). New York: Academic Press.

Stoel-Gammon, C. (1989). Prespeech and early speech development of two late talkers. *First Language, 9,* 207–224.

Stoel-Gammon, C. (1992). Prelinguistic vocal development: Measurement and predictions. In C.A. Ferguson, L. Menn, & C. Stoel-Gammon (Eds.), *Phonological development: Models, research, implications* (pp. 439–456). Parkton, MD: York Press.

Thal, D., Tobias, S., & Morrison, D. (1991). Language and gesture in late talkers: A 1-year follow-up. *Journal of Speech and Hearing Research, 34,* 604–612.

Vihman, M., & Greenlee, M. (1987). Individual differences in phonological development: Ages one and three years. *Journal of Speech and Hearing Research, 30,* 503–521.

Warren, S.F., Yoder, P.J., Gazdag, G.E., Kim, K., & Jones, H.A. (1993). Facilitating prelinguistic communication skills in young children with developmental delay. *Journal of Speech and Hearing Research, 36,* 83–97.

Wetherby, A.M., Cain, D.H., Yonclas, D.G., & Walker, V.G. (1988). Analysis of intentional communication of normal children from the prelinguistic to the multiword stage. *Journal of Speech and Hearing Research, 31*, 240–252.

Wetherby, A.M., & Prizant, B.M. (1992). Profiling young children's communicative competence. In S.F. Warren & J. Reichle (Eds.), *Communication and language intervention series: Vol 1. Causes and effects in communication and language intervention* (pp. 217–253). Baltimore: Paul H. Brookes Publishing Co.

Wetherby, A.M., & Prizant, B.M. (1993). *Communication and Symbolic Behavior Scales manual: Normed edition.* Chicago: Riverside.

Wetherby, A.M., & Prutting, C. (1984). Profiles of communicative and cognitive-social abilities in autistic children. *Journal of Speech and Hearing Research, 27*, 364–377.

Whitehurst, G.J., Smith, M., Fischel, J.F., Arnold, D.S., & Lonigan, C.J. (1991). The continuity of babble and speech in children with specific expressive language delay. *Journal of Speech and Hearing Research, 34*, 1121–1129.

Wilcox, M.J. (1992). Enhancing initial communication skills in young children with developmental disabilities through partner programming. *Seminars in Speech and Language, 13*(3), 194–212.

Yoder, P.J., & Munson, L.J. (1995). The social correlates of coordinated attention to adult and objects in mother–infant interaction. *First Language, 15*, 219–230.

Yoder, P.J., Warren, S.F., & Hull, L. (1995). Predicting children's response to prelinguistic communication intervention. *Journal of Early Intervention, 19*(1), 74–84.

Yoder, P.J., Warren, S.F., Kim, K., & Gazdag, G.E. (1994). Facilitating prelinguistic communication skills in young children with developmental delay II: Systematic replication and extension. *Journal of Speech and Hearing Research, 37*, 841–851.

Zimmerman, I.L., Steiner, V.G., & Pond, R.E. (1992). *Preschool Language Scale–3* (PLS–3). San Antonio, TX: The Psychological Corporation.

4

Phonological Assessment
Using a Hierarchical Framework

Carol Stoel-Gammon

FOR MANY YEARS, THE GOAL of phonological assessment was to determine which phonemes a child had acquired. Group studies of phonemic acquisition served as the basis of a set of norms, providing an age at which typically developing children master each of the phonemes of English (e.g., Prather, Hedrick, & Kern, 1975; Templin, 1957). Such norms were then used to document the order of acquisition of phonemes in English; they often are employed by speech-language pathologists as one of the major tools for determining whether a child exhibits a delayed or deviant pattern in phonological acquisition.

Two unstated assumptions regarding the phoneme are fundamental to this approach to phonological assessment: 1) the phoneme constitutes the unit of acquisition in child speech, and 2) there is a typical order of phonemic acquisition for children acquiring English. These assumptions, however, are unfounded. The unit of acquisition appears to be words or syllables at the early stages of development and phoneme by position or features later (Stoel-Gammon & Dunn, 1985).

A drawback of phonological analysis in terms of phonemes is that this approach ignores contextual effects that may influence production of target consonants and vowels. Yet it is well documented (Grunwell, 1987; Ingram, 1989; Stoel-Gammon & Dunn, 1985) that, in child speech, production of a phoneme may vary considerably as a result of a number of phenomena:

1. Position within the word: Most phonemes are produced more accurately when they occur in word-initial position.
2. Word length: Pronunciation tends to be less accurate in longer words.
3. Position of stress: Phonemes in stressed syllables tend to be produced more accurately than those in unstressed syllables.
4. Phonetic environment: Phoneme production may be influenced by neighboring consonants or vowels.
5. Grammatical role: Phonemes in content words tend to be produced more accurately than in function words.

For children in the early stages of language acquisition or for children with severe phonological disorders, an analysis based on the phonological patterns occurring in words, syllables, or features, as well as in segments (i.e., phonemes), provides a more complete characterization of the phonological system. An approach referred to as *nonlinear phonology* offers a useful framework for examining the relationships among various aspects of phonology by positing a hierarchical organization of words, syllables, segments, and features. (See Bernhardt & Stoel-Gammon, 1994, for a description of nonlinear phonology.)

Figure 1 illustrates the way in which the word *candy* can be decomposed into progressively smaller units, or levels. The first division is into syllables. For this analysis, factors related to *syllable level* include the number of syllables in a word as well as placement of stress in words of more than one syllable. Thus, *candy* is divided into two syllables with stress on the first syllable. The next level in the hierarchy focuses on the structure of each syllable, dividing it into an *onset* and a *rhyme*. The onset includes the initial consonant(s). In Figure 1, the consonant /k/ of *candy* constitutes the onset of the first syllable; the consonant /d/ forms the onset of the second syllable. The rhyme is composed of a vowel and any following consonant(s). For *candy*, the vowel /æ/ and the consonant /n/ form the rhyme of the first syllable; the rhyme in the second syllable is formed by the

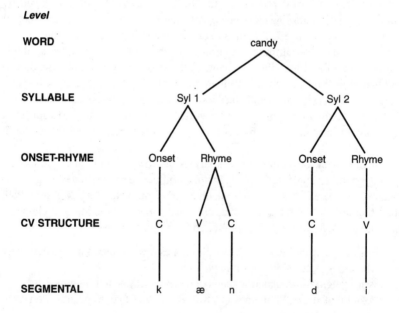

FEATURE (phonetic features of each segment)

Figure 1.   Hierarchical representation of the word *candy*.

vowel /i/. (In English, all syllables must have a rhyme. Syllable onsets are optional: Vowel-initial words, such as *into* and *around*, have initial syllables with no onset. If present, an onset contains from one to three consonants; the word *spring*, for example, has an onset of three consonants.)

The *onset-rhyme level* is composed of consonant (C) and vowel (V) constituents, forming the *CV structure level*. In Figure 1, the first syllable of *candy* is closed, CVC; the second syllable is open, CV.

Descending through the hierarchy, the *segmental level* links each C or V with the specific consonant and vowel sounds that form the word. This level is the closest to the traditional "phoneme" level. Finally, the *feature level* breaks down the speech sounds into phonetic features. In this chapter, traditional consonantal features of place, manner, and voicing are used. In some phonological theories (see Goldsmith, 1990), segments are decomposed into a hierarchically organized set of features.

APPLYING A HIERARCHICAL FRAMEWORK TO CHILD SPEECH

Table 1 presents a hierarchical phonological analysis of 30 words produced by Joey, a typically developing 17-month-old in the "single word" stage of language acquisition. Joey has a vocabulary of about 50 words and a relatively simple phonological system. The data and analyses in Table 1 are arranged as follows:

Column 1: orthographic transcription of the target word

Column 2: broad phonetic transcription of Joey's production

Column 3: the number of syllables and the stress pattern in Joey's production, with stressed syllables indicated by "S" and unstressed syllables by "s"

Column 4: the accuracy of Joey's production in terms of number of syllables and location of stress, with overall accuracy indicated at the bottom of the column

Column 5: analysis of Joey's production in terms of CV structure

Column 6: the accuracy of Joey's production in terms of CV structure, with overall accuracy indicated at the bottom of the column

Column 7: the initial consonant in Joey's production, with vowel-initial productions indicated by "NA"

Column 8: the accuracy of the initial consonant in Joey's production compared with the target form, with overall accuracy indicated at the bottom of the column

Column 9: the final consonant in Joey's production, with vowel-final production indicated by "NA"

Column 10: the accuracy of the final consonant in Joey's production compared with the target form, with overall accuracy indicated at the bottom of the column

Column 11: comments on Joey's production

Table 1. Joey's speech sample: Phonetic transcription and hierarchical analysis

Columns

Number	1 Target	2 Joey's production	3 Syllables and stress	4 Accuracy	5 CV structure	6 Accuracy	7 Initial consonant	8 Accuracy	9 Final consonant	10 Accuracy	11 Comments
1	Eye	aɪ	S	✓	VV	✓	NA		NA		
2	Bye	baɪ	S	✓	CVV	✓	b	✓	NA		
3	No	no	S	✓	CV	✓	n	✓	NA		
4	Hi	haɪ	S	✓	CVV	✓	h	✓	NA		
5	Up	ʌp	S	✓	VC	✓	NA		p	✓	
6	Ball	ba	S	✓	CV	✗	b	✓	∅	(x)	
7	Bath	bæf	S	✓	CVC	✓	b	✓	f	✗	
8	Book	bʊk	S	✓	CVC	✓	b	✓	k	✓	
9	Down	daʊn	S	✓	CVVC	✓	d	✓	n	✓	
10	Duck	dʌk	S	✓	CVC	✓	d	✓	k	✓	
11	Nose	nos	S	✓	CVC	✓	n	✓	s	✗	
12	Shoes	dus	S	✓	CVC	✓	d	✗	s	✗	
13	Juice	dus	S	✓	CVC	✓	d	✗	s	✓	
14	Car	ka	S	✓	CV	✗	k	✓	∅	(x)	
15	Keys	kis	S	✓	CVC	✓	k	✓	s	✗	

#	Word	Target										
16	Hot	hat	S	✓	CVC	✓	h	✓	t	✓		
17	Apple	'æpu	S-s	✓	VCV	X	NA		u	(x)		
18	Baby	'bebi	S-s	✓	CVCV	✓	b	✓	NA			
19	Birdie	'bʊdi	S-s	✓	CVCV	✓	b	✓	NA			
20	Daddy	'dædi	S-s	✓	CVCV	✓	d	✓	NA			
21	Doggie	'gagi	S-s	✓	CVCV	✓	g	X	NA			Assim
22	Mommy	'mami	S-s	✓	CVCV	✓	m	✓	NA			
23	Kitty	'kiki	S-s	✓	CVCV	✓	k	✓	NA			
24	Cookie	'kʊki	S-s	✓	CVCV	✓	k	✓	u	(x)		Assim
25	Bottle	'babu	S-s	✓	CVCV	✓	b	✓	NA			
26	Cracker	'kækʌ	S-s	✓	CVCV	X	k	✓	N			
27	Balloon	bə'wun	S-s	✓	CVCV	X	b	✓	∅	✓		Assim
28	Night-night	'nanaɪ	S-s	✓	CVCVV	✓	n	✓	NA	(x)		
29	Banana	'næns	S-s	X	CVCV	(x)	n	(x)	NA			
30	Peekaboo	'bibu	S-s	X	CVCV	(x)	b	X	NA			
	Accuracy			28/30 (93%)		22/30 (73%)		22/27 (81%)		7/16 (43%)		

Note: Matches between Joey's production and the target form are indicated by a check (✓) in the appropriate column. Mismatches are indicated by "X" if the error occurred at the level in question and by "(x)" if the error resulted from an error at a higher level in the hierarchy.

Analysis Perspectives

A child's speech can be analyzed from two basic perspectives. In an *independent analysis*, the child's word productions are described in terms of the features, segments, syllable shapes, and word structures that actually occur. The analysis focuses on the presence or absence of particular constituent types, independent of the adult model. There is no attempt to evaluate the accuracy of the productions or to describe the nature of the errors.

The second perspective for analyzing a child's productions, and the one that is most often adopted, is referred to as a *relational analysis* because it focuses on the relationship between the adult's targets and the child's productions (Stoel-Gammon & Dunn, 1985). This approach is the basis for determining which of the child's forms accurately match the adult model (yielding an assessment of correct productions) and which do not. The mismatches between the adult form and the child production can then be described in terms of differences at the level of syllables, segments, or features. Because they provide complementary perspectives on the developing phonological system, both independent and relational analyses should be used to provide a comprehensive assessment of a child's speech patterns.

Analysis of Joey's Productions Using a Hierarchical Framework
Independent and relational analyses of the data in Table 1 yield a set of statements regarding Joey's phonological patterns, characterizing his output at each level in the hierarchy. The relationships *between* various levels in the hierarchy also are examined, providing additional insights into the nature of Joey's phonological patterns. The data in Table 1 show that relations among hierarchical levels were manifested in several domains, the most obvious being the relationship between his *CV structures* and his *segmental* accuracy. For example, when Joey attempted to produce the target CVC of *ball* (#6) or *car* (#14), the final consonant was "in error" at the segmental level, not necessarily because of an inability to produce the /l/ or /r/ consonant but because of an error (or mismatch) at a higher level in the hierarchy, the CV structure level.

Number of Syllables and Word Stress (Columns 3 and 4) An independent analysis revealed that all of Joey's words had one or two syllables. Two-syllable words were stressed on the first syllable in all cases but one, *balloon* (#27). A relational analysis indicated that Joey's productions were highly accurate in terms of number of syllables and placement of stress: 93% of his forms matched the adult target word for these parameters. Three-syllable target words, *banana* (#29) and *peekaboo* (#30), were rendered inaccurately; in both cases, they were reduced to two syllables through omission of an unstressed syllable.

Onset-Rhyme and CV Structure Analysis (Columns 5 and 6) An independent analysis revealed that Joey's productions were very simple in terms of the onset-rhyme level (see Figure 1). His syllables were formed with either no onset, as in the words *eye* (#1) and *up* (#5), or with a single consonant, as in *shoes* [dus]

(#12) or *daddy* ['dædi] (#20). Syllable rhymes consisted of a single vowel, as in *ball* [ba] (#6); a diphthong (i.e., complex vowel), as in *bye* [baɪ] (#2); a vowel followed by a consonant, as in *book* [bʊk] (#8); or a diphthongized vowel followed by a consonant, as in *down* [daʊn] (#9). There were no productions containing a consonant cluster as an onset or as part of the rhyme.

At the word level, Joey produced CV structures that ranged from a single diphthong, VV, to open and closed monosyllables, CV and CVC, to disyllabic words of alternating consonants and vowels, CVCV. A relational analysis indicated that Joey's productions were relatively accurate in terms of CV structure (73% accuracy), with all but eight words conforming to the structure of the target. Three cases involved the segment /l/: The final /l/ of *ball* (#6) was omitted (simplification of the rhyme) and the syllabic /l/ at the end of *apple* (#17) and *bottle* (#25) was vocalized (i.e., became a vowel). The syllable onset was simplified in the word *cracker* (#26) through deletion of /r/ in the cluster /kr/; final /r/ was deleted in *car* (#14).

The remaining CV structure errors were deletion of an unstressed syllable in the words *banana* (#29) and *peekaboo* (#30). Although the CV structure of these three-syllable words was indeed incorrect, the errors were a direct consequence of alterations at a higher level in the hierarchy and thus differ from the other CV structure errors identified in the preceding paragraph.

Initial Consonants: Segmental and Featural Analysis (Columns 7 and 8) The inventory of consonants in word-initial position is analyzed in two ways: first at the level of *segments*, then in terms of the articulatory features of *place of articulation, manner of articulation,* and *voicing.*

An independent analysis revealed that Joey's consonantal repertoire in word-initial position was relatively limited. In terms of segments, the sample contained at least one instance of [b, d, k, g, m, n, h] in word-initial position. Of these, [b, d, k, n] occurred more than twice. In terms of features, Joey's inventory included the *manner* features of stops, nasals, and a glottal fricative but no supraglottal fricatives, affricates, liquids, or glides. *Place* of articulation features included labial, alveolar, velar, and glottal; labiodentals, interdentals, and palatals were missing, in part because they were infrequent in the target forms. Both voiced and voiceless consonants occurred in the sample.

A relational analysis indicated that consonantal onsets in word-initial position generally matched the adult model, with an accuracy rate of 81%. Errors included substituting [d] for the palatal affricate in *juice* (#13) and for the palatal fricative in *shoes* (#12), and producing [g] at the onset of *doggie* (#21), presumably because of the influence of the medial /g/ (see Intersegmental Relationships on p. 87). Given that /b/ was produced accurately in a number of other words, the error on /b/ of *banana* should be attributed to deletion of the unstressed syllable at a higher level in the hierarchy rather than to any difficulty with the segment per se.

Place features of target consonants in *word-initial position* generally were accurate. The errors involved voicing and manner of articulation. Palatal affricates and fricatives were produced as alveolar stops (e.g., shoes [dus] [#12]; juice [dus] [#13]). Voiceless consonants, except /k/, all were voiced.

Final Consonants: Segmental and Featural Analysis (Columns 9 and 10)
An independent analysis revealed that the repertoire of final consonants demonstrated in Joey's sample was quite small because many of the target words ended in a vowel. The consonants [p, t, k, n, f, s] occurred in at least one word. Only [s, k, n] appeared more than once. *Manner* and *voicing* features present in final consonants included nasals, voiceless stops, and voiceless fricatives. All three major *place* of articulation features—bilabial (including labiodental), alveolar, and velar—were present.

A relational analysis indicated that Joey's accuracy rate for production of final consonants was 43%, with 7 of a possible 16 consonants matching the adult target. More than half of the errors in production of final consonants resulted from mismatches at the CV structure level. Substitutions of one consonant for another (indicated by "X" in Column 10) accounted for the remaining four errors.

The phonetic features of Joey's final consonants were correct in terms of *place* of articulation in all words except *bath* (#7), which was produced with a labiodental, rather than an interdental, fricative. *Manner* of articulation of target stops, nasals, and fricatives was correct, but target liquids (i.e., /l/ and /r/) were either omitted or rendered as vowels. *Voicing* errors occurred only on the voiced fricative /z/, which was produced as its voiceless counterpart in *nose* (#11), *shoes* (#12), and *keys* (#15).

Summary   The results of this analysis of Joey's speech sample are summarized with a set of statements regarding the independent and relational analyses of the various levels in the phonological hierarchy:

1. Joey was highly accurate in producing the *number of syllables and stress patterns* of the target words, with an accuracy rate of 93%. The only errors occurred on three-syllable words, which were reduced to two syllables.

2. In terms of *CV structure*, Joey's word productions conformed to a basic pattern of alternating consonants and vowels. He produced no consonant sequences, and he generally favored open syllables in word-final position, particularly when the final consonant was a liquid. His accuracy rate at the CV structure level was 73%.

3. In *word-initial position*, Joey accurately produced the place of articulation of all target consonants except palatals; manner classes of target stops and nasals also were accurately produced. Target fricative and affricates were substituted with stops. Voiced stops predominated in word-initial positions, often substituting for voiceless targets although the voicing of initial /k/ was consistently correct. The overall accuracy rate for initial consonants was 81%.

4. In *word-final positions*, place and manner of articulation of target stops, nasals, and fricatives generally were accurate; target liquids were deleted or

rendered as vowels. All obstruents in final position were voiceless. Accuracy of word-final consonants was 43%, with more than half of the errors attributed to alterations at the CV structure level.

If Joey's speech sample were analyzed exclusively at the level of phonemes, then the assessment would be based entirely on his productions at the segmental level. In word-initial position, Joey produced the consonants [b, d, k, m, n, h] as matches to the adult; in final position, the phones [p, t, k, n, s] occurred as matches. The only consonants occurring in both sets were [k] and [n], suggesting that these two (and [h], which cannot occur in word-final positions) are the only consonants that should be classified as phonemes in Joey's speech. This type of analysis yields only limited information about Joey's phonological system. The framework used previously, in which Joey's productions are described at several levels in the phonological hierarchy, provides a more complete picture.

Hierarchical Relationships

An example of the phonological patterns occurring *between* levels in the hierarchy can be illustrated using Joey's production of the word *car*. As shown in Figure 2, Joey's production matched the target form at the word, syllable, and onset-rhyme levels but differed from the target at the CV structure level. In the

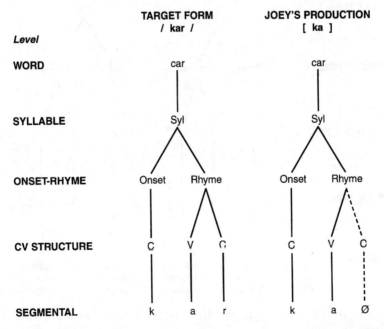

Figure 2.   Hierarchical representation of *car:* Target form and Joey's production. (Dashed lines indicate missing elements at the CV structure and, consequently, the segmental levels.)

target form, the rhyme branched, consisting of a vowel /a/ and a consonant /r/; in Joey's production, the rhyme consisted of only the vowel /a/. The mismatch between the two forms at this level necessarily created a mismatch at the segmental level.

In contrast, comparison of the target form and Joey's production of the word *nose* shows that the mismatch occurred at a different level. Figure 3 shows that Joey's production matched the target form at the syllable, onset-rhyme, and CV structure levels. It is only at the segmental and featural levels that a difference occurred: Joey altered the *voicing* feature of the final consonant, producing [s] for target /z/.

The examples in Figures 2 and 3 illustrate the primary advantage of using a hierarchical approach to phonological analysis. Joey made an error in the final consonant of both examples; however, the error occurred at the CV structure level for the word *car* and the segmental/featural level for *nose*. Highlighting the

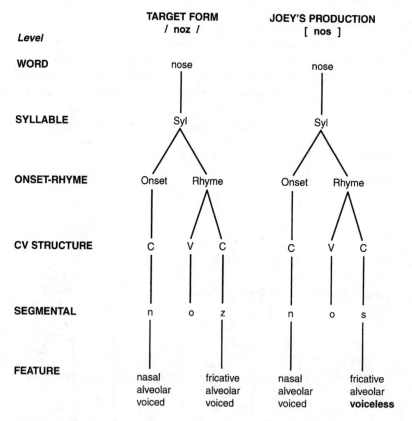

Figure 3.   Hierarchical representation of *nose:* Target form and Joey's production. (Bold print indicates feature error.)

differences in level at which an error occurs is particularly important in the analysis of phonological systems of children with phonological disorders because different treatment programs should be implemented for errors at different levels.

Intersegmental Relationships

In addition to the analyses presented previously, it is important to examine possible interactions *within* each level. In children's productions, interactions often occur at the level of segments, typically between consonants across an intervening vowel or between neighboring consonants and vowels. In cases of consonants influencing each other, one consonant in the word usually takes on features of another consonant, a process referred to as *consonant harmony*, or *assimilation* (Stoel-Gammon & Stemberger, 1994; Vihman, 1978). In consonant–vowel interactions, the place of articulation of the consonant is usually influenced by the place of articulation of the vowel (Gierut, Cho, & Dinnsen, 1993; Levelt, 1994).

In the data set presented in Table 1, there is evidence of consonant assimilation in several of the two-syllable words. In each case, alterations were made to the target form so that the first and second consonants in Joey's productions were identical:

#21. *doggie* ['gagi]
#23. *kitty* ['kiki]
#25. *bottle* ['babu]

A number of other CVCV(V) words in the sample also conform to the pattern; in these instances, the target words, not just the child's productions, have the same consonant in initial and medial position:

#18. *baby* ['bebi]
#20. *daddy* ['dædi]
#22. *mommy* ['mami]
#24. *cookie* ['kʊki]
#26. *cracker* ['kækʌ]
#28. *night-night* [nanaɪ]
#29. *banana* ['nænə]
#30. *peekaboo* ['bibu]

Although Joey produced a number of CVC words with two different consonants (see, e.g., *bath* [#7], *book* [#8], *duck* [#10], *juice* [#13]), the only multisyllabic words with nonidentical consonants were *birdie* [bʊdi] (#19) and *balloon* [bə'wun] (#27). The prevalence of this pattern suggests that Joey had a preference for two-syllable forms in which the consonants were the same. This preference appeared in the selection of words in his lexicon as well as in those productions in which he assimilated one consonant to another.

APPLYING A HIERARCHICAL
FRAMEWORK TO DISORDERED PHONOLOGY

This section presents a data set of a child with a phonological disorder and analyzes it using the same format as in the analysis of Joey's speech. Clinical implications of the analysis are presented, and the phonological systems of the two children are compared.

Table 2 presents a hierarchical phonological analysis of 30 words produced by Bobby when he was 4 years to 4 years and 2 months old. (The data set is adapted from Appendix B in Crary and Hunt, 1983.) Bobby was assessed as having normal hearing, adequate structure and function of the speech mechanism, and typical intelligence; he was enrolled in a clinical program for "delayed speech development." The information in Table 2 is arranged in the same way as in Table 1, with individual columns for the target words; Bobby's productions; and analyses of his productions in terms of number of syllables and placement of stress, CV structure, and initial and final consonants.

Analysis of Bobby's Productions Using a Hierarchical Framework

Independent and relational analyses of the data in Table 2 are summarized by the following statements, starting with the highest level in the hierarchy and moving to the lowest.

Number of Syllables and Word Stress (Columns 3 and 4) An independent analysis revealed that Bobby produced words that were one, two, or three syllables long. All multisyllabic words were stressed on the first syllable.

A relational analysis indicated that Bobby's productions were highly accurate in terms of number of syllables and placement of stress: 93% of his forms matched the features of the adult target word. There were only two words in error: The two-syllable target *open* (#18) was reduced to one syllable, and the three-syllable form *policeman* (#29) was reduced to two syllables with stress on the first syllable.

Onset-Rhyme and CV Structure Analysis (Columns 5 and 6) An independent analysis revealed that Bobby's sample contained a limited range of CV structures with words formed of alternating Cs and Vs predominating. There were no complex onsets in word-initial position (i.e., no consonant clusters) and only two cases of word-final consonants.

A relational analysis indicated that Bobby's accuracy rate for CV structures was very low; only 10% of his productions matched the target. The most frequent error types were omission of the word-final consonant and omission of a consonant in a consonant sequence. In some cases, both types of errors occurred in the same word (e.g., *grass* pronounced [dæ] [#15]; *driving* as ['daʔi] [#27]).

Initial Consonants: Segmental and Featural Analysis (Columns 7 and 8) An independent analysis revealed that Bobby's consonantal repertoire in word-initial position included 9 phones: [p, b, t, d, m, n, h, w, j]. Of these, [p, b, t, d, m, n, h, w] occurred twice. The voicing and manner features that were present included voiced and voiceless stops, nasals, and glides and voiceless fricatives. Place of articulation was limited to labial, alveolar, and glottal consonants.

A relational analysis indicated that Bobby's accuracy rate for initial consonants was 57%. Three errors resulted from deletions at the CV structure level; these are indicated by "(x)" in Column 8. Other errors involved changes at the level of features:

1. All target velar consonants changed place of articulation from velar to alveolar, resulting in [t] for /k/ and [d] for /g/ as in *cup* produced as [tʌ] (#4), *car* as [ta] (#10), and *grass* as [dæ] (#15).

2. Supraglottal fricatives /s, θ, ð/ in *sun* (#3), *three* (#9), and *this* (#13), respectively, were rendered as the glottal fricative [h]. This substitution changed the place of articulation of the target while it maintained the manner.

Final Consonants: Segmental and Featural Analysis (Columns 9 and 10) An independent analysis revealed that Bobby's sample contained only two consonants in word-final position—an alveolar stop [t] in his production of *push* [pʊt] (#14) and a glottal stop [ʔ] as the final consonant in his production of *open* (#18) pronounced as [oʔ].

A relational analysis indicated that the accuracy rate for production of final consonants was 0% with all but one of the errors resulting from final-consonant deletion at the CV structure level. In the remaining case, place and manner of articulation of the voiceless palatal fricative /ʃ/ in the word *push* (#14) were altered; Joey produced the word with voiceless alveolar stop [t] in final position.

Summary The phonological patterns of Bobby's productions are summarized with a set of statements regarding the analysis at each level in the phonological hierarchy:

1. Bobby was highly accurate in matching the adult target at the level of *number of syllables and stress patterns*. His accuracy rate was 93% with only two errors at this level: *open* (#18) pronounced as [oʔ]; and *policeman* (#29) reduced to two syllables, ['pimæ], with stress on the first syllable.

2. In terms of *CV structure*, Bobby's productions conformed to a basic pattern of alternating CV syllables regardless of the pattern of the target form. Consonant sequences were reduced to single consonants, and syllable-final consonants were omitted; consequently, his accuracy rate at this level was only 10%.

3. In *word-initial position*, accuracy of consonant production was 57%. Bobby matched the target *place, manner,* and *voicing* features for words beginning with labial and alveolar stops or nasals. Target velar stops were consistently rendered as alveolars, and most target fricatives were substituted with [h].

Table 2. Bobby's speech sample: Phonetic transcription and hierarchical analysis

	1	2	3	Columns							
				4	5	6	7	8	9	10	11
Number	Target	Bobby's production	Syllables and stress	Accuracy	CV structure	Accuracy	Initial consonant	Accuracy	Final consonant	Accuracy	Comments
1	Boy	bɔɪ	S	✓	CVV	✓	b	✓	NA		
2	Dog	dɔ	S	✓	CV	X	d	✓	∅	(x)	
3	Sun	hʌ	S	✓	CV	X	h	X	∅	(x)	
4	Cup	tʌ	S	✓	CV	X	t	X	∅	(x)	
5	Hand	hæ	S	✓	CV	X	h	✓	∅	(x)	
6	Nice	naɪ	S	✓	CVV	X	n	✓	∅	(x)	
7	Box	ba	S	✓	CV	X	b	✓	∅	(x)	
8	Moon	mu	S	✓	CV	X	m	✓	∅	(x)	
9	Three	hi	S	✓	CV	X	h	X	NA		
10	Car	ta	S	✓	CV	X	t	X	∅	(x)	
11	Want	wa	S	✓	CV	X	w	(x)	∅	(x)	
12	Skate	te	S	✓	CV	X	t	X	∅	(x)	
13	This	hi	S	✓	CV	X	h	X	∅	(x)	
14	Push	pʊt	S	✓	CVC	✓	p	✓	t	X	
15	Grass	dæ	S	✓	CV	X	d	X	∅	(x)	

16	Mouth	maʊ	S	✓	CVV	X	m	✓	∅	(x)	Assim
17	Can't	tæ	S	✓	CV	X	t	X	∅	(x)ʳ	Assim
18	Open	oʔ	S	X	VC	(x)	NA	✓	∅	(x)	
19	All gone	'ɔdɔ:	S-s	✓	VCV	X	NA	✓	∅	(x)	
20	Pretty	'pipi	S-s	✓	CVCV	✓	p	(x)	NA		Assim
21	Yellow	'jɛjɛ	S-s	✓	CVCV	X	j	X	NA		Assim
22	Water	'aʔaː	S-s	✓	VCV	X	∅	(x)	NA		
23	Cactus	'tætə	S-s	✓	CVCV	X	t	X	∅	(x)	
24	Hotdog	'hadɔ	S-s	✓	CVCV	X	h	✓	∅	(x)	
25	Baseball	'bebɔ	S-s	✓	CVCV	X	b	✓	∅	(x)	Assim
26	Cupboard	'ʌtə	S-s	✓	CVCV	X	t	✓	∅	(x)	
27	Driving	'daʔi	S-s	✓	CVCV	X	d	X	∅	(x)	
28	Snowman	'nomæ	S-s	✓	CVCV	X	n	(x)	NA		Assim
29	Policeman	'pimæ	S-s	X	CVCV	(x)	p	✓	∅	(x)	
30	Bulldozer	'bobota	S-s-s	✓	CVCVCV	X	b	✓	NA		Assim
	Accuracy			28/30 (93%)		3/30 (10%)		16/28 (57%)		0/23 (0%)	

Note: Matches between Bobby's production and the target form are indicated by a check (✓) in the appropriate column. Mismatches are indicated by "X" if the error occurred at the level in question and by "(x)" if the error resulted from an error at a higher level in the hierarchy.

4. Bobby's accuracy level for production of *final consonants* was 0%. Consonants in word-final position were greatly affected by alterations at the CV level: Of 23 words with a final consonant in the target form, Bobby omitted the consonant in 22 of his productions. In the one case in which a final consonant was produced, an error occurred at the segmental/featural level.

As in the previous case, an assessment of Bobby's phonemic system would be limited to analyzing his productions at the segmental level and, once again, would be relatively uninformative. His sample included accurate productions of eight consonants in word-initial position: [p, b, d, m, n, h, w, j]. All of these would be candidates for phonemes if they occurred in other word positions. However, there were no correct productions of consonant phonemes in word-final position. The two consonants that did appear in this position, [t] in the word *push* (#14) and *open* (#18) (produced as [oʔ]), did not match the adult model and thus their phonemic status is questionable. In essence, then, it is not possible to talk about Bobby's phonemic repertoire without explicit mention of word position and/or CV structure.

Hierarchical Relationships

The previous summary clearly indicates that Bobby's primary problems occurred at the *onset-rhyme* and *CV structure* levels. Specifically, his major difficulty was producing forms in which the rhyme of the syllable branched to include a final consonant. Word-final target consonants were omitted in all productions but one (see Table 2, Columns 9 and 10), and syllable-final consonants within the word were omitted without exception (see words #23, #24, #25, #29, and #30). In all, 22 of the 23 errors in production of final consonants (Columns 9 and 10) resulted from changes at the CV level.

In addition to deletion of syllable-final consonants, Bobby's productions were characterized by a failure to include more than one consonant in the onset of syllables. He consistently reduced initial consonant clusters to a single consonant; in some cases, this led to errors in the productions of initial consonants. For example, the initial /s/ of *skate* (#12) and of *snowman* (#28) was in error because it was omitted. Bobby's changes at the CV structure level, particularly his failure to produce consonants at the end of syllables and consonant clusters as syllable onsets, had consequences on his performance at the segmental and featural levels.

Intersegmental Relationships

Examination of intersegmental relationships in the data set presented in Table 2 reveals a pattern of consonant assimilation in several of the two-syllable words. Like Joey, Bobby often altered the target form so that the first and second consonants in his productions were identical:

#20. *pretty* ['pipi]
#21. *yellow* ['jɛjɛ]

#26. *cupboard* ['tʌtə]
#30. *bulldozer* ['bobota]

As a result of consonant assimilations and/or deletions of final consonants, only three of Bobby's words had more than one supraglottal place of articulation:

#14. *push* [pʊt]
#28. *snowman* ['nomæ]
#30. *bulldozer* ['bobota]

In all other productions containing two consonants, the consonants were either identical or one was a glottal (see Table 2, #23, #24, #25, #27, and #28). Thus, the data in Table 2 suggest that Bobby had difficulty producing consonants at more than one supraglottal place of articulation within a single word.

COMPARING THE HIERARCHICAL PHONOLOGICAL ANALYSES

The hierarchical phonological analyses presented in this chapter can be compared to identify similarities and differences in the phonological systems of Joey, age 17 months, and Bobby, age 4 years. Despite the substantial age difference, the phonologies of the two children are similar in many respects.

Syllable and stress level: Both children produced relatively simple forms in terms of number of syllables: Bobby's longest word had three syllables; Joey's longest had two syllables. All multisyllabic forms were produced with stress on the initial syllable, except for Joey's rendition of *balloon*. Accuracy levels for the number of syllables and placement of stress were high; for both children, 28 of the 30 words in the sample (93%) matched the target forms.

CV structure level: Both boys displayed a strong tendency to produce words composed of alternating Cs and Vs. Joey's sample included open (CV) and closed (CVC) monosyllables, whereas Bobby's words were formed exclusively of open syllables. Consequently, Joey's accuracy rate for the CV structure level was 73%; Bobby's was 10%. This difference can be attributed, in part, to the relatively simple CV structures of the target words in Joey's sample, as would be expected for a child at 17 months. Bobby's sample, in contrast, contained a greater number of words with consonant clusters and closed syllables, thereby increasing the possible number of errors at the CV structure level.

Initial consonants: Both children had a limited set of consonants in word-initial position, predominantly stops and nasals. Joey produced consonants at the three major places of articulation: labial, alveolar, and velar. Bobby produced only labial and alveolar (and glottal) consonants. Joey's inventory of initial consonants lacked voiceless obstruents, whereas Bobby's included both voiced and voiceless stops. In terms of accuracy, Joey's productions matched the initial consonant of the target form in 81% of the cases; Bobby's accuracy was 57%. As in the CV structure analysis, Bobby's reduced accuracy results from the greater diversity of onset consonants in the target words in his sample.

Final consonants: Joey's inventory of final consonants was limited to voiceless obstruents and a single nasal. Liquid consonants (/l/ and /r/) in final position either were omitted or were produced as vowels; his accuracy rate for final consonants was 43%. Bobby had little opportunity to produce final consonants because of his pattern of deleting syllable-final consonants at the CV structure level. His accuracy rate for final consonants was 0%.

Intersegmental relationships: Both children displayed a tendency to produce disyllabic words in which the consonants were the same. In some cases, this pattern occurred in the target form and simply was maintained in the child's production (e.g., *mommy, daddy, cookie* in Joey's sample; *baseball* in Bobby's sample). In other cases, one of the consonants in the word assimilated to the other, yielding inaccurate forms such as ['pipi] for *pretty* (Bobby, see Table 2, #20) and ['babu] for *bottle* (Joey, see Table 1, #25).

The analysis of Bobby's speech sample, coupled with the previous comparisons, suggests that Bobby had a serious phonological disorder. At the age of 4 years, his CV structures and inventory of final consonants were more limited than those of a 17-month-old. His major difficulties were in two areas. First, and most important, his productions were limited to the simplest syllable structures, with no consonant clusters and rare occurrences of consonants in the rhyme. A program of phonological remediation aimed at expanding the range of CV structures would be appropriate. Second, his inventory of consonants in word-initial, as well as word-final, position was well below age-level expectations. In this domain, intervention would be directed toward increasing the range of place and manner classes to include velar consonants, voiced and voiceless supraglottal fricatives, and liquids. Efforts also would be directed toward eliminating the consonant assimilation pattern that prevented him from producing consonants at different places of articulation within a word.

CONCLUSION

If the relationships between language acquisition and phonology are considered in the comparisons of Joey and Bobby, the differences between them become more apparent. (See Stoel-Gammon & Stone, 1991, for a discussion of the interface between phonology and other aspects of language.) On the one hand was Joey, a typically developing toddler of 17 months. He had a vocabulary of about 50 words, spoke in one-word utterances, and displayed phonological patterns that were commensurate with his general linguistic level. Although he made many errors, his speech was relatively intelligible, in part because the linguistic content of his utterances was simple.

On the other hand was Bobby, a child with nearly typical productive language skills. Like other children his age, he spoke in multiword sentences, had a vocabulary of a thousand or more words, and talked about a wide variety of topics. His phonology, however, resembled that of a child of 18–20 months, with extremely limited CV structures and a small consonantal inventory. Because his phonology was inadequate to support the linguistic structures he used, his speech would be highly unintelligible. The mismatch between his phonology and other aspects of his language development created an overall system best described as "deviant" rather than "delayed," as the relationship between language and phonology does not mirror that of a younger, typically developing child.

The hierarchical phonological analyses presented provide a framework for comparing different aspects of the boys' productive phonological systems, revealing similarities at a number of levels. Taken from a larger perspective, however, the phonology–language relationships are quite different: For Joey, language and phonology were commensurate and both were within typical range; for Bobby, phonology lagged far behind language, creating a situation in which phonological intervention clearly was needed.

REFERENCES

Bernhardt, B., & Stoel-Gammon, C. (1994). Nonlinear phonology: Introduction and clinical application. *Journal of Speech and Hearing Research, 37,* 123–143.

Crary, M., & Hunt, T.L. (1983). CV to CVC: A case report of a child with open syllables. *Topics in Language Disorders, 3,* 157–180.

Gierut, J., Cho, M.-H., & Dinnsen, D. (1993). Geometric accounts of consonant–vowel interactions in developing systems. *Clinical Linguistics and Phonetics, 7,* 219–236.

Goldsmith, J. (1990). *Autosegmental and metrical phonology.* New York: Garland Press.

Grunwell, P. (1987). *Clinical phonology* (2nd ed.). London: Croom Helm.

Ingram, D. (1989). *Phonological disability in children* (2nd ed.). London: Cole & Whurr.

Levelt, C.C. (1994). *On the acquisition of place.* The Hague: Holland Academic Graphics.

Prather, E.M., Hedrick, D.L., & Kern, C.A. (1975). Articulation development in children aged two to four years. *Journal of Speech and Hearing Disorders, 40,* 179–191.

Stoel-Gammon, C., & Dunn, C. (1985). *Normal and disordered phonology in children.* Austin, TX: PRO-ED.

Stoel-Gammon, C., & Stemberger, J.P. (1994). Consonant harmony and underspecification in child speech. In M. Yavas (Ed.), *First and second language phonology* (pp. 63–80). San Diego: Singular Publishing Group.

Stoel-Gammon, C., & Stone, J. (1991). Assessing phonology in young children. *Clinics in Communication Disorders, 1,* 25–39.

Templin, M. (1957). Certain language skills in children: Their development and interrelationships. *Institute of Child Welfare Monographs, 26.*

Vihman, M.M. (1978). Consonant harmony: Its scope and function in child language. In J.H. Greenberg (Ed.), *Universals of human language* (Vol. 2, pp. 281–334). Stanford, CA: Stanford University Press.

5

Linguistic Theory
and the Assessment of Grammar

Laurence B. Leonard and Julia A. Eyer

Pᴿᴼᴮᴸᴱᴹˢ ᵂᴵᵀᴴ ᴳᴿᴬᴹᴹᴬᴿ ᴄᴼᴺˢᵀᴵᵀᵁᵀᴱ ᴬ significant part of the language difficulties present in many groups of children with communication disorders. This
chapter outlines how the assessment of these grammatical problems can be use-
fully guided by linguistic theory. The theoretical framework illustrated in this
chapter is *principles and parameters*. Following a review of certain details of
this framework is an examination of its contribution to identifying several types
of grammatical impairments.

PRINCIPLES AND PARAMETERS

The principles-and-parameters framework has its roots in previous versions of
transformational grammar. Although this framework borrows much of its nota-
tion from these previous approaches, it differs from them in many respects. A
problem with the previous approaches is that they were too powerful; although
they contained rules that could generate grammars present in natural languages,
these rules also generated grammars that are highly implausible. The solutions to
this problem have evolved since the early 1980s and owe much to the proposals
of Chomsky (1981, 1986). During the 1980s, the framework that evolved was
dubbed *government and binding* theory. This term has given way to *principles
and parameters* because the latter best captures the essence of this framework.

The primary goal of the principles-and-parameters approach is to explain
how language is learned. What the child learns presumably must be constrained
in such a way that only those variations present in natural languages are considered; hypotheses that are alien to human languages are never entertained. The
constraints that are responsible for this are termed *principles*. Although all principles are, by definition, consistent with human languages, those that apply to all
human languages are said to be part of *Universal Grammar.*

Preparation of this chapter was supported in part by National Institutes of Health research
grant #DC00458 and National Institutes of Health training grant #DC00030. The authors wish to
thank Lisa M. Bedore, Bernard Grela, and the editors of this volume for their helpful suggestions.

It is not sufficient to have principles that limit a child's hypotheses to those details that appear in the world's languages. Languages differ a great deal from one another. The framework also must demonstrate how children can acquire very different languages so quickly. This is possible because languages do not differ haphazardly but rather in sets of characteristics that vary systematically from language to language; there are *parameters* along which languages vary. For example, languages vary according to whether the verbs in the language are always inflected. Languages requiring verb inflections also are those that allow grammatical subjects to be omitted and/or moved to different positions in the sentence depending on the discourse. According to this framework, the child requires only minimal exposure to sentences containing verbs to settle on the proper value for this parameter. Once the value of the parameter is set, the hypotheses about the language that the child must entertain are dramatically reduced.

Underlying Structure

In the principles-and-parameters framework, as in its predecessors, a distinction is made between the underlying structure of a sentence and its surface form. The underlying structure provides the abstract representation of a sentence; it is here that the grammatical relationships of the sentence are specified. The underlying structure is related to the surface form of the sentence through highly con- strained movement rules. For English, the underlying structure takes the general form shown in (1).

(1)

The categories shown in (1) can be divided into lexical categories and func- tional categories. Examples of lexical categories are the familiar noun (*N*) and verb (*V*) and their maximal phrasal projections noun phrase (*NP*) and verb phrase (*VP*). Other examples of lexical categories, though not represented here, include adjective (*A*) and preposition (*P*) and their phrasal projections *AP* and *PP*. The functional categories shown in (1) are complementizer (*C* or *COMP*) and inflection (*I* or *INFL*) and their phrasal projections *CP* and *IP*.

All phrasal projections have the same structure, illustrated in (2).

(2)

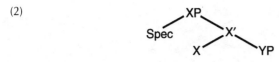

For example, the phrasal projection *VP* shown in (1) branches into a specifier (*Spec*) and an intermediate category *V'.* This, in turn, branches into *V,* considered to be the head, and another phrasal projection, *NP.* One of the fundamental aspects of this framework is that different kinds of phrases (e.g., *NP, VP, PP*) have a common underlying structure.

The intermediate categories, such as *N'* and *V',* are perhaps the least familiar. The necessity of having such categories is that units larger than a word but smaller than a phrase are sometimes operative in the grammar. For example, in the sentence *Bob chose this high-calorie meal rather than that one,* the word *one* can stand for "high-calorie meal" (*Bob chose this high-calorie meal rather than that high-calorie meal*). Yet *high-calorie meal* is not a grammatical unit, as evidenced in the ungrammatical sentence **Bob chose high-calorie meal.*

This chapter focuses on only a few of the details of the principles-and-parameters framework that have relevance to the assessment of grammar in children with communication disorders. Emphasis is placed on the status of the two functional categories shown in (1)—*I* and *C* and their phrasal projections *IP* and *CP.*

The I-System

The properties of grammar that are associated with *I* and *IP* sometimes are referred to collectively as the *I-system.* To illustrate these properties, consider the differences between the utterances in (3) and (4), produced by Child 1 and Child 2, respectively.

(3)   She's eating apple   They like to eat pizza
      Jill poured juice   Mommy can drink coffee
      You're hurting me   He wants milk
      I'll find it   Mommy not want book

(4)   This in big truck   Me want a toy
      Take out cookies   Put milk on table
      Me take it   Them get pencils
      No want pancake

The two children differ in their grammatical development. Child 1 appears to be more advanced in at least two respects: Her utterances are somewhat longer on average, and the grammatical morphemes she uses (e.g., regular past *-ed,* third singular *-s,* auxiliary *is* and *are*) are considered to be later-developing forms than the grammatical morphemes used by Child 2 (noun plural *-s, in, on*). This difference is profound from the standpoint of principles and parameters. The I-system in (5) illustrates this point.

(5)

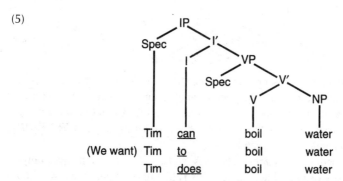

	Tim	can	boil	water
(We want)	Tim	to	boil	water
	Tim	does	boil	water

Modal auxiliaries such as *can* (and *will, could, should,* etc.) and infinitival *to* presumably are base generated (generated in the underlying structure) in the head *I* position of *IP*. If *I* is finite—that is, if it carries tense and agreement features—then it is filled with a modal (as in "Tim *can* boil water"). If *I* is infinitival, then the *I* position is occupied by *to* ("We want Tim *to* boil water"). If *I* is underlyingly empty, then its tense and agreement features can be discharged by filling *I* with the dummy auxiliary *do* ("Tim *does* boil water"). Only Child 1 showed elements of this type. These are illustrated in (6).

(6)

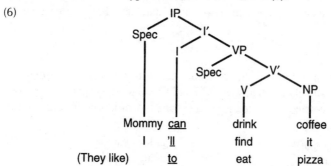

	Mommy	can	drink	coffee
	I	'll	find	it
(They like)		to	eat	pizza

It also is possible to fill an underlyingly empty *I* through movement of auxiliary or copula *be* from the head *V* position in *VP,* as in (7).

(7)

	Tim	is	boiling	water

Again, Child 1 provides examples of such elements in her speech, as shown in (8); Child 2, by contrast, provides no evidence along these lines.

(8)

```
            IP
          /    \
      Spec      I'
        |      /  \
        I     /    VP
        |    /    /   \
        |   /  Spec    V'
        |  /    |     /  \
        | /     V    /    NP
        |       |   /      |
       She     's  eating  apple
       You     're hurting  me
```

If the structure contains no auxiliary in *VP*, and *I* is underlyingly empty, then the tense and agreement features of *I* can be discharged onto the head *V* in the form of an inflection. This is shown in (9).

(9)

```
            IP
          /    \
      Spec      I'
        |      /  \
        I     /    VP
        |    /    /   \
        |   /  Spec    V'
        |  /    |     /  \
        | /     V →  /    NP
        |       |   /      |
       Tim    boils      water
```

The two examples of this type present in Child 1's speech are provided in (10). Evidence of inflections is lacking in Child 2's speech.

(10)

```
            IP
          /    \
      Spec      I'
        |      /  \
        I     /    VP
             /    /   \
          Spec    V'
            |    /  \
            V   /    NP
            |  /      |
           Jill      juice
           He        milk
          poured
          wants
```

The role of the I-system is not limited to details traditionally associated with verbs. The grammatical subject (e.g., "Tim") appears in the specifier position of *IP* in (5)–(10). The subject occupies this position through movement from the specifier position of *VP*. As a result of this movement, the subject assumes a position in which it can receive nominative case assigned by *I*. An example is shown in (11).

(11)

```
            IP
        Spec    I'
              I    VP
            Spec   V'
                 V    NP
        He  can  boil  water
```

Nominative case is evident in the speech of Child 1 but not in that of Child 2. Some of the clearest examples from Child 1 are shown in (12).

(12)

```
            IP
        Spec    I'
              I    VP
            Spec   V'
                 V    NP
        She  's   eating  apple
        He        wants   milk
        I    'll  find    it
```

A review of the differences between Child 1 and Child 2 shows that only Child 1 provided evidence of modal auxiliaries, infinitival *to,* auxiliaries *is* and *are,* verb inflections *-s* and *-ed,* and nominative case. These elements constitute many of the grammatical elements that make up the I-system. In contrast, Child 2 used certain grammatical morphemes, but they were not elements associated with the I-system. Consequently, it can be argued that this child provides evidence of a grammar made up of lexical categories only. Radford (1990) proposed that utterances such as those of Child 2 can be handled by an underlying structure such as (13); that is, grammatical subjects in the child's grammar are still in the specifier position of *VP* rather than of *IP* and thus not in a position to receive nominative case. In addition, the verb has no access to an I-system and is therefore free of tense and agreement features.

(13)

```
          VP
      Spec    V'
           V    NP
      Them get  pencils
```

A more subtle difference exists between the two children that relates to the I-system. Both children produced utterances with negatives; Child 1 said *Mommy not want book,* and Child 2 produced *No want pancake.* In the principles-and-parameters framework, negative particles presumably appear between *IP* and *VP,* as in (14).

(14)

```
              IP
          /      \
       Spec        I'
        |        /    \
        |       I     NegP
        |       |    /    \
        |       |  Neg     VP
        |       |   |    /    \
        |       |   |  Spec    V'
        |       |   |   |    /    \
        |       |   |   |   V      NP
        |       |   |   |   |      |
       She     is  not    watching  him
```

Once an I-system is in place, children manage to use utterances in which the grammatical subject is to the left of the negative particle (e.g., *She not watching him*) even if children are not yet consistent in their use of auxiliaries. This is possible because of the presence of the specifier position in *IP,* which serves as the landing site (i.e., the final position after movement) of the subject. Child 1's utterance *Mommy not want book* is an example of this type, as illustrated in (15). For children with no I-system, there is no means by which the subject can appear to the left of the negative particle.

(15)

```
              IP
          /      \
       Spec        I'
        |        /    \
        |       I     NegP
        |       |    /    \
        |       |  Neg     VP
        |       |   |    /    \
        |       |   |  Spec    V'
        |       |   |   |    /    \
        |       |   |   |   V      NP
        |       |   |   |   |      |
      Mommy        not    want    book
```

The differences between Child 1 and Child 2 might reflect very different underlying grammars, at least to the extent that spontaneous speech is any indication. Child 1's speech showed clear evidence of an I-system, whereas Child 2's speech provided evidence only of lexical categories.

The C-System

The second functional category system appearing in (1) is the *C-system,* given its name because of the grammatical properties associated with *C* and its phrasal projection *CP.* In English, the C-system is most relevant for questions and certain types of complex sentences. The importance of the C-system is illustrated by contrasting utterances produced by Child 3 and Child 4 in (16) and (17), respectively.

(16) Do you want tea?   What Daddy buying?
     I wonder if they like popcorn   Are you watching me?

(17) Mommy's watching TV?   Who is making noise?
     What fell off the table?   You're going home?

The differences between Child 3 and Child 4 are less obvious than those between Child 1 and Child 2. Both children ask yes–no as well as wh- questions, and both show evidence of auxiliary forms. However, the status of these questions might be quite different. To see how, examine the structure in (1) with details pertaining to questions filled in. This is shown in (18) and (19).

(18)

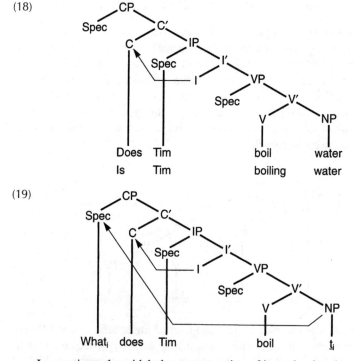

In questions, the widely known operation of inversion involves the copula or auxiliary form moving from the *I* position to the *C* position; this is illustrated in both (18) and (19). Wh- movement, shown in (19), involves the wh- word moving from its base position to the specifier position in *CP*. Also shown in (19) is that the wh- word, moved from *NP*, left a "trace" (*t*) coindexed with itself; the coindexing is indicated by $_i$.

Child 3 produced utterances conforming to the structures in (18) and (19). These are shown in (20) and (21), respectively.

(20)

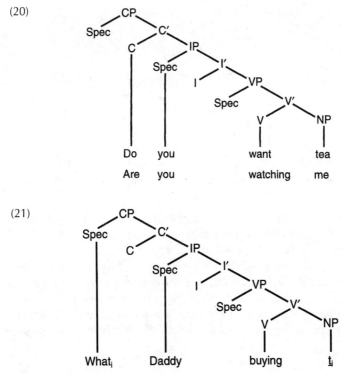

(21)

The yes–no questions in (20) seem to involve movement (of auxiliary *do* and auxiliary *are*) to C. The child's wh- question in (21), though not yet adult-like, seems to involve a C-system because the wh- word appears to the left of the subject. Presumably, it resides in the specifier position of *CP* even though the *C* position was never occupied.

The evidence for a C-system in Child 4's questions is less convincing. This child used yes–no questions that were probably acceptable in casual speech; however, because the auxiliary *is* and *are* forms were produced in declarative word order, there was no movement to *C* and, consequently, no evidence of any category to the left of *IP*. Child 4 also produced wh- questions. However, upon closer examination of these questions, the wh- words appear to be occupying the grammatical subject slot (*Who is making noise? The dog is making noise*), which is located in *IP*. So, again, it is possible that *CP* does not exist in the child's grammar.

Another important function of the C-system is illustrated in (22). The C-system provides a location for overt complementizers such as *that* and *if*. Specifically, such complementizers are base generated in the *C* position. When Child 3 produced *I wonder if they like popcorn,* as shown in (16), she provided evidence that her grammar possessed this position.

(22)

| | (She thinks) | that | Tim | can | boil | water |
| | (She wonders) | if | Tim | can | boil | water |

The utterances produced by Child 3 and Child 4 suggest very different underlying grammars. Child 3's grammar appears to possess a C-system; Child 4's grammar provided no evidence of this sort.

Although the I-system and the C-system are but two constructs within the broader principles-and-parameters framework, they might be central to the assessment of grammar in children with language disorders. The next section illustrates this point by reviewing several accounts of grammatical impairments with an eye toward the possible role of these two functional category systems.

ACCOUNTS OF GRAMMATICAL IMPAIRMENTS IN CHILDREN WITH SPECIFIC LANGUAGE IMPAIRMENT

Among the groups of children experiencing difficulties with grammar are those who are labeled as having *specific language impairment* (SLI). Children with SLI have language problems that are not clearly associated with other factors. Their hearing is within normal limits, and they show no signs of obvious neurological impairment. They also score at age-appropriate levels on nonverbal tests of intelligence, although subtle cognitive limitations sometimes can be found on close inspection. These children show a mild to moderate degree of difficulty in producing many aspects of language; however, grammar often is one of the more serious areas of difficulty. For example, even when children with SLI are matched with younger, typically developing children according to mean length of utterance, the children with SLI often are found to make less use of grammatical morphemes and sometimes to demonstrate a more restricted range of syntactic structures (see reviews in Johnston, 1988; Leonard, 1989; and Rice, 1991). Since 1990, several investigators have offered possible explanations for the serious grammatical impairments observed in many children with SLI. Three of these are reviewed, with an emphasis on the possible role played by functional categories.

Slow Development of Functional Categories

Based on proposals that typically developing children's early grammars lack functional categories (e.g., Guilfoyle & Noonan, 1992; Radford, 1990), Eyer and Leonard (1995), Guilfoyle, Allen, and Moss (1991), and Loeb and Leonard (1991) have suggested that children with SLI might be especially delayed in the development of functional categories. Although other aspects of grammar might be slow to develop in these children, functional categories show an extraordinary delay in their appearance. Loeb and Leonard (1991) focused their proposal on the I-system in particular; the proposals of Eyer and Leonard (1995) and Guilfoyle et al. (1991) are more far-reaching, dealing with all functional categories.

Exploring whether a child with SLI has delayed development of functional categories requires examining the child's control of the grammatical elements associated with the functional categories of interest. For the I-system, this would include the modal auxiliaries, auxiliary *do,* auxiliary *be,* copula *be,* infinitival *to,* finite verb inflections *-ed* and *-s,* and nominative case pronouns. For the C-system, examination would be directed toward the child's control of copula and auxiliary inversion in both yes–no and wh- questions, and complementizers such as *that* and *if.*

Children with language problems typically experience difficulties with many areas of language; for difficulties with functional categories to be clinically meaningful, then, such difficulties would have to exceed those observed in other areas. Accordingly, it would be necessary to examine the child's control of grammatical elements that are not closely tied to functional categories. For example, if a child were experiencing special difficulties with the I-system, then the child's control of noun plural *-s* would be expected to be closer to age expectations (even if still subpar) than the finite verb inflections (third singular *-s,* past *-ed*). If the C-system were problematic, then the diversity of argument structures reflected in the child's speech would be closer to age level than would the child's control of complementizers and auxiliary inversion. For example, the child might use the double-object construction (e.g., *Mommy give me some milk*), sentences with oblique arguments (e.g., "on the table" in *Daddy put that on the table*), and sentences with verb complements (e.g., *Mommy need fix the car*), yet produce questions in which neither the wh- word nor an auxiliary appears to the left of the subject (e.g., *Why going?, Daddy's on the roof?*).

The proposal that functional categories are especially slow in development could be translated in one of two ways. First, the functional categories may be initially absent from the underlying grammar. Second, the functional categories may be present in the underlying grammar but the grammatical elements that are associated with these categories (e.g., modals, copula *be,* auxiliary inversion, complementizers) are especially slow to appear. In either case, these elements would be expected to appear eventually, though their development might be protracted. A problem of this type, then, would manifest in degree of control of the elements, not necessarily in the total absence of such elements.

Extended Optionality of Infinitives

Wexler (1994) has proposed that typically developing children initially pass through a stage during which they alternate between using finite verb inflections and using infinitives (i.e., nonfinite verb forms) in contexts requiring the former. In a language such as English, this means alternating between forms such as regular past -ed and the bare stem (e.g., *Sally jumped* and *Sally jump*). (Although infinitival *to* does not appear in these alternations, the bare stem can still be taken to be nonfinite, as evidenced in appropriate utterances such as *I saw Sally jump;* one does not say **I saw Sally jumped.*) This alternation does not represent simple free variation between finite and nonfinite forms because children at this stage do not use finite forms in contexts requiring nonfinite forms. Thus, the children seem to know something about tense and agreement. According to Wexler, this optional use of infinitives is attributable to young children's lack of knowledge that tense marking is obligatory in main clauses. Rice, Wexler, and Cleave (1995) have argued that this optional infinitive stage is especially protracted in children with SLI.

One of the intriguing aspects of the extended optionality account is that the underlying grammar is presumed to contain *I* and *IP;* only the child's knowledge of the obligatory nature of finiteness is lacking. Therefore, when the child happens to mark finiteness, all of the details associated with finiteness in the I-system take effect. This permits ready assessment of the extended optionality account as an explanation of a child's problem with certain details of grammar. For example, if a child fails to use a finite verb form, then preverbal pronouns might not be marked for nominative case (e.g., *Him like baseball cards*). However, if a finite form is used, then preverbal pronouns should receive nominative case (*He likes baseball cards*). Similarly, because only finite elements can move to the *C* position in questions, a nonfinite copula form would never appear to the left of the subject in a question. Thus, *Laura be sad?* might be produced, but *Be Laura sad?* would not. Another important feature of this account is the expectation that if a finite form is used, it will be used correctly. Thus, although auxiliary *be* forms often will be absent, when they are used, *is* will appear in third-person-singular contexts, *am* in first-person-singular contexts, and so forth.

Problems with Movement

Hadley (1993) and Smith (1992) have advanced somewhat different proposals that implicate movement of elements to functional category positions as a major problem in children with SLI. In noting that auxiliary *be* forms were more difficult for children with SLI than were modal auxiliaries and, for some children, auxiliary *do* forms, Hadley suggested that these children might have difficulty with the *V*-to-*I* movement that is involved with *be*. The example shown in (7) is repeated here as (23).

(23)

```
              IP
         Spec    I'
                I    VP
                   Spec   V'
                      V      NP
         Tim    is    boiling   water
```

Both modals and *do,* by contrast, presumably are base generated in *I* and require no movement. The relevant examples in (5) are repeated here as (24).

(24)

```
              IP
         Spec    I'
                I    VP
                   Spec   V'
                      V      NP
         Tim    can    boil    water
         Tim    does   boil    water
```

Smith's (1992) proposal was concerned with wh- movement. Smith found that children with SLI had difficulties using wh- questions involving "long-distance" movement (i.e., movement of the wh- word from an embedded sentence to the specifier position of the first *CP*). The structure of this type of question is illustrated in (25).

(25)

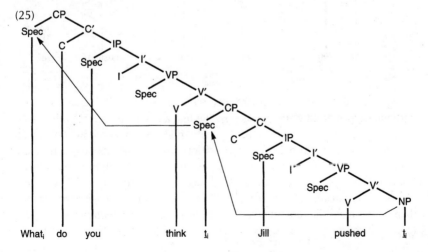

The wh- word not only leaves a trace in its original position (*NP*) but also makes an intermediate stop in the specifier position of *CP* in the embedded sentence, again leaving a trace. Smith observed that even though children with SLI could manage movement of the wh- word in such constructions, they seemed unaware that the vacated positions required no overt form. The children often produced a second wh- word in the specifier of the embedded *CP* (e.g., *What do you think what Jill pushed?*) or filled the original *NP* slot with a lexical item (e.g., *What do you think Jill pushed something?*).

If a child were suspected of having significant problems with *V*-to-*I* movement, then the child's control of auxiliary *be* should be further behind age expectations than should his or her control of auxiliaries (modals and *do*) that require no movement. If the problem concerned traces and long-distance wh- movement, then the child's control of long-distance wh- movement should lag further behind age level than should control of questions with embedded sentences that contain *CP* but involve no wh- movement, as in (26).

(26)

Although the proposals of Hadley (1993) and Smith (1992) deal with only particular types of movement, it is possible that a child's problems with movement are even more pervasive. The difficulty might be evidenced in any type of movement to a functional category position. To explore this possibility, the child's control of auxiliary inversion in yes–no questions might be examined. For example, it would be expected that the child's control of modal auxiliary inversion (e.g., *Can she run fast?*) would fall further behind age expectations than would his or her command of modal auxiliaries in a declarative position (e.g., *She can run fast*). Because modals are presumed to be base generated in the *I* position, such a comparison should provide a relatively straightforward view of the role of movement to the functional category position *C*.

The child's ability with passive constructions also might be the focus of evaluation. According to some investigators (e.g., Guilfoyle & Noonan, 1992), passives require that the theme located in the *NP* within *V'* move to the specifier position of *IP*, as in (27).

(27)

To determine whether this type of movement is especially problematic for a child, assessment might focus not only on passives but also on adjectival constructions as in *Ed was funny*. The reason for this type of comparison is that the passive involves movement in addition to the *NP* in *V'* moving to the specifier position in *IP*. Adjectival constructions serve as a control in this respect. In such constructions, the subject moves from the specifier position of *VP* to the specifier position of *IP*. An evaluation is necessary of whether the child's control of passive lags further behind age level than does his or her control of adjectival constructions.

APPLYING THEORY TO
REAL DATA: SPONTANEOUS SPEECH SAMPLES

Each of the three accounts of grammatical impairments suggests constellations of functional category elements that might be evaluated in a child's speech. Many of these elements can be gleaned from spontaneous speech data. Unfortunately, even though these elements are highly diagnostic, a judgment as to their status in the child's grammar cannot be rendered simply on whether they appear in the child's speech. A variety of criteria must be considered before a decision can be made.

Frequency Criteria

The mere presence of some detail in the child's speech does not necessarily constitute evidence for the grammatical capacity with which it is usually associated. The detail might have been learned in an unanalyzed fashion as part of a larger unit. Adopting a frequency criterion can significantly reduce the likelihood that such examples unduly influence the conclusions drawn about the child's grammar. For example, if a particular grammatical form is required to appear in at least five utterances, then the likelihood that the form is unanalyzed would be lower.

However, a simple count of the number of utterances containing the form is not sufficient. Certainly, no clinician would credit a child with the third-person-singular verb inflection if this form appeared only in *Thar she blows*, no matter how frequently this utterance were produced. Similarly, not much more certainty can be established if the form appeared frequently but only in an utterance such as *Daddy works late*. The frequency criterion should be based on nonidentical utterances containing the form. The utterances in (28), for example, would constitute more convincing evidence that the third-person-singular inflection is represented in the child's grammar. It would be unlikely that all of these instances of -*s* were unanalyzed.

(28) Mommy likes to run
      He likes me
      Tammy wants my apple juice
      Sammy plays baseball
      Daddy talks funny

Diversity Criteria

The strength of the evidence reflected in (28) does not rest solely on the presence of -*s* in five distinct utterances. This inflection appeared with four different verbs—*like, want, play,* and *talk*. If -*s* appeared only with a single verb, then the possibility might remain that the verb plus inflection was actually learned as a single lexical item. If some criterion for lexical diversity also were required, then this possibility would be greatly reduced.

There is another way in which diversity criteria might be used. As a type of shorthand, terms such as "modal auxiliaries," "auxiliary *be*," and "copula *be*" often are used. However, it is difficult to be certain when exactly auxiliary *be* is acquired. It may be when the child uses auxiliary *is* a number of times, or it may be when *are* and *am* (and *was* and *were*) forms also are used. It would seem that five instances of *is* and five instances of *are* would constitute stronger evidence for the attainment of auxiliary *be* than would 10 instances of *is*, for example.

Contrasts

Frequency and diversity criteria are not sufficient to conclude that the child has knowledge of a functional category element. Consider the productions in (29).

(29) Mommy likes donuts   Mommy like flowers
      Maggie wants bottle   We wants milk
      Daddy snores   Grandpa snore
      Mickey tells jokes   These fits

Although the child produces the third-person-singular -*s* inflection with five different verbs, there is no evidence that -*s* is used contrastively (i.e., to mark third-person singular in particular). Productions such as *We wants milk and *These fits suggest that the child has no knowledge of the agreement functions that this inflection serves. The problem does not rest with the absence of -s in *Mommy like flowers and *Grandpa snore. Provided that the child meets some reasonable frequency and diversity criteria and uses -s only in appropriate contexts, the absence of this inflection does not mean the absence of knowledge; only the degree of control of this inflection is in question.

The notion of contrast also is applicable in the case of auxiliary verbs. Assume that the only elements of I reflected in a child's speech were the auxiliary + negative don't and the modal auxiliary can. The limitation of this evidence is that these forms provide no indication of control of tense or agreement, one of the primary functions of I. Stronger evidence of I would be if the two forms were, for example, don't and doesn't, with the latter appearing only in appropriate (third-person-singular) contexts. In this case, there would be a contrast in agreement. If the child's forms were can and could, then there would be a contrast in tense, provided that could appeared only in past contexts. Note that such criteria allow for the possibility that utterances such as *She don't go there alternate with those such as She doesn't see it in the child's speech. Provided that doesn't occurs only in third-person-singular contexts, the presence of don't in some contexts requiring doesn't speaks only to the degree of the child's control of the form.

Overregularization

If a child were to use a particular grammatical inflection 20 times with 14 different verbs only in grammatical contexts that required the inflection, then evidence for the child's knowledge of this element would be considerable. Nevertheless, the possibility would remain that the child had learned the inflection on a rote basis, lexical item by lexical item, by taking careful note of the contexts in which the inflection appeared and did not appear. For this reason, documentation of the child's use of a grammatical element in contexts unlikely to be heard in the speech of others would be extremely valuable. The quintessential case of such use is evidenced in overregularization, whereby the child produces an inflection with a stem that requires an irregular form, as in *throwed for threw. Such use probably indicates that the regular past inflection is part of the child's underlying grammar. The frequency with which overregularization occurs is less critical, assuming that the child occasionally uses the -ed inflection with verbs requiring it.

Commission Errors as Converging Evidence

In a language such as English, developmental level often is determined on the basis of the presence versus absence of a grammatical element. When the element is absent, a less-advanced stage of development is assumed. However, errors of commission also can be used as evidence for an earlier developmental level. One example of this is when negative words such as *no* or *not* appear to the left of the grammatical subject, as in *No Paula drink that*. As noted previously, according to some theorists, utterances such as *Paula drink that* might reflect a grammar composed of lexical categories only, as shown in (13). Only later does the grammar expand to accommodate functional categories. Utterances such as *No Paula drink that* would be consistent with this view; that is, the appearance of *Paula* to the right of *no* suggests that there was no constituent available to the left of the negative particle (viz, *IP*) into which *Paula* could move. Such evidence is quite strong, given that it reflects word order that varies from the order in the target language.

Commission Errors as Counterevidence

Just as commission errors can serve as supportive evidence for particular accounts of grammatical impairment, they also can be used to argue against such accounts. Consider the utterance *Mommy not likes candy*. For the extended optionality account, such an utterance would be problematic. According to this account, if the option selected is [+ finite], then tense and agreement features must be expressed to the left of the negative term. These features cannot be moved from *I* to *V* (in the form of an inflection), given the presence of negation between the two. According to this account, then, the utterance should take the form *Mommy doesn't like candy*. If tense and agreement features are not present to the left of *not,* then an inflection must not appear (*Mommy not like candy*), reflecting a [– finite] selection.

Parsimony

There are occasions in which the data supporting an account are far from compelling but might be chosen over alternative explanations on the basis of parsimony. Consider the utterances in (30).

> (30) a. You can't eat cats!
> b. Mommy don't drive me
> c. Karen pushed me
> d. Paula sewed my dress
> e. Let's see if the toys in here
> f. Why birds eat worms?
> g. How Daddy do that?

The utterances in (30a)–(30d) contain elements associated with an I-system; those in (30e)–(30g) contain elements associated with a C-system. However, some scholars might be quick to point out ways in which these utterances can be explained without the necessity of functional categories. For example, it might be argued that 1) *can't* and *don't* simply were learned as lexical alternatives to *not,* 2) *-ed* was learned as a (nonfinite) participle (equivalent to "has push*ed*" without the auxiliary), 3) *Let's see if* was learned as an unanalyzed whole, and 4) both

NegP and fronted wh- words developed through adjunction with (attachment to) *VP*, as in (31) and (32) (see Radford, 1990).

(31)

```
              VP
         ╱    ╲
       Spec    VP
             ╱   ╲
           NegP    V'
                 ╱   ╲
                V      NP
                │      │
              You can't  eat    cats
              Mommy don't drive me
```

(32)

```
              VP
         ╱    ╲
       Spec    VP
             ╱   ╲
           Spec    V'
                 ╱   ╲
                V      NP
                │      │
              Why birds  eat    worms
              How Daddy  do     that
```

Although such an account of the facts is highly plausible, the four types of factors that must be invoked render it rather unattractive. A more parsimonious alternative is that the child's underlying grammar possessed the structure evidenced in adult grammar, functional categories and all.

The relative utility of these seven types of criteria undoubtedly varies as a function of the particular grammatical elements under examination. Together, however, they should provide a comprehensive picture of the status of any given element in the child's grammar.

APPLYING THEORY TO
REAL DATA: SPECIFICALLY DESIGNED TASKS

Some of the grammatical forms that can be especially helpful in evaluating particular hypotheses occur with low frequency even in the spontaneous speech of adults. To assess the child's use of such forms, tasks must be devised that provide natural contexts for the forms. This state of affairs actually can be turned to the examiner's advantage by allowing him or her to test predictions about the nature of the child's grammatical impairment.

Consider the following example: Some investigators have proposed that early wh- questions do not reflect evidence of a C-system but are, instead, base-generated adjuncts in sentence-initial position, much as in (32). These questions are then reorganized with the wh- words in the specifier position of *CP* as soon as children learn lexical complementizers such as *that* and *if* in (33).

(33) Mommy knows that I'm smart
I wonder if it's raining

A related, but more refined, proposal is that this process might proceed lexical item by lexical item, such that the movement of a particular wh- word to *CP* in a matrix clause (e.g., *What do you hear?*) depends upon the child's registering the same wh- word in embedded questions (e.g., *Do you know what she wants?*) (see de Villiers, 1992). This particular proposal requires that the child note instances of a sentence-internal lexical item occupying the specifier position of *CP,* as shown in (34).

(34)

Given the problems that wh- questions pose for children with language disorders, it is important to determine whether such problems are related to difficulties with lexical complementizers, thus reflecting a more general problem with the C-system. Of course, utterances with complementizers are not frequent in spontaneous speech. For this reason, specific tasks might be designed. For example, the examiner could use the child as an intermediary in requesting information from a puppet that served as witness to some event. An illustration is shown in (35).

(35) Examiner: Let's go over to our farm. Oh, look, the water is pink now. Why? Mr. Puppet was here. Maybe he knows. Go ask him. Ask him if he knows.
Child: You know why water is pink?

The activity can be extended so that the child asks a number of questions of the puppet, ensuring a sufficient test of the child's ability to use forms that require an embedded *CP.*[1]

----

[1]A helpful review of tasks that can be used to elicit these and many other grammatical structures can be found in McDaniel, Cairns, and McKee (in press).

Specifically designed tasks are especially useful in assessing the child's comprehension of grammatical details. Consider, for example, the evaluation of the child's understanding of passive constructions. A truth-value judgment task might be employed in this case (e.g., Crain, 1986). The examiner acts out some event using toy figures, and another experimenter manipulates and talks for a puppet. Following each event, the puppet "says" what just transpired. The child's task is to judge whether the sentence produced by the puppet is an accurate description of what happened. (The task is sometimes embellished, such as by allowing the child to feed the puppet a cookie if the description is accurate and a rag if the description misportrays the event.) So, if the event focused on a toy bear figure and this figure were suddenly kissed by a duck, then the puppet might produce a passive sentence that either correctly describes the event ("The bear was kissed by the duck") or incorrectly describes it ("The duck was kissed by the bear").

APPLICATIONS BEYOND STANDARD ENGLISH

A major strength of the principles-and-parameters framework is that its goals are to explain at once the universal properties of language and the differences that occur between languages. Consider how this dual concern might be applied to the assessment of grammatical impairments in a language other than standard English. In Spanish, as in English, an I-system and a C-system are presumed to be represented in the mature underlying grammar. It is possible, therefore, that a Spanish-speaking child's problems with grammar can be attributed to difficulties with functional categories. Indeed, each of the accounts of grammatical impairments discussed previously could, in principle, hold for Spanish as well as for English.

However, the differences in the structure of Spanish and English mean that grammatical difficulties attributable to the same source will manifest themselves in somewhat different ways in the two languages. In Spanish, for example, verbs must be inflected; bare stems do not appear. Therefore, if a child's grammar lacks an I-system, then the child will use what appears to be an inflected form. However, it is inflected only in appearance; it is actually a default form that lacks tense and agreement features. The form typically used as a default is the third-person singular. An example appears in (36).

(36)

"Mommy eat cookie"

To ascertain whether the third-person singular actually reflects a finite form or is merely a default form, it would be necessary to assess the child's use of other inflections, such as first-person singular and third-person plural. Utterances such as those in (37) would suggest the availability of an I-system; those in (38) would suggest that an I-system was not operative. The grammatical subjects in these examples are placed in parentheses simply to indicate that they can be omitted in most speaking contexts.

(37) (Yo) como galleta   "(I) eat cookie"
     (Ellos) comen galleta   "(They) eat cookie"

(38) (Yo) come galleta
     (Ellos) come galleta

In many languages, there are grammatical elements associated with functional categories that are not present in English. Spanish is no exception. For example, when direct-object pronouns are employed to refer to objects or people clearly established from the context, clitics are used. Unlike their noun counterparts, direct-object clitics move from their original position after the finite verb to a position in front of the verb. The new position presumably is in *I*. The example in (39) illustrates that the clitic *lo* ("it") moves from the *NP* in *V'* to the *I* position.[2] This means that children whose grammatical impairments are related to the I-system frequently might omit direct objects.

(39)

lo vemos
"(We) see it"

To ensure that these omissions are not related to a more general problem with direct objects, the same children might be asked to describe events in which the direct object constitutes a new element in the situation. For example, the child might be asked to describe a sequence of pictures in which a monkey takes several bananas in succession and then takes a peach. In this context, "peach" (*durazno* in Spanish) is likely to be expressed in noun form and would occupy the *NP* position in *V'.* Because this position is not a functional category position, omission would not be likely.

Clitics also could be used to determine whether a child's grammatical impairments were related to lack of knowledge that finiteness is obligatory in main clauses. Only a finite *I* can license a clitic in preverb position. Thus, when

---

[2]The finite verb *vemos* also appears under *I*. In Spanish, it is presumed that verbs receive tense and agreement features by moving from *V* to *I*. This point is not central to the examples used here.

the child fails to use a finite form—for example, when the child simply chooses the default third-person singular regardless of appropriateness—clitics should not precede the verb. However, when the child seems to express finiteness by virtue of using the correct inflected form, clitics should be much more likely to appear.

CONCLUSION

This chapter has examined how two functional category systems in the principles-and-parameters framework—the I-system and the C-system—might prove useful in assessing grammar in children with communication disorders. Problems related to these systems might account for a wide variety of grammatical difficulties, whether the problem revolves around whole functional category systems or around specific details, such as movement to functional category positions or knowledge that finite verbs are obligatory in main clauses.

Even with a theoretical framework as a guide to assessment, it is necessary to adopt criteria for determining whether a child is credited with control of some grammatical detail. Seven such criteria were discussed: frequency, diversity, contrasts, overregularization, commission errors as converging evidence, commission errors as counterevidence, and parsimony. Some of the theoretically relevant grammatical structures might best be assessed through the use of specifically designed tasks; this is especially true for structures that occur infrequently in spontaneous speech and for the assessment of comprehension more generally.

The chapter emphasized the assessment of grammatical problems in standard English, but the framework lends itself to the study of other languages and dialects. A few examples were provided in Spanish for illustration. The same questions can be pursued in Spanish as in English, but the grammatical difficulties of the children might manifest themselves in different ways. Many aspects of the principles-and-parameters framework could not be included because of space constraints; nevertheless, the information that was presented illustrates that language assessment can benefit from a theoretical framework of this type.

REFERENCES

Chomsky, N. (1981). *Lectures on government and binding.* Dordrecht, The Netherlands: Foris.
Chomsky, N. (1986). *Barriers.* Cambridge: MIT Press.
Crain, S. (1986, October). *On the developmental autonomy of syntax.* Paper presented at the Boston University Conference on Language Development, Boston.
de Villiers, J. (1992). On the acquisition of functional categories: A general commentary. In J. Meisel (Ed.), *The acquisition of verb placement* (pp. 423–443). Dordrecht, The Netherlands: Kluwer.
Eyer, J., & Leonard, L. (1995). Functional categories and specific language impairment: A case study. *Language Acquisition, 4,* 177–203.

Guilfoyle, E., Allen, S., & Moss, S. (1991, October). *Specific language impairment and the maturation of functional categories.* Paper presented at the Boston University Conference on Language Development, Boston.

Guilfoyle, E., & Noonan, M. (1992). Functional categories and language acquisition. *Canadian Journal of Linguistics, 37,* 241–272.

Hadley, P. (1993). *A longitudinal investigation of the auxiliary system in children with specific language impairment.* Unpublished doctoral dissertation, University of Kansas, Lawrence.

Johnston, J. (1988). Specific language disorders in the child. In N. Lass, J. Northern, L. McReynolds, & D. Yoder (Eds.), *Handbook of speech-language pathology and audiology* (pp. 685–715). Baltimore: University Park Press.

Leonard, L. (1989). Language learnability and specific language impairment in children. *Applied Psycholinguistics, 10,* 179–202.

Loeb, D., & Leonard, L. (1991). Subject case marking and verb morphology in normally developing and specifically language-impaired children. *Journal of Speech and Hearing Research, 34,* 340–346.

McDaniel, D., Cairns, H., & McKee, C. (in press). *Methods for assessing children's syntax.* Cambridge: MIT Press.

Radford, A. (1990). *Syntactic theory and the acquisition of English syntax.* Oxford, England: Blackwell.

Rice, M.L. (1991). Children with specific language impairment: Toward a model of teachability. In N.A. Krasnegor, D.M. Rumbaugh, R.L. Schiefelbusch, & M. Studdert-Kennedy (Eds.), *Biological and behavioral determinants of language development* (pp. 447–480). Hillsdale, NJ: Lawrence Erlbaum Associates.

Rice, M.L., Wexler, K., & Cleave, P. (1995). Specific language impairment as a period of extended optional infinitive. *Journal of Speech and Hearing Research, 38,* 850–863.

Smith, K. (1992, January). *The acquisition of long-distance wh- questions in normal and specifically language-impaired children.* Paper presented at the meeting of the Linguistic Society of America, Philadelphia.

Wexler, K. (1994). Optional infinitives, head movement, and the economy of derivations. In D. Lightfoot & N. Hornstein (Eds.), *Verb movement* (pp. 305–350). Cambridge, England: Cambridge University Press.

6

Evaluating Narrative Discourse Skills

Allyssa McCabe

DISCOURSE REFERS TO SENTENCES CONNECTED by a topic or theme. Many researchers (e.g., Bruner, 1986) split discourse into two categories—narrative and what is variously termed paradigmatic (Bruner, 1986), explanatory (Beals & Snow, 1994), or expository. Narratives usually concern real or pretend memories of something that happened and usually are, therefore, recounted in the past tense. However, there also are hypothetical, future-tense narratives and others given in the historical present tense. Narratives often contain a chronological sequence of events, but they also can contain a single event or can skip around in time (McCabe, 1991a). Expository discourse refers to explanations, lectures, or descriptions—often given in the present tense and often centered around a topic or theme. Following is an example of narrative discourse by Nick, a typical European American, 6-year-old boy:

NICK: Hi Alice. I broke my arm. It was, well, um, well, um, um, the day, 2 days ago. I was climbing the the tree and I, well see, I went towards the *low* branch and I and I I got caught with my baving suit? I dangled my hands down and they got bent because it was like this hard surface under it? Then they bent like in two triangles. But luckily it was my *left* arm that broke.

FAMILY FRIEND: Was your family with you when you broke it?

NICK: What? *No.* Only my *mom* was. My mom was in the shower, so I *screamed* for Jessica, and Jessica goed told my mom.

FAMILY FRIEND: Did you go see Dr. Vincent?

NICK: I *don't* have Dr. Vincent. I had to go to the hospital and get mm, it was much more worser than you think because I had to get, go into the operation room and I had to get my, and I had to take um anesthesia and I had to fall, fall, fall asleep and they bended my arm back and I have my cast on.... Do you want to sign my cast?

This narrative contrasts with the following examples of expository talk by Liliana, a typical European American, 6-year-old girl:

LILIANA   [after finishing *Charlotte's Web,* crying]: All the people in the whole world know that spiders die, so why do they have to put it in a book?

BROTHER: Mine [granola bar] is bigger.
LILIANA: No, if it was fat and you turned it skinnier, it would be bigger.
MOTHER: What do you mean "bigger"?
LILIANA: If you took this bar and you bited teeny bites out of the side, it would turn taller. And if [brother's] was turned skinnier and mine turned skinnier, then mine would still be littler than [brother's].

Discourse is an extraordinarily contextualized, profoundly social activity reflecting many factors and affecting many aspects of a person's life. One must consider the influence of the interviewer, aspects of the situation, kind of discourse being assessed, demographics of the speaker, and analyses used for assessment before drawing any conclusions about the normalcy of speakers. Failure to consider key variables such as the cultural background of an individual and possible overuse of the familiar fictional storytelling paradigm could result in misdiagnosing difference as impairment or impairment as competence.

Because it is difficult to truly assess comprehension and production of discourse other than in a trivial or misleading way, it is critical to underscore how many aspects of a person's life will be affected by impaired discourse abilities. Two of the most affected aspects are literacy acquisition and the conduct of social relationships. Numerous studies have documented that impairments in early discourse production predict difficulties in the acquisition of literacy (e.g., Bishop & Edmundson, 1987; De Hirsch, Jansky, & Langford, 1966; Dickinson & Snow, 1987; Feagans, 1982; Feagans & Short, 1984, 1986; Graybeal, 1981; Griffith, Ripich, & Dastoli, 1986; Hansen, 1978; Johnston, 1982; Levi, Musatti, Piredda, & Sechi, 1984; Liles, 1985; Michaels, 1981; Roth & Spekman, 1986; Scarborough & Dobrich, 1990; Weaver & Dickinson, 1982; see Dickinson & McCabe, 1991, for review). Studies also have documented the ways in which children's impaired discourse abilities result in negative perceptions of their personalities (Hemphill & Siperstein, 1990) or even ostracism (Rice, 1991) by their peers. Thus, discourse impairments, if present, must be identified and addressed.

The goal of identifying discourse-level impairments is to ascertain whether an individual has difficulty on the discourse level of language that is independent of word-finding difficulties and impairments of syntax and morphology. Struggling to find words and/or producing many ungrammatical sentences may impinge upon the coherence of discourse production, but they are not necessarily discourse-level impairments.

Furthermore, true discourse-level difficulties involve impairments in the *form* of discourse rather than in the *content* of what is said; children may tell lies or otherwise disturbing narratives, but if they do so in good form, then they should not be considered as having discourse-level difficulties. They might even be said to exhibit discourse prowess because of their ability to conjure up plausible stories without having experienced real events.

CRITICAL VARIABLES FOR ASSESSING NARRATIVE DISCOURSE

When assessing the narrative discourse produced by children, it is necessary to consider the authenticity of the discourse that has been elicited. Several variables affect the child's production: 1) influence of the interviewer, 2) aspects of the situation, 3) kind of discourse assessed, and 4) aspects of individuals interviewed.

Influence of the Interviewer

In many ways, interviewers are responsible for the kind and quality of the discourse they elicit (Mishler, 1986). Children talk very differently to peers than they do to adults (Labov, 1972), sometimes telling longer and more complex narratives to adults than to other children (Umiker-Sebeok, 1979). Furthermore, they tell longer, more explicit narratives to adults who have not shared their narrated experiences than they do to adults who have shared those experiences and therefore do not require as much information to make sense of the narration (Menig-Peterson, 1975). Also, children are more accurate in reporting experiences to a friendly, or "reinforcing," adult than to a distant one (Goodman, Bottoms, Schwartz-Kenney, & Rudy, 1991).

Interviewers may want to engage in conversational exchanges with children, even to the point of telling children short narratives of their own. Interviewers should avoid leading questions, such as the ones asked by the family friend in the narrative at the beginning of this chapter. If children are asked leading questions to which they do not know the answer (e.g., "Who was there?"), they may fall back on their knowledge of general events rather than focus on the distinctive aspects of some experience that held most meaning to them (Hudson & Shapiro, 1991). Interviewers should, instead, rely on relatively neutral responses to children's answers; otherwise, the children's independent discourse abilities will be obviated. It is wise to involve children in tasks, such as art projects, to minimize their self-consciousness. Interviewers should not rush the production of discourse. (See McCabe & Rollins, 1994, for further explanation of procedures found to be effective in eliciting narrative discourse from children.) These are only a few of the ways in which interviewers must be conscientious about the procedure they use to elicit discourse; otherwise, discourse obtained will be more representative of an interviewer's skill than of a child's narrative abilities.

Aspects of the Situation

Discourse produced in an obviously test-like situation differs from that produced in freely flowing conversations. For example, children produce more coherent personal narratives at an earlier age in informal conversational contexts than when they are explicitly asked to produce a narrative (Hudson & Shapiro, 1991). Specifically, when children produce narratives in spontaneous, ongoing conversation, they more frequently use summaries or abstracts (e.g., "I remember when my brother got a sliver" [Peterson & McCabe, 1983, p. 74]) or other ways of introducing a narrative (e.g., "Do you know what? Every single tree fell down on our house" [Peterson & McCabe, 1983, p. 196]). These introductory devices are necessary in ongoing conversation to capture a listener's attention. In an experimental context, however, the experimenter is already attending to the subject (Hudson & Shapiro, 1991), so no such device is needed.

Kind of Discourse Assessed

Expository versus Narrative   Although there are many possible typologies of discourse, the most basic split seems to be between narrative and expository discourse, as was mentioned previously. (See McCabe, 1991b, for further discussion.) There are further typologies of both narrative (e.g., Preece, 1987) and nonnarrative discourse (e.g., Beals & Snow, 1994; Newkirk, 1987). Some researchers argue that narrative is a primary means of making sense of experience (e.g., Egan, 1987; Wells, 1985), yet others argue that informational, nonstory forms are just as accessible as story forms (e.g., Pappas, 1993). In studies that compare the two forms, however, elementary school–age students generally have less control of informational, expository forms than of narrative forms (e.g., Hidi & Hildyard, 1983; Langer, 1986). In contrast to this early superiority in the narrative genre, one study found that kindergartners were just as advanced in pretend, or "emergent," readings of information books as they were in pretend readings of stories (Pappas, 1993). At 14 years of age, the superiority of narrative over expository performance actually has been found to reverse, so that reports are a more elaborated genre than stories (Langer, 1986). However, if *children's* discourse is to be evaluated, some form of narrative should be included in the evaluation process. Evaluators also may want to assess other forms of discourse, such as explanations. But sole reliance on nonnarrative discourse risks underestimating children's discourse capabilities. (See Menig-Peterson & McCabe, 1978, for further discussion of this issue.)

Genres of Narrative   The majority of published work on discourse analysis actually is on the production or retelling of fictional stories, a form of discourse that children rarely engage in spontaneously (Preece, 1987) and, perhaps for that reason, a form that is less well developed in preschool children than is the narration of personal experiences (Hudson & Shapiro, 1991). Thus, this chapter centers primarily on narratives of real past personal experiences. Narratives of past personal experiences are produced spontaneously by children in all known cultures; although enormous variation in the form of personal narratives in various cultures has been documented (McCabe, 1996; Schieffelin & Eisenberg, 1984), children from all cultures sampled through 1995 have found the production of personal narratives in conversations with adults (who did not share those experiences) to be a reasonable, familiar task (McCabe, 1996).

Comprehension versus Production Issues   Issues of comprehension are not easily separated from production capabilities in discourse assessment. Many investigations and assessments of discourse ask children to retell a story to assess their oral or written expression (e.g., Semel, Wiig, & Secord, 1989); unfortunately, retelling a story can be affected by both comprehension and production factors. Abundant memory research documents that comprehension processes can both improve and distort the recall of stories. (See Bransford, 1979, for further discussion.) Using memory tasks to assess comprehension could be complicated by a child's inability to express his or her understanding and remembrance of a story because of word-finding difficulties or laryngitis, for example. Conversely, a child with echolalia could parrot a story, producing all of the main points and details, without understanding the story any more than a tape recorder could be said to understand stories it records. Most tasks purporting to assess discourse by asking children to produce a narrative in response to some fixed stimulus (e.g., a picture or previously told story) are simultaneously assessing comprehension and production.

There are, however, approaches to assessing discourse that simply focus on the production of stories and make no claims about comprehension abilities (e.g., McCabe & Rollins, 1994). What is needed, as is examined in more detail at the end of this chapter, is some means of assessing comprehension without involving production capabilities.

Aspects of Individuals Interviewed

There are numerous typical individual sources of variation in discourse. These factors must be considered carefully before attempting to diagnose difficulty.

Age   The age of the child being interviewed must be considered before anything else because there is a regular developmental progression in the form of discourse production. Documentation of this course of development is so abundant that a full review would be beyond the scope of this chapter. Key findings are that the onset of narration about personal experiences occurs somewhere between the ages of 2 and 3 years in the context of conversations with parents about past events (e.g., Eisenberg, 1985; McCabe & Peterson, 1991; Sachs, 1979). The length of children's spontaneous narratives increases between the ages of 3 and 5 years, and children come to include more elements of a good narrative on their own (e.g., Umiker-Sebeok, 1979). When children first tell longer narratives, they tend to compromise a strict linear delivery, but by 5 years of age, children almost always tell well-sequenced, chronological recapitulations of past experiences if their culture values this practice (Peterson & McCabe, 1983). At 6, children tell a complete, if simple, personal narrative (Peterson & McCabe, 1983), much like the narrative about the broken arm at the beginning of this chapter. Older children continue to develop narrative skill, clustering orientative comments at the outset of their narrative where such comments are of greatest use to listeners (Menig-Peterson & McCabe, 1978).

At 6 or 7 years of age, however, children are more canonical than either idiosyncratic adults or their younger, less-mature peers (Berman, in press); in many ways, 6-year-olds meet the basic requirements of good storytelling. Not only do they tell personal narratives that are well formed in terms of high-point analysis, but also their narratives often are judged to be complete episodes using story grammar analysis (Peterson & McCabe, 1983), which means that they include information about setting, events that precipitate some problem to be solved or goal to be achieved, motivating states of protagonist(s), attempts to solve problems or reach goals, consequences of those efforts, and reactions to those consequences. By age 9, however, 28% of children's productions are too complicated to be adequately described using this notion of a canonical complete sequence (based on Peterson & McCabe, 1983).

Although children begin to incorporate the plans and motives of real people into their personal narratives around the age of 4, they take quite a bit longer to do so when telling or retelling fictional stories (Hudson & Shapiro, 1991). In fact, fictional stories are not said to be logically and coherently causally plotted until fifth grade (Stein, 1988). Preschool fiction has been found to omit many key elements (Applebee, 1978; Botvin & Sutton-Smith, 1977; Nelson & Gruendel, 1986); younger children use fewer expressive options because they cannot conceive of the full range of possible perspectives to be encoded or fully assess the listener's viewpoint, and they do not command the full range of formal linguistic devices (Berman & Slobin, 1994). In some genres of fictional narrative production, children shift from early evaluative centering on single actions to more developed orientation to a past or future point in a hierarchically ordered narrative structure, relating parts of the narrative to the construction of the whole and revealing insights of actors' motivations with regard to the narrative in its entirety (Bamberg, 1994).

Gender Much information is available on the ways in which men and women and boys and girls comport themselves differently in discourse (e.g., McCabe & Lipscomb, 1988; Tannen, 1990). Specifically, girls respond to more narrative prompts and produce more and longer narratives than do boys (Peterson & McCabe, 1983). Their longest narratives are longer than those of boys (Peterson & McCabe, 1983). These gender differences in talkativeness are typical (Hyde & Linn, 1988). Of greater interest is that girls are more inclined to recall what was said in the past than are boys (Ely & McCabe, 1993). For the purpose of assessing discourse, then, boys may be harder to interview than girls simply because they are boys.

Culture Culture affects almost every aspect of the assessment situation, including body language, eye contact between evaluator and child, and potential stereotypes and racism on the part of both evaluator and child. As Seymour (1986) pointed out, the variety of cultural groups in the United States and the poor educational skills among so many children from various ethnic groups make it very difficult for educators always to distinguish typical language behavior from atypical language behavior. He also pointed out that the problem is exacerbated by "the fact that the educator and the child are often of different cultural backgrounds, and by the absence of normative data on minority children" (p. 54). This chapter focuses only on the impact of culture on the production and comprehension of discourse—narrative differences. However, difficulties in distinguishing narrative differences from narrative impairments abound. (See Gutierrez-Clellen & Quinn, 1993, for review.)

Production Numerous cultural differences in various aspects of discourse have been documented. With respect to children's production of narrative discourse alone, many dimensions of cultural variation have been documented (e.g., Watson, 1975). Whereas European North American children tend to tell stories about one experience at a time, African American, Japanese American, and Latino children more frequently discuss multiple experiences in one narrative. Although children of all cultures studied through 1995 refer to action (e.g., "I ripped my pants"), description ("It was wax"), and evaluation ("It was a big old hole"), cultures differ in the relative attention children pay to these basic components of personal narrative. Compared with Latino, Japanese American, and African American children, European North American children pay less attention to evaluation and more attention to action sequences in their oral personal narratives (McCabe, 1996; Minami & McCabe, 1991; Rodino, Gimbert, Perez, Craddock-Willis, & McCabe, 1991). These are only a few of the differences and a few of the cultures about which distinctive narrative form and/or practices have been documented. There are numerous other cultural groups about which very little is known of their distinctive discourse practices. Evaluators must be extremely cautious in evaluating children from cultures other than those about which there is extensive normative information available regarding discourse form in order to avoid misdiagnosing cultural differences as individual impairments.

Comprehension The manner in which individuals produce stories affects their comprehension of stories they hear. Long ago, a British psychologist, F.C. Bartlett (1932), presented a North American Indian folktale to British citizens of various ages and had them recall the tale repeatedly. Over these retellings, Bartlett noticed that his subjects omitted much information and reshaped other information—substituting words more familiar to them, leaving out some enigmatic things, and putting in other information—essentially making the tale into something closer to an English tale than to the original North American Indian one.

Bartlett's (1932) experiment has been corroborated by subsequent studies. Adult readers wrote better summaries of stories for which they had an appropriate set of expectations, or schema, than of stories from a different culture; and repeated retellings of a North American Indian story that deviated from English-speaking, Caucasian college students' own schemas resulted in poor performance (Kintsch & Greene, 1978). Foreign scripts were misremembered to be more like North American scripts by North American subjects (Harris, Lee, Hensley, & Schoen, 1988). Americans and illiterate and schooled villagers in Botswana recalled stories (themes and episodes) from their own culture better than they recalled stories from the other one (Dube, 1982). Palauan and American 11th-grade readers read culturally familiar and unfamiliar passages in their own language. Students used different, more efficient strategies when confronted by texts from their own culture than when confronted by texts from a different culture—texts that did not meet their expectations. Students also recalled significantly more ideas and elaborations and produced fewer distortions for the culturally familiar passage than for the unfamiliar passage (Pritchard, 1990). Of most relevance is that when preschool children of different ethnic backgrounds are asked to retell the same story, they do so in distinctive ways. Specifically, while the total number of phrases spoken by Puerto Rican children did not differ from that spoken by African American children, the nature of what they recalled was quite different; Puerto Rican children recalled far more description and far less action than did African American children (John & Berney, 1968). Similarly, when Ponam elementary school children were asked to retell two stories from the European tradition, they recalled more propositions from both, including substantially more factual details (e.g., settings, initiating events, attempts, outcomes) than did American children. However, they omitted many of the constituents (e.g., affect, consequence, resolution, moral) required for their recalls to meet good story grammar standards (Invernizzi & Abouzeid, 1995).

What all of these studies mean is that children, as well as adults, comprehend and remember more of stories that conform to the kind of stories they have heard at home. To ask children from non-European North American backgrounds to recall European-based stories and then to score these stories using story grammar, which is based on the analysis of Russian folktales (Propp, 1968), is to put them at a double disadvantage. Cultural differences in storytelling traditions almost certainly will be misdiagnosed as impairments of comprehension.

Socioeconomic Status   The effects of socioeconomic status on maternal speech to children have been well documented. (See Hoff-Ginsberg, 1994, for review.) Such effects, however, have been found to be associated primarily with lexical development and not necessarily with discourse skill (Hoff-Ginsberg, 1994). In fact, the socioeconomic effects that have been documented and interpreted as discourse-level effects essentially pertain to word specificity. Specifically, low-income individuals of all ages frequently are said to use more unspecified pronouns (see Hemphill, 1989). This may be due, in part, to an overall socialization to the importance of collaborative meaning construction—of being able to count on others to contribute both actively (i.e., via insertions) or passively (i.e., figuring out what unspecified pronouns mean) to discourse. Emphasizing that listeners fill in what is left unsaid by speakers contrasts to a middle-class focus on individual, relatively explicit monologues delivered to silent and passive audiences (Hemphill, 1989). Perhaps also associated with lower-class, tacit collaboration is less facility in the use of specific referent words.

Family Issues Children echo their parents in the kinds of information they include in their narratives. If parents talk at length with 2-year-olds about past experiences, then their children will narrate at length on their own to other adults a year and a half or several years later (McCabe & Peterson, 1990, 1991). There also are more specific echoes. If parents habitually ask their children questions about the context of experiences (e.g., who, what, when, where), then their children later spontaneously provide more such orientation than do children whose parents ask few such questions (Fivush, 1991; Peterson & McCabe, 1992, 1994). If parents emphasize the sequence of actions that occurred during past experiences, then children later emphasize actions (Peterson & McCabe, 1992). If parents repeatedly ask their children about *why* things happened the way they did or talk about causality themselves, then children subsequently provide more causal information than do children whose parents do not pay much attention to causality in past experiences (Fivush, 1991; McCabe & Peterson, in press). Finally, parents who focus on past conversations (as opposed to actions) have children who do the same (Ely, Gleason, & McCabe, 1996). For the purposes of assessing discourse difficulty, then, evaluators must keep in mind that difficulties may lie in the input children have received rather than in their inherent cognitive limitations.

APPROACHES TO ASSESSMENT

Formal Assessments

Few formal assessments of language competence address the issue of assessing difficulties in discourse production. None of the formal assessments that make such an effort attempts to do so for children younger than 5 years of age. For older children, a few formal language tests ask children to make up a story about a picture or pictures (e.g., Detroit Test of Learning Aptitude–III [Hammill, 1991]; Reynell Developmental Language Scales [Reynell, 1985]; Test of Word-Finding in Discourse [German & Simon, 1991]) or to retell a fictional story orally (Test of Adolescent Language–2 [Hammill, Brown, Larsen, & Wiederholt, 1987]; Preschool Language Scale–3 [Zimmerman, Steiner, & Pond, 1992]) or in written form (Clinical Evaluation of Language Fundamentals–Revised [Semel et al., 1989]). These tests assess difficulties in word finding (German & Simon, 1991); sequencing (e.g., Hammill et al., 1987; Semel et al., 1989); presenting a story with a clear beginning, middle, and end (Hammill et al., 1987; Semel et al., 1989); and representing a clear and resolved problem-solving episode (i.e., producing a good structure by story grammar standards [Hammill et al., 1987; Semel et al., 1989]). In view of the aforementioned considerations posed by cultural differences in storytelling traditions and forms, however, the usefulness of tests for these features of storytelling for children from backgrounds other than European North American would seem limited, with considerable potential for misdiagnosing difference as impairment. In short, all formal assessments reviewed operate using a European-based definition of what makes a good story.

Research-Based Informal Assessments

Informal clinical assessments of narrative skill have been offered by various research paradigms. Researchers, like test makers, usually have used fictional stories to assess the narrative skills of young children. Researchers often have scored children's productions or retellings for the extent to which these display story grammar structure; that is, children were evaluated on the basis of the extent to which their stories began with information about the setting of the story and proceeded to tell how some problem was encountered and subsequently resolved. Surprisingly, much research has established that school-age children with learning disabilities do not have problems with story grammar structure per se (Graybeal, 1981; Griffith et al., 1986; Johnston, 1982; Jordan, Murdoch, & Buttsworth, 1991; McConaughy, 1985; Merritt & Liles, 1989; Ripich & Griffith, 1988; Roth & Spekman, 1986; Weaver & Dickinson, 1982); that is, children with dyslexia, specific language impairment (SLI), and brain injury seem quite capable of reporting problem-solving episodes.

Some researchers (e.g., Jordan et al., 1991) have attributed their failure to find differences in the story grammar analysis of narrative production by children with language impairment and with typical development to mean that narrative is not impaired in the former. Such a conclusion is not warranted for several reasons. First, those findings simply could be interpreted as showing that story grammar analysis was insensitive to the difficulties of the various challenged populations. Second, as was mentioned previously, children seldom spontaneously make up oral fictional stories for adults, nor do they often retell fictional stories in everyday life (Preece, 1987), so perhaps the performance of typical children was considerably constrained.

Compared with stories composed by children themselves, story retelling in response to a picture results in longer, more detailed productions that more frequently contain complete story grammar episodes (Liles, Coelho, Duffy, & Zalagens, 1989; Merritt & Liles, 1989). However, children both with and without language impairment often become confused and exhibit word-finding difficulties as they generate a story around a picture stimulus, so that reliable scoring is difficult. It is not surprising that many studies that found no differences between typically achieving children and children diagnosed as having SLI or learning disabilities used story retelling as a means of eliciting narratives (e.g., Graybeal, 1981; Griffith et al., 1986; Hansen, 1978; McConaughy, 1985; Ripich & Griffith, 1988; Strong & Shaver, 1991; Weaver & Dickinson, 1982). Neither group had much practice on such tasks, and so neither was superior. But it is quite problem-

atic that available formal means of assessing narrative skill ask children to generate stories in response to pictures or to retell stories rather than ask them to
produce the kind of discourse forms with which they have extensive experience.
A few studies have taken somewhat different approaches either to scoring (Liles,
1985) or to scoring and collecting genres of discourse (Hemphill et al., 1994)
and have documented problematic cohesion (e.g., Liles, 1985) and shorter, less
task-focused talk, with less fully differentiated use of such genre features as
openings and tense by children who show atypical language development
(Hemphill et al., 1994).

A New Approach

Mindful of all the factors previously detailed, McCabe and her colleagues have
begun to investigate assessment for identifying and intervening with impairments in oral narrative production. One of their goals is to find methods that are
applicable for preschool children, for whom early intervention would be desirable. Another goal is to provide methodology that will be appropriate for children from non-European cultural backgrounds.

*High-Point Analysis: Assessment for Identifying Discourse Pro-
duction Impairments* McCabe and Rollins (1994) proposed a method of
collecting and analyzing oral narratives produced in conversation that would
serve as a first step toward identifying discourse-level difficulties in children age
3½–9 years. They provided information concerning preschool narrative development in typically developing, European North American, English-speaking children that was based on previous work McCabe had done with Peterson (McCabe
& Peterson, 1991; Peterson & McCabe, 1983). Peterson and McCabe analyzed
personal narratives of young children using several forms of narrative analysis to
describe the developmental sequence of narrative macrostructure. Using what
they have termed *high-point analysis,* McCabe and Peterson found the developmental sequence summarized in Table 1. At 3½ years, children tend to combine

Table 1. Results from McCabe and Peterson's high-point analysis for European North
American, English-speaking children[a]: The percentage of structural types at each age

Age (years)	Two-event	Leap frog	End at a high point	Classic	Chrono-logical[c]	Misc.[c]
3½	63.3[b]	10	3	3	20	
4	15	29[b]	2	12	23	18
5	10	4	29[b]	21	25	10
6	10	6	23	35[b]	15	10
7	2	0	17	48[b]	25	8
8	0	0	17	62[b]	21	0
9	6	0	17	58[b]	13	6

Adapted from McCabe and Peterson (in press) and Peterson and McCabe (1983).

[a] Ten children were assessed at age 3½ (McCabe & Peterson, 1991), and 16 children were assessed at
each of the other age groups (Peterson & McCabe, 1983).

[b] Most common structure produced by children at each age.

[c] Narrative type found at all ages.

only two events even in their longest narratives, a form that McCabe and Peterson have termed a *two-event narrative,* as in the following example:

N: I go to Janie's school
and da man had a white rabbit.

By age 4, children's narratives tend to consist of more than two events, but 4-year-olds often narrate events out of sequence in what McCabe and Peterson have termed a *leap-frog narrative.* Leap-frog narratives often omit some events necessary for the listener to fully understand some experience, as in the following narrative by a 4-year-old girl[1]:

E: When I go home I have to visit my aunt who's in the hospital. She broke both of her legs. And she has to have them kind of hung up, suspended from the ceiling with those little wires.
B: She had to have cast on.
E: That's right.
B: My sister had, she's had. She broke a arm when she fell in those mini-bike.
E: Tell me about what happened.
B: She broke her arm. She had, she went to the doctor, so I, my dad gave me spanking, and I
E: Your dad gave you what?
B: A spanking to me.
E: A spanking?
B: Yeah. And she had to go to the doctor to get a cast on. She had to go get it, get it off and, and it didn't break again.
E: And then it didn't break again?
B: No. She still got it off. She can't play anymore.
E: She can't play anymore?
B: She can't play we, she can play rest of us now... Mm, she has cast on. When she was home. When she came back and she, and she, and she hadda go back and, take off the cast.
E: She had to go back and take off the cast?
B: Yeah. The doctor.

By age 5, children rarely have trouble sequencing events in oral narratives. Five-year-olds do, however, tend to end their narratives prematurely, dwelling on a climactic event at the end of their narration in what is called an *end-at-a-high-point narrative:*

E: Did you ever go to the doctor's office?
D: Uh-uh. No, yes, over Dr. Graham's house, night.
E: You went there? What happened?

---

[1] E = experimenter; taken from Peterson and McCabe (1983).

D: Nothing. Just I sticked around and he told me to come in first and then he, and, that's all I had to do. And taked me out, out, and and he put me in the doctor office. And I had a cold.

E: You did?

D: Last night.

E: Right.

D: And I, I was scared to come in. And he didn't shot me or nothing.

E: He didn't shot you or anything?

D: Uh-uh. He didn't even shot me.

E: He didn't shot you?

D: He gave me them, them tiny pills too, just like you. That's only reason I had.

Six-year-olds tell well-formed narratives that orient a listener to who, what, and where something happened; reiterate a sequence of events that builds to some sort of climax or high point; and then go on to resolve themselves by telling how things turned out. That is, children age 6 and older often tell what is called a *classic narrative,* as in the broken-arm narrative at the outset of this chapter. The child begins with an abstract ("I broke my arm") that summarizes the story to follow. He then orients the listener about when the accident occurred and the activity that he was doing at the time (e.g., "climbing the tree"). He builds up to a high point—clearly marked by the evaluative phrase: "Then they bent like in two triangles. But luckily it was my *left* arm that broke." The child subsequently resolves the narrative by detailing what happened afterward—how he got help and what happened at the hospital. He brings the conversation out of narration of past events into the present by concluding with a coda: "Do you want to sign my cast?"

Although there is a developmental sequence of narrative macrostructure from two past events to leap-frog to end-at-a-high-point to classic narrative structure, not all personal-event narratives fall along this developmental continuum, as is also shown in Table 1. On the contrary, chronological narratives are produced by children and adults of all ages.

In the clinical adaptation of the method that Peterson and McCabe used (McCabe & Rollins, 1994), clinicians were asked to elicit personal narratives from children, transcribe these narratives, and answer a series of questions (e.g., "Are there two past-tense events?" "Is there a high point?") to arrive at a global scoring of the child's longest, most complex personal narrative. They could then compare specific productions to age-norms (see Table 1) to determine whether children's discourse was typical or atypical compared with the discourse of their peers.

Dependency Analysis: Assessment for Intervention with Discourse Production Impairments   Once clinicians have assessed the existence of true discourse-level disability, they must pinpoint which of the many aspects of connected discourse is problematic for a particular child or children with particular kinds of narrative impairments. McCabe and other colleagues have completed a series of pilot studies that compare typical with atypical narrative production. The purpose of the first such study (Bliss, Miranda, & McCabe, 1994; Miranda, 1993) was to delineate more precisely qualitative and quantitative differences between narrative abilities of children diagnosed with SLI on the word and syntax levels and typically achieving comparison children. Ten English-speaking, European North American boys in each group were interviewed about real past experiences, using a conversational elicitation technique (Peterson & McCabe, 1983). A total of 94 discourses (47 discourses from each group, in which each discourse consisted of related narratives) were transcribed and analyzed reliably using dependency analysis (Deese, 1984; Peterson & McCabe, 1983), an approach that compares the child's staged order of propositions with a chronological one and, in this process, articulates propositions that are implied rather than explicit. A number of comparisons were made, the most important of which were that 1) discourses of children with SLI left proportionately more information implicit, requiring listeners to fill this in for themselves; and 2) the average correlation between staged and chronological order of propositions was .88 for children with SLI versus .96 for typically achieving children, which was a statistically significant difference. In addition, children with SLI engaged in a kind of pseudodevelopment of their narratives, shifting to general scripts of their day or their capabilities rather than providing information about some specific event that occurred in the past. Surprisingly, children with SLI told as many events as did their typical peers, and a possible sequence could be constructed from the events they did narrate. However, children with SLI did not tell the kind of autonomous narrative (i.e., one that makes few demands on listeners or readers) that would lead to a favorable prognosis for their development of full literacy. The following narrative by a 9-year-old boy diagnosed with SLI would be classified as the kind of leap-frog form of typically achieving 4-year-olds; it exemplifies the findings described previously:

E: Last week, I had a sore throat. I went to the doctor and I had to get a shot. Have you ever gotten a shot at the doctor's?

J: Yeah.

E: Tell me about it.

J: I was losing my voice, I was having asthma attack real bad. So, my friend go it and he got to me while I was coughing in the middle of the night, and he got a shot right on my leg and I had to take my tonsils out, I didn't like it. And....

E: You had to get your tonsils out?

J: That's what the doctor said.

E: And then what happened?

J: I went into the hospital for a week. And...because a I had a real bad asthma thing, and they just put me in the hospital for a week. And and I and I broke my knee.

E: You broke your knee?

J: Yeah. While I was ridin' my bike, I was jumpin on a curb and and I was
     it was I was slidin' through the air, and it looks like I broke my knee. I
     couldn't move nothin'.

E: What happened?

J: My mom took me to the hospital and said um, said uh…the doctor said we
     he might be, we might be, we're going to…he has to do, can't ride his bike
     in the street, I can't ride my bike in the street anymore. Cause uh I get hurt.
     My friend David had a car accident.

E: He did?

J: Yeah, and he um he's in the hospital right now be…and (pause) he stopped
     and said I forgot. He said uh, they said uh, he can't he couldn't he can't, they
     put a metal thing on his head. He will not talk. He's deaf now.

E: He's deaf?

J: Uh-uh. And they, they're gonna take it off soon. So they did, not he can talk
     now. And doin' O.K. now, they took it off already. Uh…my friend, my
     mom's friend works in a hospital and in somewhere in Roseville. I forgot
     what's her name (pause). That's all I can think of.

The second such study (Biddle, 1994; Biddle, McCabe, & Bliss, in press)
described a similar fine-grained dependency analysis that differentiated the discourse difficulties experienced by children and adults who have traumatic brain
injuries (TBI) compared with peers who do not have injuries. Children and
adults with TBI were significantly more dysfluent than were matched controls
and left unstated many propositions necessary for the adequate comprehension
of their narrative. In addition, individuals with TBI were significantly more repe-
titious than were their peers. The following narrative from a 7-year-old girl with
TBI exemplifies characteristic repetitiousness and a lack of specific elaboration.
For example, listeners are left to guess whether the two stings happened on the
same occasion, and they were not informed about exactly when either happened,
quite a contrast to the broken-arm narrative by a younger boy at the outset of this
chapter ("It was…2 days ago"):

F: I got stung on the same place twice. One time I was running home because I
     was playing with my neighbor. Her name is Helen. I was in my bare feet.
     And I got my foot stung. The next time, I got my toe stung. We had like
     cement steps that were going up to where we park. There was a beehive. I
     was stepping on a step. And it stung me again.

Such studies establish the existence of true discourse-level difficulties in
these special populations. The analyses themselves also function as a guide to
the kind of interventions to implement with atypical children in general and any
one child in particular. For example, both groups need clinical focus on becoming more explicit in their discourse. Ordering propositions appears quite difficult
for children with SLI, whereas repetitiousness is a key issue for individuals with

TBI. Within each group was substantial individual variation, so these assorted aspects of discourse would be of varying salience for any particular atypically developing child.

Needs in Assessing Discourse

Much work remains to be done to provide normative discourse production data on children of all ages from various cultures and ethnicities in the United States and in other countries. Specific information is needed on how children with identifiable special needs (e.g., mental retardation) at all of these ages and from all of these backgrounds compare with their typically achieving peers. Methodologies for collecting and scoring production, however, are at least in place.

Also needed is a well-conceived means of assessing children's comprehension of discourse apart from any of their productive capacities—something analogous to the Peabody Picture Vocabulary Test for use with discourse comprehension. Children's ability to follow various commands (a common component of many assessment batteries) is not necessarily indicative of their ability to comprehend much longer segments of logically connected discourse. There are available means of determining a child's ability to answer a few "what," "where," and "why" questions about short, artificial passages that they hear or read (Semel, Wiig, & Secord, 1987). However, children still need to *produce* answers as long as phrases or even sentences and include diverse vocabulary items, so word-finding problems might very well impair their ability to show discourse-level comprehension. Moreover, the passages do not include material that is non-European in form; in view of the fact that there is much documentation of cultural differences in comprehension (reviewed previously), this would seem problematic.

CONCLUSION

Although it is difficult to accurately diagnose discourse-level difficulties, it is essential to do so. Discourse difficulties impair the smooth acquisition of literacy and conduct of human relationships. Efforts to assess the production of narrative discourse exist, and some progress has been made in this arena; however, much work remains to be done. Efforts to assess the comprehension of discourse are even more scant and problematic. Researchers must see these gaps as opportunities.

REFERENCES

Applebee, A.N. (1978). *The child's concept of story.* Chicago: University of Chicago Press.

Bamberg, M. (1994). Development of linguistic forms: German. In R.A. Berman & D.I. Slobin (Eds.), *Relating events in narrative: A crosslinguistic developmental study* (pp. 189–238). Hillsdale, NJ: Lawrence Erlbaum Associates.

Bartlett, F.C. (1932). *Remembering*. Cambridge, England: Cambridge University Press.

Beals, D.E., & Snow, C.E. (1994). "Thunder is when the angels are upstairs bowling": Narratives and explanations at the dinner table. *Journal of Narrative and Life History*, 4(4), 331–352.

Berman, R. (in press). Narrative competence and storytelling performance: How children tell stories from different perspectives and in different contexts. *Journal of Narrative and Life History*, 5(4).

Berman, R.A., & Slobin, D.I. (1994). Introduction. In R.A. Berman & D.I. Slobin (Eds.), *Relating events in narrative: A crosslinguistic developmental study* (pp. 1–35). Hillsdale, NJ: Lawrence Erlbaum Associates.

Biddle, K.R. (1994). *Narrative skills following traumatic brain injury in children and adults*. Unpublished qualifying paper, Tufts University, Medford, MA.

Biddle, K.R., McCabe, A., & Bliss, L.S. (in press). Narrative skills following traumatic brain injury in children and adults. *Journal of Communication Disorders*.

Bishop, D.V.M., & Edmundson, A. (1987). Language-impaired 4-year-olds: Distinguishing transient from persistent impairment. *Journal of Speech and Hearing Disorders*, 52, 156–173.

Bliss, L.S., McCabe, A., & Miranda, E. (1994, November). *Jumping around and leaving things out: A comparison of narrative skills in specific language impaired and normally achieving boys*. Miniseminar presented at the Annual Convention of the American Speech-Language-Hearing Association, New Orleans.

Botvin, G.N., & Sutton-Smith, B. (1977). The development of structural complexity in children's fantasy narratives. *Developmental Psychology*, 1, 377–388.

Bransford, J.D. (1979). *Human cognition: Learning, understanding, and remembering*. Belmont, CA: Wadsworth.

Bruner, J. (1986). *Actual minds, possible worlds*. Cambridge, MA: Harvard University Press.

Deese, J. (1984). *Thought into speech: The psychology of a language*. Englewood Cliffs, NJ: Prentice Hall.

De Hirsch, K., Jansky, J.J., & Langford, W.S. (1966). *Predicting reading failure*. New York: Harper and Row.

Dickinson, D.K., & McCabe, A. (1991). A social interactionist account of language and literacy development. In J. Kavanaugh (Ed.), *The language continuums* (pp. 1–40). Parkton, MD: York Press.

Dickinson, D.K., & Snow, C.E. (1987). Interrelationships among prereading and oral language skills in kindergartners from two social classes. *Early Childhood Research Quarterly*, 2, 1–25.

Dube, E.F. (1982). Literacy, cultural familiarity, and "intelligence" as determinants of story recall. In U. Neisser (Ed.), *Memory observed* (pp. 274–292). San Francisco: Freeman & Co.

Egan, K. (1987). Literacy and the oral foundation of education. *Harvard Educational Review*, 57, 445–472.

Eisenberg, A.R. (1985). Learning to describe past experiences in conversation. *Discourse Processes*, 8, 177–204.

Ely, R., Gleason, J.B., & McCabe, A. (1996). "Why didn't you talk to your mommy, honey?" Parents' and children's talk about talk. *Research on Language and Social Interaction*, 29(1), 7–26.

Ely, R., & McCabe, A. (1993). Remembered voices. *Journal of Child Language*, 20(3), 671–696.

Feagans, L. (1982). The development and importance of narratives for school adaptation. In L. Feagans & D. Farran (Eds.), *The language of children reared in poverty* (pp. 95–116). New York: Academic Press.

Feagans, L., & Short, E.J. (1984). Developmental differences in the comprehension and production of narratives by reading disabled and normally achieving children. *Child Development, 55,* 1727–1736.

Feagans, L., & Short, E.J. (1986). Referential communication and reading performance in learning disabled children over a three-year period. *Developmental Psychology, 22,* 177–283.

Fivush, R. (1991). The social construction of personal narratives. *Merrill-Palmer Quarterly, 37*(1), 59–81.

German, D.J., & Simon, E. (1991). Analysis of children's word-finding skills in discourse. *Journal of Speech and Hearing Research, 34,* 309–316.

Goodman, G.S., Bottoms, B.L., Schwartz-Kenney, B.M., & Rudy, L. (1991). Children's testimony about a stressful event: Improving children's reports. *Journal of Narrative and Life History, 1*(1), 69–99.

Graybeal, C.M. (1981). Memory for stories in language-impaired children. *Applied Psycholinguistics, 2,* 269–283.

Griffith, P.L., Ripich, D.N., & Dastoli, S.L. (1986). Story structure, cohesion, and propositions in story recalls by learning disabled and non-disabled children. *Journal of Psycholinguistic Research, 15*(6), 539–549.

Gutierrez-Clellen, V.F., & Quinn, R. (1993). Assessing narratives of children from diverse cultural/linguistic groups. *Language, Speech, and Hearing Services in Schools, 24,* 2–9.

Hammill, D.D. (1991). *Detroit Test of Learning Aptitude–III.* Austin, TX: PRO-ED.

Hammill, D.D., Brown, V.L., Larsen, S.C., & Wiederholt, J.L. (1987). *Test of Adolescent Language (TOAL–2).* Austin, TX: PRO-ED.

Hansen, C.L. (1978). Story retelling used with average and learning disabled readers as a measure of reading comprehension. *Learning Disability Quarterly, 1,* 62–69.

Harris, R.J., Lee, D.J., Hensley, D.L., & Schoen, L.M. (1988). The effect of cultural script knowledge on memory for stories over time. *Discourse Processes, 11,* 413–431.

Hemphill, L. (1989). Topic development, syntax, and social class. *Discourse Processes, 12*(3), 267–286.

Hemphill, L., Feldman, H.M., Camp, L., Griffin, T.M., Miranda, A.B., & Wolf, D.P. (1994). Developmental changes in narrative and non-narrative discourse in children with and without brain injury. *Journal of Communication Disorders, 27,* 107–133.

Hemphill, L., & Siperstein, G. (1990). Conversational competence and peer response to mildly retarded children. *Journal of Educational Psychology, 82,* 128–134.

Hidi, S.E., & Hildyard, A. (1983). The comparison of oral and written productions in two discourse types. *Discourse Processes, 6,* 91–105.

Hoff-Ginsberg, E. (1994, April). *Home language development and oral language development: The effects of socioeconomic status and birth order.* Paper presented at the American Educational Research Association meetings as part of a strand of sessions on "Predicting literacy outcomes for low-income children: A world wide perspective, Part 1—Effects of home interventions on literacy and language development," New Orleans.

Hudson, J.A., & Shapiro, L.A. (1991). From knowing to telling: The development of children's scripts, stories, and personal narratives. In C. Peterson & A. McCabe (Eds.), *Developing narrative structure* (pp. 89–136). Hillsdale, NJ: Lawrence Erlbaum Associates.

Hyde, J., & Linn, M.C. (1988). Gender differences in verbal ability: A meta-analysis. *Psychological Bulletin, 104,* 53–69.

Invernizzi, M.A., & Abouzeid, M.P. (1995). One story map does not fit all: A cross-cultural analysis of children's written story retellings. *Journal of Narrative and Life History, 5*(1), 1–20.

John, V.P., & Berney, J.D. (1968). Analysis of story retelling as a measure of the effects of ethnic content in stories. In J. Helmuth (Ed.), *The disadvantaged child: Head Start and early intervention* (Vol. 2, pp. 259–287). New York: Brunner/Mazel.

Johnston, J.R. (1982). Narratives: A new look at communication problems in older language-disordered children. *Language, Speech, and Hearing Services in Schools, 13,* 144–155.

Jordan, F.M., Murdoch, B.E., & Buttsworth, D.L. (1991). Closed-head-injured children's performance on narrative tasks. *Journal of Speech and Hearing Research, 34,* 572–582.

Kintsch, W., & Greene, E. (1978). The role of culture-specific schemata in the comprehension and recall of stories. *Discourse Processes, 1,* 1–13.

Labov, W. (1972). *Language in the inner city.* Philadelphia: University of Pennsylvania Press.

Langer, J. (1986). *Children reading and writing: Structures and strategies.* Norwood, NJ: Ablex.

Levi, G., Musatti, L., Piredda, L., & Sechi, E. (1984). Cognitive and linguistic strategies in children with reading disabilities in an oral storytelling test. *Journal of Learning Disabilities, 17*(7), 406–410.

Liles, B.Z. (1985). Cohesion in the narratives of normal and language-disordered children. *Journal of Speech and Hearing Research, 28,* 123–133.

Liles, B.Z., Coelho, C.A., Duffy, R.J., & Zalagens, M.R. (1989). Effects of elicitation procedures on the narratives of normal and closed head-injured adults. *Journal of Speech and Hearing Disorders, 54,* 356–366.

McCabe, A. (1991a). Editorial. *Journal of Narrative and Life History, 1*(1), 1–2.

McCabe, A. (1991b). Narrative structure as a way of understanding narratives. In A. McCabe & C. Peterson (Eds.), *Developing narrative structure* (pp. i–xi). Hillsdale, NJ: Lawrence Erlbaum Associates.

McCabe, A. (1996). *Chameleon readers: Teaching children to appreciate all kinds of good stories.* New York: McGraw-Hill.

McCabe, A., & Lipscomb, T. (1988). The development of sex differences in verbal aggression. *Merrill-Palmer Quarterly, 34*(4), 389–401.

McCabe, A., & Peterson, C. (1990, July). *Keep them talking: Parental styles of interviewing and subsequent child narrative skill.* Paper presented at the Fifth International Congress for the Study of Child Language, Budapest, Hungary.

McCabe, A., & Peterson, C. (1991). Getting the story: A longitudinal study of parental styles in eliciting oral personal narratives and developing narrative skill. In A. McCabe & C. Peterson (Eds.), *Developing narrative structure* (pp. 217–253). Hillsdale, NJ: Lawrence Erlbaum Associates.

McCabe, A., & Peterson, C. (in press). "Why did he push you?": Parental scaffolding of causal language about the past. In J. Costermans & M. Fayol (Eds.), *Processing interclausal relationships in the production and comprehension of text.* Hillsdale, NJ: Lawrence Erlbaum Associates.

McCabe, A., & Rollins, P.R. (1994). Assessment of preschool narrative skills: Prerequisite for literacy. *American Journal of Speech-Language Pathology: A Journal of Clinical Practice, 4,* 45–56.

McConaughy, S.H. (1985). Good and poor readers' comprehension of story structure across different input and output modalities. *Reading Research Quarterly, XX*(2), 219–232.

Menig-Peterson, C. (1975). The modification of communicative behavior in preschool-aged children as a function of the listener's perspective. *Child Development, 46,* 1015–1018.

Menig-Peterson, C., & McCabe, A. (1978). Children's orientation of a listener to the context of their narratives. *Developmental Psychology, 74,* 582–592.

Merritt, D.D., & Liles, B.Z. (1989). Narrative analysis: Clinical applications of story generation and story retelling. *Journal of Speech and Hearing Disorders, 54,* 429–438.

Michaels, S. (1981). "Sharing time": Children's narrative styles and differential access to literacy. *Language in Society, 10,* 423–442.

Minami, M., & McCabe, A. (1991). *Haiku* as a discourse regulation device: A stanza analysis of Japanese children's personal narratives. *Language in Society, 20*(4), 577–599.

Miranda, E. (1993). *Dependency analysis of narrative discourse in language-impaired and nonimpaired children.* Unpublished qualifying paper, Harvard University, Cambridge, MA.

Mishler, E. (1986). *Research interviewing: Context and narrative.* Cambridge, MA: Harvard University Press.

Nelson, K., & Gruendel, J.M. (1986). Children's scripts. In K. Nelson (Ed.), *Event knowledge: Structure and function in development* (pp. 21–46). Hillsdale, NJ: Lawrence Erlbaum Associates.

Newkirk, T. (1987). The non-narrative writing of young children. *Research in the Teaching of English, 21*(2), 121–143.

Pappas, C.C. (1993). Is narrative "primary"? Some insights from kindergarteners' pretend readings of stories and information books. *Journal of Reading Behavior, 25*(1), 97–129.

Peterson, C., & McCabe, A. (1983). *Developmental psycholinguistics: Three ways of looking at a child's narrative.* New York: Plenum.

Peterson, C., & McCabe, A. (1992). Style differences in eliciting personal experience narratives: Are they related to differences in how children structure narratives? *First Language, 12,* 299–321.

Peterson, C., & McCabe, A. (1994). A social interactionist account of developing narrative orientation. *Developmental Psychology, 30*(6), 937–948.

Preece, A. (1987). The range of narrative forms conversationally produced by young children. *Journal of Child Language, 14,* 353–373.

Pritchard, R. (1990). The effects of cultural schemata on reading processing strategies. *Reading Research Quarterly, 25*(4), 273–295.

Propp, V. (1968/1928). *Morphology of the folktale.* Austin: University of Texas Press.

Reynell, J. (1985). *Reynell Developmental Language Scales.* Los Angeles: Webster Psychological Services.

Rice, M. (1991). Social interactions of speech- and language-impaired children. *Journal of Speech and Hearing Research, 34*(6), 1299–1307.

Ripich, D.N., & Griffith, P.L. (1988). Narrative abilities of children with learning disabilities and nondisabled children: Story structure, cohesion, and propositions. *Journal of Learning Disabilities, 21*(3), 165–173.

Rodino, A.M., Gimbert, C., Perez, C., Craddock-Willis, K., & McCabe, A. (1991, October). *"Getting your point across": Contrastive sequencing in low-income African-American and Latino children's personal narratives.* Paper presented at the 16th Annual Boston University Conference on Language Development, Boston.

Roth, F.P., & Spekman, N.J. (1986). Narrative discourse: Spontaneously generated stories of learning-disabled and normally achieving students. *Journal of Speech and Hearing Disorder, 51,* 8–23.

Sachs, J. (1979). Topic selection in parent–child discourse. *Discourse Processes, 2,* 145–153.

Scarborough, H.S., & Dobrich, W. (1990). Development of children with early language delay. *Journal of Speech and Hearing Research, 33,* 70–83.

Schieffelin, B.B., & Eisenberg, A.R. (1984). Cultural variation in children's conversations. In R.L. Schiefelbusch & J. Pickar (Eds.), *The acquisition of communicative competence* (pp. 378–420). Baltimore: University Park Press.

Semel, E., Wiig, E.H., & Secord, W. (1987). *Clinical Evaluation of Language Fundamentals–Revised.* San Antonio, TX: The Psychological Corporation.

Semel, E., Wiig, E.H., & Secord, W. (1989). *Clinical Evaluation of Language Fundamentals–Revised Screening Test.* San Antonio, TX: The Psychological Corporation.

Seymour, H.R. (1986). Alternative strategies for the teaching of language to minority individuals. In *Concerns for minority groups in communication disorders (ASHA Reports #16,* pp. 52–57). Rockville, MD: American Speech-Language-Hearing Association.

Stein, N. (1988). The development of children's storytelling skill. In M.B. Franklin & S. Barten (Eds.), *Child language: A book of readings* (pp. 282–297). New York: Oxford University Press.

Strong, C.J., & Shaver, J.P. (1991). Stability of cohesion in the spoken narratives of language-impaired and normally developing school-aged children. *Journal of Speech and Hearing Research, 34,* 95–111.

Tannen, D. (1990). *You just don't understand.* New York: Ballantine Books.

Umiker-Sebeok, D.J. (1979). Preschool children's intraconversational narratives. *Journal of Child Language, 6,* 91–109.

Watson, K.A. (1975). Transferable communicative routines: Strategies in group identity in two speech events. *Language in Society, 4,* 53–72.

Weaver, P.A., & Dickinson, D.K. (1982). Scratching below the surface structure: Exploring the usefulness of story grammars. *Discourse Processes, 5,* 225–243.

Wells, G. (1985). Preschool literacy-related activities and success in school. In D. Olson, N. Torrance, & A. Hildyard (Eds.), *Literacy, language and learning* (pp. 229–256). New York: Cambridge University Press.

Zimmerman, I., Steiner, V., & Pond, R. (1992). *Preschool Language Scale–3 (PLS-3).* San Antonio, TX: The Psychological Corporation.

7

Cognitive Referencing in Language Assessment

Kevin N. Cole and Marc E. Fey

T HE CONCEPT OF LANGUAGE IMPAIRMENT seems, on the surface, to be fairly straightforward. It might be assumed, for example, that children can be judged to have speech and/or language impairment when they are exhibiting or are at risk for problems in educational, social, or cognitive development or in psychosocial adjustment because of difficulty understanding or using sounds, words, sentences, or other units of language. Children who fit this characterization would be considered appropriate candidates for the services of a speech-language pathologist (SLP).

In practice, identifying children as having language impairment is anything but simple or straightforward. Descriptions of three hypothetical children illustrate the problem that is the topic of this chapter. Three children, Newt, Jesse, and Bill, were born on the same day and have very similar family makeup, comparable and uneventful medical histories, the same school experience, and no significant emotional or behavior problems. Newt and Jesse exhibit receptive and expressive morphosyntactic and lexical semantic (i.e., vocabulary) scores 2 standard deviations below the mean for their age on norm-referenced tests. These scores and the problems they represent for these children at home and in the classroom are confirmed by parent report and clinical observation.

In contrast, Bill's scores on the standardized tests were well within the typical range. His teacher, however, has complained that Bill is forever chattering in class and that he often makes little sense. He is particularly interested in his electronic games at home and is reluctant to talk about anything else, even when the class is reviewing a science assignment or a story they have just read. Consequently, Bill's classmates view him as "weird," and he has not developed any real friends at school.

Based on the information available on these children, an SLP made the following decisions: Newt was judged to have language impairment and to be an appropriate candidate for language intervention. Jesse and Bill, however, were not considered to have language impairments and, consequently, were not viewed as appropriate candidates for language intervention.

How can these children, each of whom has demonstrated difficulties in communication with language that is affecting performance in school, be evaluated so differently? One possibility is that this clinician's decision was based on a procedure called *cognitive referencing*. Using a model of cognitive referencing, a developmental language impairment can be identified only after considering the child's nonverbal cognitive abilities. There are two versions of the model. The first, which most often is seen in research on language impairments, requires performance IQ to be within the average range, regardless of the severity of the language delay when compared with the child's chronological age. The average range usually is interpreted as a standard score on a nonverbal performance scale of 85 or greater, although many investigators and clinicians extend this criterion to a low of 80 (Aram, Morris, & Hall, 1992; Tomblin & Buckwalter, 1994). The second version of the model is more common in eligibility criteria for speech-language services. This model, which typically is applied after the first, requires language abilities to be significantly lower than other nonverbal cognitive abilities, usually by some predetermined amount, such as 1 or 2 standard deviation units (see Aram et al., 1992), or an age interval, such as 1 year (Stark & Tallal, 1981). The basic assumption underlying either model of cognitive referencing is that the language impairments exhibited by children with no intelligence–language discrepancy and/or with below-average intelligence are etiologically, symptomatically, and/or neurologically different from those of children who have average intelligence and language scores that are lower than expected based on nonverbal intelligence. If this assumption is true, then children with lower intelligence might have different prognoses and/or would require different intervention programs than would children who have average intelligence and who exhibit an intelligence–language discrepancy.

The preceding hypothetical example illustrates the impact that cognitive referencing can have on clinical decision making. Newt received a score of 92 on an IQ test, which is consistent with his adaptive behavior. Thus, when referenced to his measured cognitive abilities, Newt's language still appears to be markedly impaired. In contrast, Jesse scored 73 on the IQ test. Jesse's language is consistent with expectations based on IQ test performance; thus, using the cognitive referencing model, he would not be judged to have a language-learning problem that would qualify him for speech-language services, even though his language ability is significantly delayed for a child his age.

Bill's situation is slightly different. His language test scores were well within the typical range. Thus, there is no discrepancy between his language as evaluated on these tests and his average IQ of 105. In this case, the clinician recognized that his problems with language involved the context and use of language rather than its form. Because the standardized language tests administered were insensitive to this type of semantic pragmatic impairment, however, the clinician was left with no standard scores that could be used to document a discrepancy between Bill's language and his cognitive performance. Therefore, she chose not to identify him as a student in need of speech-language services.

In 31 of the 50 states, departments of special education require clinicians to consider not only the child's performance on language measures but also the relationship between cognitive ability and language development (Casby, 1992). Thus, to qualify for SLP services through the public schools in many of these states, children first must demonstrate an impairment in performance with reference to their age. Then, they must exhibit cognitive abilities that are significantly higher than their language performance or that are within the typical range of intelligence. There are many ways in which these guidelines and policies can be administered. In some cases, such as with Jesse and Bill, it may be extremely difficult to enroll a child in intervention when the predetermined guidelines, based on a standard norm-referenced test battery, are not met. In other cases, clinicians may have some latitude in implementing the guidelines and may include professional judgment in addition to information derived from standardized tests.

Regardless of how they are applied, however, these policies have at their core some critical assumptions about language, how language performance can be measured, the relationship of language development to cognitive development, and the effectiveness of language intervention. If these assumptions are questionable, then the guidelines on which they are based should be questioned as well. This chapter examines the theoretical underpinnings for caseload triage based on cognitive referencing and reviews empirical investigations into the practice.

VARIANTS OF COGNITION–LANGUAGE MODELS

Cognitive referencing is based on a theory that holds that cognitive ability sets an upper limit for language ability. This underlying assumption is referred to as the *cognitive hypothesis* (Cromer, 1976; Miller, 1981; Sinclair, 1973). Several models of the relationship between language and cognitive development have emerged, and extensive reviews of differing accounts of the relationship are available (e.g., Rice, 1983). The "strong" cognitive hypothesis (Cromer, 1974) asserts that nonverbal intellectual ability is essentially all that is needed for language to develop. It is both necessary and sufficient to account for the facts of language development. A weaker version of the cognitive hypothesis (Cromer, 1976) asserts that certain nonverbal attainments are necessary for the child to reach related language milestones but that they are not sufficient. Additional mental abilities specifically related to language also would need to develop for language to be learned. An alternative to the cognitive hypothesis, the *correlational hypothesis*, maintains that linguistic achievements, as well as attainments in nonverbal cognitive domains (e.g., the development of the object concept, causality, the ability to assume the perspective of others), are constrained by the same underlying intellectual capacity. Performance in any of these domains may exceed performance in any other domain at a given point in development, but abilities across domains always are expected to be correlated because they all are governed by the same underlying intellectual capacity. This type of model makes it possible for some cognitive advances to appear first in language performance and only later in nonverbal tasks. In contrast, in a modular model of the mind, some cognitive systems, including language, are assumed to be highly encapsulated, developing and functioning independent of other systems. For example, agreement between subjects and verbs (e.g., *I go* versus *She goes*) or even the notions of subject, verb, and object seem to have no clear parallels outside the language system. In this view of the mind, some aspects of language development largely are disassociated from other aspects of development except in instances of extreme intellectual impairment (Chomsky, 1980; Cromer, 1988; Gardner, 1983; Pinker, 1994; see also the discussion in Kamhi, 1992).

Clearly, the direction and amount of influence between cognitive ability and language development vary greatly across theoretical models. A detailed discussion of these variant accounts of the relationship between nonverbal cognition and language is beyond the scope of this chapter. It is sufficient to note that despite the widespread appeal of the strong cognitive hypothesis, other theoretical perspectives permit and even predict circumstances in which 1) knowledge in the language domain is acquired and expressed prior to acquisition and expression of that knowledge in other domains, and 2) there are no direct correlates of some types of linguistic knowledge in any other cognitive system.

CLINICAL IMPLICATIONS OF THE
DISCREPANCY MODEL OF COGNITIVE REFERENCING

Belief in the strong cognitive hypothesis has led some researchers to conclude that children with relatively equal delays in nonverbal intelligence and language development are poor candidates for language intervention delivered by an SLP (Chapman & Miller, 1980; Lyngaas, Nyberg, Hoekenga, & Gruenewald, 1983; Owens & House, 1984). Consequently, if children without cognition–language discrepancies are recommended for intervention, then they may be given lower priority for treatment by the SLP (Fey, 1986).

If the underlying assumptions of the cognitive referencing model are accurate, and only children with nonverbal cognitive skills developed beyond their language skills can benefit from intervention delivered by an SLP, then the model could serve three important purposes. First, it would allocate services only to children who can benefit from the intervention, saving both money and the limited time of SLPs in the schools. This is not insignificant considering the shortage of SLPs in the schools (Wolery et al., 1994). Second, if the model is accurate, then it would prevent wasting the time of students with equally delayed language and cognitive skills on language intervention that would not be effective. The student's instruction time could be better spent on more appropriate learning tasks, thus maximizing the child's educational program. Third, if the assumptions on which it is based are accurate, then cognitive referencing would spare caregivers the emotional hardship of dealing with their child's failure to respond to intervention when the prognosis for a positive response to intervention is very poor. Unfortunately, the cost of being wrong with respect to the assumptions of the model of cognitive referencing is enormous. Most important, if the model is inappropriate, then a large number of children who would benefit from language intervention by SLPs might not be served.

APPLICATIONS OF COGNITIVE REFERENCING IN RESEARCH

In addition to being used for determining service eligibility in schools, cognitive referencing in various forms also has been used to select subgroups of children for research in language development and disorders. Research on language disorders frequently includes only children exhibiting a specific language impairment (SLI) profile (Cole, Schwartz, Notari, Dale, & Mills, 1995; Watkins & Rice, 1994). To qualify for inclusion in most of these studies, then, children must meet a standard IQ criterion (usually above 85), have delayed language development with respect to a standard criterion (e.g., below 85), and exhibit no apparent physical or emotional cause for the unexpectedly low performance in language. These criteria, however, still permit the inclusion of children who do not exhibit a significant discrepancy between nonverbal IQ and measured language performance (Camarata & Swisher, 1990). For example, a child could qualify in many studies with an IQ of 85 and language standard scores as high as 84. Researchers assume that children with language impairments and higher cognitive abilities may differ in meaningful ways from children with language impairments who have lower cognitive abilities. Because of this assumption, they often examine only children with profiles of normal nonverbal cognition and low language, effectively excluding children with below-average IQs regardless of the extent of their language impairments.

When control groups are included in studies of children fitting the SLI profile, they generally consist of children developing typically who are matched for either language development (usually measured in mean length of utterance [MLU]) or chronological age. Children with delayed language skills who also exhibit below-average cognitive ability are seldom included in research with children who fit an SLI profile.

Given the critical nature of the assumption that children with language impairments who have IQ discrepancies are fundamentally different from children who have low achievement (e.g., scores on language tests) and low IQ, it is remarkable that there has been so little experimental attention devoted to the assumption's verification. (See Stanovich, 1994, for a discussion of this point in reading disabilities.) This predicament has been redressed with respect to the roughly analogous situation in the area of reading disabilities. Several studies have examined whether children with reading impairments who have IQ–reading discrepancies are different on a variety of cognitive tasks from children with reading disabilities who have no discrepancies (Fletcher, Francis, Rourke, Shaywitz, & Shaywitz, 1992; Pennington, Gilger, Olson, & DeFries, 1992; Stanovich & Siegel, 1994). This research generally has shown that children in both groups have impairments in the ability to decode and spell novel words using phonetic cues (i.e., phonological coding tasks), even when they are compared with younger, typical readers who are matched on a general measure of reading performance (Stanovich & Siegel, 1994). There is virtually no evidence that these impairments, which are presumed to be at the foundation of the children's reading difficulties, are greater among children who exhibit an IQ–reading discrepancy than among poor readers who have low IQs that are commensurate with their reading performance. Typically, there have been few differences between these groups of poor readers on a wide range of cognitive tasks (Fletcher et al., 1992). When differences have been observed, they generally are small and appear on tasks that fall outside of the core of phonological coding tasks (Stanovich & Siegel, 1994). Similarly, there is no difference between these groups in the extent to which their problems are inherited. Thus, although they may differ in IQ and on their performance of some cognitive tasks unrelated to phonological coding, children from these two groups of poor readers appear to be neither etiologically nor behaviorally distinct. Instead, performance on phonological coding tasks (e.g., reading unfamiliar or nonsense words) predicts poor reading performance independent of intelligence, at least as it is measured by IQ tests. On the basis of this evidence, Stanovich (1994) and others have suggested that phonological coding skills and the phonological awareness abilities presumed to underlie them are representative of a cognitive module that is relatively unaffected by other cognitive developments and operations.

It is unclear whether children with language impairments ascertained by a discrepancy between IQ and language scores have language problems that are fundamentally different from those of children with language impairments who have no such discrepancy. This assumption is at the core of the cognitive referencing model, however, and as shown, it has broad implications for clinical service. Research in this area will be fundamental to understanding children's language impairments. Clinicians cannot wait for the outcomes of this research, however. Fortunately, there are many existing factors that render cognitive referencing untenable as a method of determining who should receive speech-language services.

THEORETICAL, EMPIRICAL, AND LEGAL CHALLENGES TO USING COGNITIVE REFERENCING

Theoretical Challenges

As noted previously, the discrepancy model of cognitive referencing is based on the cognitive hypothesis, which contends that nonverbal cognition drives language, including semantic and morphosyntactic development (Sinclair, 1973). If the model is correct, then children should not have language skills developed beyond their cognitive abilities. This prediction has been strongly challenged.

A challenge to the theoretical model that cognition sets the upper limits for language is the double disassociation between cognition and language development in children. The first type of disassociation between language and cognition is evident in children with SLI. Not even the staunchest supporters of the view that language is a product of some general cognitive capacities rather than of an autonomous mental domain or module deny that many children with language impairments perform exceedingly poorly in language by comparison with their performance on at least some other cognitive tasks (e.g., Johnston, 1994). The strong cognitive hypothesis does not predict and cannot account for such a cognition–language relationship.

The second type of disassociation of language and cognition, however, seriously challenges even the weak cognitive hypothesis. This form of disassociation is seen in children who have developed language beyond their nonverbal cognitive abilities. This is evident in specific disorders, such as Williams syndrome (Thal, Bates, & Bellugi, 1989), in which morphosyntactic abilities may exceed expectations based on cognitive and pragmatic performance, and Down syndrome (Chapman, 1995; Chapman, Schwartz, & Kay-Raining Bird, 1991), in which lexical comprehension may far exceed expectations based on performance in other cognitive and linguistic domains. These findings are very compatible with modular explanations of language development in which certain linguistic components (e.g., syntax, the lexicon) or linguistic processes (e.g., comprehension, production) function relatively independent of one another and of some other cognitive functions once believed to be central to language development.

A second, more practical, challenge to cognitive referencing is defining intelligence and identifying appropriate ways to measure it. Stanovich (1991) contended, "One would be hard pressed to find a concept more controversial than intelligence in all of psychology!" (p. 9). Despite not having a clear understanding or agreement regarding what intelligence is, it is the benchmark for the diagnosis of language disability.

Even if there were agreement about what is meant by intelligence, the challenges in accurately assessing the domain are formidable. Sattler (1988) summarized potential limitations of intelligence testing: 1) the tests sample only a limited number of conditions under which intelligent behavior is revealed, 2) IQ tests often are misused as measures of innate capacity, 3) the single IQ does not do justice to the multidimensional nature of intelligence, 4) IQ testing is limited in predicting nonacademic intellectual activity because the standard question format does not capture the demands of real-life situations, 5) IQ tests are culturally biased against ethnic groups, and 6) original and novel responses are penalized.

Thus, the clinical use of the cognitive referencing model is challenged to the degree that there is no agreement on what is meant by intelligence, and there is no standard for measuring it. Furthermore, it is not difficult to conceive that some specific nonverbal cognitive attainments are prerequisite to or at least highly correlated with other specific linguistic milestones, suggesting shared underlying cognitive mechanisms across domains. Even so, it is unclear why one would expect scores on nonverbal intelligence tests, which tend to be heavily loaded with visual-perceptual tasks in the preschool years (Johnston, 1982; Kamhi, Minor, & Mauer, 1990), to tap the types of cognitive abilities on which these specific cognition–language relationships may be based (Lahey, 1990).

Theorists and researchers can and should wrestle with the constructs of intelligence, the relationship of intellectual development to language development, and the best methods for measuring intelligence despite current problems in definition and measurement. Such inquiries should lead to the refinement of these constructs of language and cognition and to the development of more appropriate measurement tools in each domain. However, the definition and measurement problems associated with IQ tests raise serious questions about using these tests in formulas for making decisions about who has language impairment and who needs and can profit most from language intervention.

Unfortunately, the definition and measurement problems associated with intelligence also can be found in the language domain. The problems in each area are compounded when comparisons across domains are made on the basis of IQ and language test scores (Lahey, 1990).

Cole, Dale, and Mills (1992) examined whether cognitive referencing categorizations were stable over time. Specifically, they examined whether young children (3–7 years old) with delayed language, who were categorized as eligible or ineligible for intervention (using a discrepancy formula based on the relationship between their language test scores and IQ scores), would remain in the same category during an 8-month period (1 school year). Results indicated that children generally did not stay in the same categories during this time period. For example, when the McCarthy Scales of Children's Abilities (MSCA) (McCarthy, 1972) and the Peabody Picture Vocabulary Test–Revised (PPVT–R) (Dunn & Dunn, 1981) were used to develop the cognition–language profile, approximately 70% of the eligible group changed from eligible to not eligible, and 13% of the not-eligible group changed from not eligible to eligible. When the MSCA and the Test of Early Language Development (TELD) (Hresko, Reid, & Hammill, 1981) were used to develop profiles, 90% of the eligible group changed to not eligible, and 7% of the not-eligible group changed to eligible.

In a related study, Cole et al. (1995) examined the stability of SLI profiles over 1 school year. Children's classification into either SLI or developmental lag language impairment (DLLI) groups showed poor stability, with children changing categories frequently in both directions over time.

The results of both of these studies indicate that for a large percentage of children with delayed language, the relationship between IQ and language quotient changes substantially between yearly assessments. It is possible that these changes reflect the natural response of children with language impairments to effective intervention programs. If so, the cognitive referencing model would predict that the eligible students (those with higher IQs and delayed language) might become ineligible as a result of greater improvement in language performance during the year, with fairly stable IQ scores at pretest and posttest periods. Instead, in both of the studies, a drop in IQ for students selected for high IQ was accompanied by an increase in language performance. Both of these changes from pretest to posttest could have been the result of regression to the mean. Whether or not this is the case, the results of these studies provide no support for the predictions of the cognitive referencing model.

Poor test–retest reliability of cognition–language profiles is one source of instability that makes cognitive referencing difficult to implement. Another possible source of variability is in agreement of various test profiles. For example, does a profile battery consisting of the MSCA and the PPVT–R identify the same children as eligible (or not eligible) for services as does the Columbia Mental Maturity Scale (CMMS) (Burgemeister, Blum, & Lorge, 1972) and the TELD? Cole, Mills, and Kelley (1994) tested this hypothesis based on a cognitive referencing model. Twenty-six children were administered the MSCA and the CMMS (a nonverbal IQ test). In addition to using the complete MSCA IQ score, the researchers used the Perceptual-Performance section of the test to reduce the language load of the cognitive assessment. Language tests included the Test for Auditory Comprehension of Language–Revised (TACL–R) (Elaborated Sentences and Grammatical Morphemes subtests) (Carrow-Woolfolk, 1985), the PPVT–R, and the TELD. Each language test was used in conjunction with the three IQ measures (the MSCA total test, the MSCA Perceptual-Performance subtest, and the CMMS). The extremes in eligibility classification that resulted are shocking. Some profiles identified as few as 4 of 26 children as eligible under a cognitive referencing triage model, while other measures identified only 4 of the 26 children as *not eligible*.

Aram et al. (1992) reported similar findings in a study in which different IQ–language discrepancy criteria using a standardized test battery were compared with the clinical judgments of expert clinicians in the field of developmental language disorders. Regardless of the discrepancy formula used, 40%–60% of the children determined by clinicians to have language impairment were not identified by the standardized test battery. In another study, involving a comparison of very low birth weight infants and a randomly selected group of control subjects on a different battery of language and intelligence tests, almost half of the control subjects were identified as having language impairments. Even when the cutoff was changed from 1 standard deviation to 2 standard deviations below performance IQ, nearly 19% of the control subjects were determined to have language impairment. Thus, while the test battery used in the first study underidentified language impairments, the other battery grossly overidentified language problems.

The results of the studies reviewed in this section illustrate that the choice of instruments used in developing a cognition–language profile and the criteria for classifying children as having language impairment have tremendous effects on whether an IQ–language discrepancy is observed. On the basis of this evidence, the discrepancy model of cognitive referencing appears insupportable as a means of identifying children with language impairment who need clinical services.

Empirical Challenges

Perhaps the key prediction of the cognitive referencing model is that children with relatively higher intelligence will benefit from language intervention services to a greater degree than will children with lower intelligence. This prediction can be challenged on empirical grounds independent of the logical and psychometric grounds examined in the last two sections.

The prediction is two-pronged, reflecting the two versions of the cognitive referencing model. First, it might be anticipated that language intervention will be more effective for children with language impairments who have average nonverbal IQs than for children with below-average IQs. Second, even if the first prediction is proved wrong, it could still be speculated on the basis of the discrepancy model of cognitive referencing that intervention will be more effective for children who have a significant IQ–language discrepancy than for children who have nonverbal IQs that are commensurate with their language impairments. As it turns out, both of these predictions appear to be incorrect.

The first prediction was tested by Fey, Long, and Cleave (1994). These investigators evaluated the morphosyntactic performance of two groups of preschool children with language impairments drawn from a sample of children who had participated in an earlier study (Fey, Cleave, Long, & Hughes, 1993). One group of 10 children had average IQs above the standard criterion of 85 (*M* = 94.33). The other group of eight children had IQs in the borderline range of intelligence (*M* = 76.75). All of the children exhibited discrepancies between performance mental age (MA), based on the Leiter International Performance Scale (Leiter, 1979), and expressive grammar, based on the Developmental Sentence Scoring (DSS) procedure (Lee, 1974). The range of MAs and MLUs was the same for both groups, and the groups were well matched for MLU. Still, the children in the borderline-IQ group had significantly lower MAs and lower standardized comprehension scores than did the children with average IQs. This means that the gap between language and nonverbal IQ was smaller for the children in the borderline-IQ group.

These groups were compared prior to intervention on a set of DSS measures that have been shown to distinguish between children who are developing typically and those who have SLI. No differences were observed between groups on any of these measures. Then, the groups were compared on their responses to one of two models of language intervention designed to facilitate grammatical development during a 4½-month period (Fey et al., 1993). Both groups of children demonstrated significant gains from pretest to posttest on the experimental measures, but no differences in gains were observed between groups.

In the original study by Fey et al. (1993), the intervention administered by a clinician was more consistent than the intervention provided indirectly by the children's parents. Therefore, additional comparisons were made between the four children with average IQs and the five children with borderline IQs who had received clinician intervention. Surprisingly, although there were large improvements in DSS for all children, the gains were significantly greater for the children in the borderline-IQ group. Fey et al. (1994) pointed out that this difference could be spurious as a result of the large number of statistical tests that were administered. Still, the findings of this study run counter to the predictions of the cognitive referencing model. In fact, the group with lower MAs and a less-marked MA–language gap appeared to have derived even greater benefits from the clinician-administered intervention than did the MLU-matched group with average IQ and a larger MA–language discrepancy.

The findings reported by Fey et al. (1994) suggest that below-average intelligence does not preclude gains resulting from intervention for children who have a significant cognition–language discrepancy. This study does not address whether children with language performance commensurate with nonverbal intelligence can benefit from intervention as much as can children who exhibit significant gaps between nonverbal cognitive and linguistic performance. Three studies have dealt squarely with this issue.

Cole, Dale, and Mills (1990) compared the progress of children who had performance IQs at least 1 standard deviation above language performance (cognition–language discrepancy) with gains made by children with delays in nonverbal cognition that were equivalent to their delays in language development (no discrepancy). The mean age for the children was 5 years, and the intervention covered a period of 1 year. No between-group differences in gains were found for MLU, the PPVT–R, or the Preschool Language Assessment Instrument (Blank, Rose, & Berlin, 1978). Furthermore, both groups made statistically significant gains on the norm-referenced PPVT–R, suggesting that both the children with cognition–language discrepancies (mean IQ of 94) *and* the children with low performance in both domains (mean IQ of 71) made greater gains in receptive vocabulary than would be expected by maturation alone.

It is possible that the finding of no differences in response to intervention in the study of Cole et al. (1990) was the result of low statistical power because of the small number of subjects in the study (50). To investigate this possibility, Notari, Cole, and Mills (1992) reanalyzed the data from the earlier study with the addition of 48 new subjects to increase statistical power. Again, no differences in gains from pretest to posttest were found between the groups. As in the study of Cole et al. (1990), both groups demonstrated greater gains from pretest to posttest than would be predicted by maturation alone on the PPVT–R. In addition, however, both groups demonstrated gains in standard scores on the

TELD. This illustrates that the gains that could be associated with the children's intervention and educational programs were not restricted solely to receptive vocabulary.

The studies of Cole et al. (1990) and Notari et al. (1992) examined both morphosyntactic and semantic aspects of language development. Mercer (1993) explored the influence of children's cognition–language profiles on the development of pragmatic skills. She examined the pragmatic categories of initiating, turn taking, topic relevance, acknowledging, and repair strategies. Her objective was to determine whether young children with delayed language who had cognition–language discrepancies gained more from a year of language intervention that included pragmatic goals than did children who had equivalent language and nonverbal cognitive performance. She found few differences in the children's ability to benefit from pragmatic intervention based on cognitive–language profile. The few differences that were found indicated that the children with lower cognitive performance made greater gains. This, of course, is the opposite of what is predicted by the cognitive referencing model.

Legal Challenges

The clinical use of cognitive referencing faces its most formidable practical challenge not from theoretical or empirical examination but from case law regarding the intent of PL 101-476, the Individuals with Disabilities Education Act (IDEA) of 1990, and other laws providing rights and services to children with disabilities, including children with communication disorders. One such case, *Timothy W. v. Rochester, New Hampshire, School District* (1987) appears to be especially pertinent to the use of cognitive referencing. In this case, a child with severe developmental delay was denied special education services by the school district because the district predicted that the child would not be able to benefit from any intervention because of the severity of his disability. The first circuit court, deciding against the school district, emphasized that PL 91-230, the Education of the Handicapped Act (EHA) of 1970, was designed specifically for students like Timothy and that the district's prediction of Timothy's ability to significantly benefit from intervention could not be used as a means of triage. The relevance of this ruling to the practice of cognitive referencing is fairly straightforward. A child may not legally be denied services on the basis of a prediction that he or she will not benefit because of low level of functioning.

In a related case (*Polk v. Central Susquehanna Intermediate Unit*, 1988), a child with severe disabilities was provided with physical therapy, consisting of consultations twice a month with the teacher and the therapist. The third circuit court ruled that a program is not necessarily appropriate just because it provides some minimal amount of service. In addition, the court considered whether the district may have had a *policy* of refusing direct physical therapy for children with severe developmental delays. Such a policy would be a violation of the EHA's requirement to provide individualized education programs. The court determined that the district maintained a policy of underserving these children and was, therefore, out of compliance with the law.

Cases like these strongly suggest that excluding a class of children (those with lower cognitive ability) from services may violate federal laws guaranteeing free, appropriate public education to all children. Providing minimal consultative services may not be deemed an appropriate option for serving children with very low ability levels if this service model is provided to a class of children based on a prediction that they will not benefit from the level of services provided to other children.

CONCLUSION

The discussion thus far illustrates that both versions of cognitive referencing are insupportable on theoretical, psychometric, and empirical grounds as clinical methods for determining who is eligible for language intervention. Using IQ cutoffs and IQ–language discrepancy formulas as means of identifying subjects for the study of children's language impairments is similarly questionable. Given these assumptions, one might be tempted to conclude that intelligence is an extraneous variable in the study of children's language impairments. There are several reasons that this position is premature, at best, and most probably wrong.

First, there can be little question in the mind of anyone who has worked with children with developmental language delays that some children who have severe problems in the comprehension and/or use of conventional linguistic devices appear bright and capable in other respects and are sometimes ingenious in their creation of means to communicate nonverbally (see Johnston, 1994). Furthermore, there is a great deal of evidence that some children with mental retardation seem to have more severe delays in language than in other areas of functioning. This imbalance appears to be especially common among children with Down syndrome. (See Chapman, 1995, for a review.) Thus, there can be little doubt that there are children who have severe linguistic limitations in the face of much better performance in other cognitive domains. Difficulty in operationalizing the concept of SLI using existing measurement tools (e.g., IQ and language tests) may stand in the way of the clinical usefulness of this classification, but it does nothing to reduce the potential importance of the construct itself. Nor does it eliminate the relatively unexplored possibility that children who are legitimately classified as having SLI are different in etiology, neurophysiology, or phenotype from children whose language impairments are accompanied by cognitive impairments commensurate in their severity. Studies are needed in which comparisons are made of language, language learning, and nonlanguage tasks between children with language impairments who do or do not have IQ–language discrepancies. Ideally, children from both groups should cover a wide range of intelligence, at least from mental retardation requiring limited supports to the above-average range. To guard against measurement error, children should be assigned to the specific-impairment group only when the 95% confidence intervals for nonverbal IQ and language do not overlap. In such studies, it reasonably can be asked whether there are phenotypical, neurological, or etiological differences between groups. Of course, it may be shown that there are no differences on *any* variables that distinguish these groups of children. It also may be that the linguistic phenotype observed is completely independent of level of nonverbal cognition. In other words, it may be that nonverbal intelligence is of little theoretical or clinical importance in defining, studying, and planning interventions for children's language impairments. The point is that the most important questions have not yet been asked, and the relevant hypotheses have not yet been tested.

Second, even if the phenotype for developmental language impairment were independent of nonverbal intelligence, it seems unlikely that differences in intelligence will be shown to be insignificant in planning intervention programs for young children. As Lyon (1989) has pointed out, differences in intelligence may relate to factors such as the level of motivation to communicate, the ability to engage in play with peers, emotional reaction to communication failure, and task persistence especially at and below the range of mental retardation requiring intermittent supports. Similarly, there may be differences in the perceptions and reactions of parents and teachers based on the child's perceived level of nonverbal intelligence. These factors may not be related to the language impairment per se, but they could be significant variables in the child's ability to cope with or compensate for the problem or in the development of an effective and efficient program of clinical management.

Third, notwithstanding the psychometric and logical problems associated with the use of nonverbal IQ in discrepancy formulas, a number of studies have demonstrated a significant relationship between nonverbal IQ scores and language measures. For example, it has long been maintained that the correlation between mental age and language measures, such as MLU, is greater than that between age and MLU (Miller, 1981). In some cases, these correlations have been substantial. In a sample of children and youth with Down syndrome, Chapman et al. (1991) observed that chronological age and mental age together accounted for approximately 80% of the variance in scores in vocabulary and syntax comprehension. Perhaps more significant, several studies have observed a relationship between preexperimental IQ scores and language outcomes on a posttest. Bishop and Edmundson (1987) and Paul and Cohen (1984) each observed correlations between preexperimental IQ and gains on language measures sampled 1 or more years later. Furthermore, Cole, Dale, Mills, and Jenkins (1993); Friedman and Friedman (1980); and Yoder, Kaiser, and Alpert (1991) all observed aptitude by treatment interactions involving IQ. In each study, one intervention method was of greater benefit to high-functioning children than to low-functioning children. In contrast, an alternative method resulted in greater gains by the low-functioning children.

There may be a role for intelligence measurement in intervention planning for children with developmental language impairments and for children with specific language impairments. Some measure of cognitive performance is needed to examine differences and similarities in etiology and performance for children with specific language impairments and for children with developmental language impairments. More research is needed in these areas. There is, however, no support for the continuation of cognitive referencing in the forms of IQ cutoffs or IQ–language discrepancy formulas as a clinical method of caseload selection or prioritization. IQ measures may reveal something about *how* children should be served, but they do not appear to be relevant in deciding *who* should be served.

REFERENCES

Aram, D.M., Morris, R., & Hall, N.E. (1992). The validity of discrepancy criteria for identifying children with developmental language disorders. *Journal of Learning Disabilities, 25,* 549–554.

Bishop, D.V., & Edmundson, A. (1987). Language-impaired 4-year-olds: Distinguishing transient from persistent impairment. *Journal of Speech and Hearing Disorders, 52*(2), 156–173.

Blank, M., Rose, S.A., & Berlin, L.J. (1978). *Preschool Language Assessment Instrument: The language of learning in practice.* Orlando, FL: Grune & Stratton.

Burgemeister, B.B., Blum, L.H., & Lorge, I. (1972). *Columbia Mental Maturity Scale* (3rd ed.). San Antonio, TX: The Psychological Corporation.

Camarata, S., & Swisher, L. (1990). A note on intelligence assessment within studies of specific language impairment. *Journal of Speech and Hearing Research, 33,* 205–207.

Carrow-Woolfolk, E. (1985). *Test for Auditory Comprehension of Language–Revised (TACL–R).* Allen, TX: DLM Teaching Resources.

Casby, M. (1992). The cognitive hypothesis and its influence on speech-language services in the schools. *Language, Speech, and Hearing Services in Schools, 23,* 198–202.

Chapman, R.S. (1995). Language development in children and adolescents with Down syndrome. In P. Fletcher & B. MacWhinney (Eds.), *The handbook of child language* (pp. 641–663). Oxford: Blackwell.

Chapman, R.S., & Miller, J., (1980). Analyzing language and communication in the child. In R. Schiefelbusch (Ed.), *Nonspeech language and communication: Acquisition and intervention* (pp. 159–196). Baltimore: University Park Press.

Chapman, R.S., Schwartz, S.E., & Kay-Raining Bird, E. (1991). Language skills of children and adolescents with Down syndrome: I. Comprehension. *Journal of Speech and Hearing Research, 34*(5), 1106–1120.

Chomsky, N. (1980). On cognitive structures and their development: A reply to Piaget. In M. Piatelli-Palmarini (Ed.), *Language and learning: The debate between Jean Piaget and Noam Chomsky* (pp. 35–54). Cambridge, MA: Harvard University Press.

Cole, K., Dale, P., & Mills, P. (1990). Defining language delay in young children by cognitive referencing: Are we saying more than we know? *Applied Psycholinguistics, 11,* 291–302.

Cole, K., Dale, P., & Mills, P. (1992). Stability of the intelligence quotient–language quotient relation: Is discrepancy modeling based on a myth? *American Journal on Mental Retardation, 97*(2), 131–143.

Cole, K., Dale, P., Mills, P., & Jenkins, J. (1993). Interaction between early intervention curricula and student characteristics. *Exceptional Children, 60,* 17–28.

Cole, K., Mills, P., & Kelley, D. (1994). Agreement of assessment profiles used in cognitive referencing. *Language, Speech, and Hearing Services in Schools, 25,* 25–31.

Cole, K., Schwartz, I., Notari, A., Dale, P., & Mills, P. (1995). Examination of the stability of two methods of defining specific language impairment. *Applied Psycholinguistics, 16,* 103–123.

Cromer, R. (1974). The development of language and cognition: The cognitive hypothesis. In B.M. Foss (Ed.), *Normal perspectives in child development* (pp. 184–252). Baltimore: Penguin Books.

Cromer, R.F. (1976). The cognitive hypothesis of language acquisition and its implications for child language deficiency. In D. Morehead & A. Morehead (Eds.), *Normal and deficient child language* (pp. 283–333). Baltimore: University Park Press.

Cromer, R.F. (1988). The cognitive hypothesis revisited. In F. Kessel (Ed.), *The development of language and language researchers* (pp. 223–248). Hillsdale, NJ: Lawrence Erlbaum Associates.

Dunn, L.M., & Dunn, L.M. (1981). *Peabody Picture Vocabulary Test–Revised.* Circle Pines, MN: American Guidance Service.

Education of the Handicapped Act (EHA) of 1970, PL 91-230. (April 13, 1970). Title 20, U.S.C. 1400 et seq: *U.S. Statutes at Large, 84,* 121–195.

Fey, M.E. (1986). *Language intervention with young children.* San Diego: College-Hill Press.

Fey, M.E., Cleave, P.L., Long, S.H., & Hughes, D.L. (1993). Two approaches to the facilitation of grammar in language impaired children: An experimental evaluation. *Journal of Speech and Hearing Research, 36,* 141–157.

Fey, M.E., Long, S.H., & Cleave, P.L. (1994). Reconsideration of IQ criteria in the definition of specific language impairment. In R.V. Watkins & M.L. Rice (Eds.), *Communication and language intervention series: Vol. 4. Specific language impairments in children* (pp. 161–178). Baltimore: Paul H. Brookes Publishing Co.

Fletcher, J.M., Francis, D.J., Rourke, B.P., Shaywitz, S.E., & Shaywitz, B.A. (1992). The validity of discrepancy based definitions of reading disabilities. *Journal of Learning Disabilities, 25,* 555–561.

Friedman, P., & Friedman, K. (1980). Accounting for individual differences when comparing the effectiveness of remedial language teaching methods. *Applied Psycholinguistics, 1,* 151–170.

Gardner, H. (1983). *Frames of mind.* New York: Basic Books.

Hresko, W.P., Reid, K., & Hammill, D.D. (1981). *Test of Early Language Development.* Austin, TX: PRO-ED.

Individuals with Disabilities Education Act (IDEA) of 1990, PL 101-476. (October 30, 1990). Title 20, U.S.C. 1400 et seq: *U.S. Statutes at Large, 104,* 1103–1151.

Johnston, J.R. (1982). Interpreting the Leiter IQ: Performance profiles of young normal and language disordered children. *Journal of Speech and Hearing Research, 25,* 291–296.

Johnston, J.R. (1994). Cognitive abilities of children with language impairment. In R.V. Watkins & M.L. Rice (Eds.), *Communication and language intervention series: Vol. 4. Specific language impairments in children* (pp. 107–121). Baltimore: Paul H. Brookes Publishing Co.

Kamhi, A.G. (1992). Three perspectives on language processing: Interactionism, modularity, and holism. In R.S. Chapman (Ed.), *Processes in language acquisition and disorders* (pp. 45–64). St. Louis: C.V. Mosby.

Kamhi, A.G., Minor, J.S., & Mauer, D. (1990). Content analysis and intratest performance profiles on the Columbia and the TONI. *Journal of Speech and Hearing Research, 33,* 375–379.

Lahey, P. (1990). Who shall be called language impaired? Some reflections and one perspective. *Journal of Speech and Hearing Disorders, 55*, 612–620.

Lee, L. (1974). *Developmental Sentence Analysis*. Evanston, IL: Northwestern University Press.

Leiter, R. (1979). *Leiter International Performance Scale*. Chicago: Stoelting Company.

Lyngaas, K., Nyberg, B., Hoekenga, R., & Gruenewald, L. (1983). Language intervention in the multiple contexts of the public school setting. In J. Miller, D. Yoder, & R. Schiefelbusch (Eds.), *Contemporary issues in language intervention* (American Speech-Language-Hearing Association Reports, *12*, pp. 239–258). Rockville, MD: American Speech-Language-Hearing Association.

Lyon, R. (1989). IQ is irrelevant to the definition of learning disabilities: A position in search of logic and data. *Journal of Learning Disabilities, 22*, 504–506, 512.

McCarthy, D. (1972). *Manual for the McCarthy Scales of Children's Abilities*. New York: The Psychological Corporation.

Mercer, C. (1993). *Comparison of the effects of language intervention for children with differing language/cognitive profiles*. Unpublished master's thesis, University of Washington, Seattle.

Miller, J. (1981). *Assessing language production in children: Experimental procedures*. Austin, TX: PRO-ED.

Notari, A., Cole, K., & Mills, P. (1992). Cognitive referencing: The (non)relationship between theory and application. *Topics in Early Childhood Special Education, 11*, 22–38.

Owens, R., & House, L. (1984). Decision-making processes in augmentative communication. *Journal of Speech and Hearing Disorders, 49*, 18–25.

Paul, R., & Cohen, D.J. (1984). Outcomes of severe disorders of language acquisition. *Journal of Autism and Developmental Disorders, 14*, 405–421.

Pennington, B.F., Gilger, J.W., Olson, R.K., & DeFries, J.C. (1992). The external validity of age versus IQ discrepancy definitions of reading disability: Lessons from a twin study. *Journal of Learning Disabilities, 25*, 562–573.

Pinker, S. (1994). *The language instinct: How the mind creates language*. New York: William Morrow and Company.

Polk v. Central Susquehanna Intermediate Unit 16, 853 F.2d 171 (3rd Circuit, 1988).

Rice, M.L. (1983). Contemporary accounts of the cognition/language relationship: Implications for speech language clinicians. *Journal of Speech and Hearing Disorders, 48*(4), 347–359.

Sattler, J. (1988). *Assessment of children* (3rd ed.). San Diego: Sattler.

Sinclair, H. (1973). Language acquisition and cognitive development. In T. Moore (Ed.), *Cognitive development and the acquisition of language* (pp. 9–25). New York: Academic Press.

Stanovich, K. (1991). Discrepancy definitions of reading disability: Has intelligence led us astray? *Reading Research Quarterly, 26*, 7–29.

Stanovich, K. (1994). Annotation: Does dyslexia exist? *Journal of Child Psychology and Psychiatry, 35*, 579–595.

Stanovich, K., & Siegel, L.S. (1994). Phenotypic performance profile of children with reading disabilities: A regression based test of the phonological core variable difference model. *Journal of Educational Psychology, 86*, 24–53.

Stark, R.E., & Tallal, P. (1981). Selection of children with specific language deficits. *Journal of Speech and Hearing Disorders, 46*, 114–122.

Thal, D., Bates, E., & Bellugi, U. (1989). Language and cognition in two children with Williams syndrome. *Journal of Speech and Hearing Research, 32*, 489–500.

Timothy W. v. Rochester, New Hampshire, School District, Education of the Handicapped Law Review, Dec. 509:141, 1987.

Tomblin, J.B., & Buckwalter, P. (1994). Studies of genetics of specific language impairment. In R.V. Watkins & M.L. Rice (Eds.), *Communication and language intervention series: Vol. 4. Specific language impairments in children* (pp. 17–34). Baltimore: Paul H. Brookes Publishing Co.

Watkins, R.V., & Rice, M.L. (Eds.). (1994). *Communication and language intervention series: Vol. 4. Specific language impairments in children.* Baltimore: Paul H. Brookes Publishing Co.

Wolery, M., Venn, M.L., Holcombe, A., Brookfield, J., Martin, C.G., Huffman, K., Schroeder, C., & Fleming, L.A. (1994). Employment of related service personnel in preschool programs: A survey of general early educators. *Exceptional Children, 61,* 25–39.

Yoder, P.J., Kaiser, A.P., & Alpert, C.L. (1991). An exploratory study of the interaction between language teaching methods and child characteristics. *Journal of Speech and Hearing Research, 34*(1), 155–167.

8

Parent Report Assessment of Language and Communication

Philip S. Dale

HIGH TECHNOLOGY PERMEATES EVERYDAY LIFE. Microcomputers can be found in automobiles, toys, even washing machines and toasters. The study of language usage and acquisition is no exception. Among the techniques being used are computerized analysis of language samples (MacWhinney, 1995); split television monitors with a soundtrack that matches one image, for the study of language comprehension (Golinkoff, Hirsh-Pasek, Cauley, & Gordon, 1987); evoked-potential recording to detect brain responses to grammatical and semantic anomalies (Osterhout & Holcomb, 1995); and positron emission tomography (PET) and magnetic resonance imaging (MRI) to identify the brain locus of specific aspects of language processing (Frackowiak, 1994; Peterson, Fox, Posner, Mintun, & Raichle, 1988).

In contrast to those technologically complex methods, this chapter reports on the revival and improvement of a very old and "low-tech" approach to assessing early language and cognition; one that is not only practical and cost effective but also is, for certain purposes, simply *better* than the alternatives. It is *parent report:* the systematic utilization of the extensive experience of parents (and potentially other caregivers) with their children. Parent report, in the form of diary studies, is, in fact, the oldest form of child-language research. A long series of "baby biographies," including or even focusing on language, began with Dietrich Tiedemann's diary of infant behavior, which appeared in 1787 (Bar-Adon & Leopold, 1971). Perhaps the most famous and certainly one of the best is that of Darwin (1877, excerpted in Bar-Adon & Leopold, 1971). The tradition has continued into the 20th century (e.g., Dromi, 1987; Tomasello, 1992). These studies have been conducted by parent-scientists with substantial training in the observation and analysis of behavior.

Professionals concerned with assessing individual children's development also have relied on parent report, especially for purposes of initial screening. Motivation to use parent report has been greatly increased by the Education of

---

Portions of this chapter have been adapted from Fenson et al. (1993) and Fenson et al. (1994).

the Handicapped Act Amendments of 1986 (PL 99-457), which mandated increased parental involvement in developing programs for young children. There has been reluctance, however, to use parent report as the primary basis for assessment. Most parents do not have specialized training in language development and may not be sensitive to subtle aspects of language structure and use. Furthermore, a natural pride in their own child and a failure to critically test their impressions of their child's abilities may cause parents to overestimate the child's development; conversely, frustration in the case of delayed language may lead to underestimates (Dale, Bates, Reznick, & Morisset, 1989). Because of these assumptions, discrepancies between parent report and standardized professional assessment have been viewed as evidence of the inaccuracy of parent report. Thus, in both research and clinical practice, the role of parent report has been strictly limited.

Just how strong the prejudice has been against parent report as a valid measure of specific aspects of language development is illustrated vividly by the following quotation from an anonymous prepublication reviewer of Fenson et al. (1994), a monograph that included extensive evidence of the validity of a particular parent report measure:

> I must admit that my first reaction to these data was skepticism. For example, I asked myself yet again, "How could parents be sufficiently precise in their responses?" and "Was any variation which resulted a function more of the parent's personality than the child's actual capabilities?" The data contained in this monograph, however, ... clearly elevate the status of parent report data. I believe after reading this monograph that I will no longer overhear conversations (as I have in the past) at conferences where individuals dismiss [this] data set with "It's only parent report data." (Anonymous personal communication, January 1993)

This chapter reviews the state of parent report, including an examination of some quite successful instruments, drawing some general conclusions about this technique; considers the potential applications of parent report in research and clinical practice; and discusses some promising directions for developing additional measures.

WHY PARENT REPORT HAS SO MUCH PROMISE

Language assessment techniques for young children fall into three main categories. The first is structured tests. Tests require time, trained personnel, and, above all, the cooperation of the young child. Their usefulness is limited by expense and by the modest validity that most of these instruments have demonstrated prior to age 2½–3 years. The second, in many cases the "method of choice" for early assessment, is language sampling. Quality sampling requires highly trained personnel and a substantial amount of time for analysis. Even under ideal circumstances, however, the representativeness of a single sample gathered in an unfamiliar setting will be highly variable. Many pragmatic intents, such as asking for an object in the next room, refusing a parental action such as washing, or attempting to engage another child in play, are not likely to arise under these circumstances; therefore the child's mastery of the vocabulary and grammatical forms that would express those intents cannot be evaluated. Furthermore, if the child is observed while interacting with a parent, then it is the dyad that is being assessed, regardless of whether that is the goal; if the child is observed while interacting with an examiner, then validity will be influenced by the child's willingness to interact with a stranger. Thus, as valuable as language sampling can be, especially for breaking new ground in the study of language and speech and/or for when information is needed for the design of intervention, the practicality and validity may be limited for many purposes, such as large-scale screening or large-sample research projects.

Parent report, the third main category of language assessment techniques, has a number of inherent advantages over structured test and language sampling. Most important is that parent report is based on experience with the child that is not only more extensive than what any researcher or clinician can obtain but also is more representative of the child's ability. Parents have experience with children at play, during meals, while bathing, at bedtime, during tantrums—in short, with the full range of the child's life and, therefore, with the full range of language structures used in these contexts. Parents also have had opportunities to hear the child interact with other people: the other parent, grandparents, siblings, and friends. Because parent report represents an aggregation over much time and many situations, it is less influenced by performance factors such as word frequency. In a short language sample, only the higher-frequency words are likely to be observed, while many other well-learned words simply may not have the opportunity to be used. As Bates, Bretherton, and Snyder (1988) pointed out, "Parental report is likely to reflect what a child knows, whereas [a sample of] free speech reflects those forms that she is more likely to use" (p. 57).

The very fact that parent report is based on experience outside of the clinic or laboratory makes it especially suitable for many applications, such as pre-screening to help the professional select focused assessment procedures for a visit and monitoring changes in language resulting from intervention (i.e., the generalization issue). The systematic use of parent report also acts to incorporate parents into intervention or research as collaborators. This not only helps provide higher-quality information to the professional, but it also can substantially increase the motivation of the parent to continue participating in an intervention program or in a research project.

One of the most important advantages of parent report is that it makes possible the collection of data from far larger samples of children than would be possible with tests or naturalistic observation. Information from more adequate samples can benefit both clinical practice and research. Fenson et al. (1994), for example, used the norming data from the MacArthur Communicative Development Inventories (Fenson et al., 1993)—a sample of 1,803 children age 8–30 months—to address questions about variability in communicative development.

Large samples are needed to provide an accurate statistical description of extreme scores (e.g., which score corresponds to the 10th percentile). To be sure, other kinds of information also are needed to determine the cutoff for exceptionality (e.g., Should we use the 10th percentile? One and one half standard deviations? Two standard deviations?). Longitudinal studies of individual children are essential to determine whether there are substantial differences in later outcome corresponding to particular levels of early language ability, but the availability of adequate norms of the kind made possible by parent report will add enormously to interpreting the findings from those longitudinal studies. Research on questions such as environmental influences on language development also can benefit from large samples. Correlational research on these influences is hampered by the problem of multicollinearity: The predictor variables such as parental education, number of books in the home, family size, use of questions versus imperatives, frequency of semantically contingent parent responses, and so forth are likely to be intercorrelated, making it difficult to separate the effects of each of them individually. Large samples in which there is a substantial amount of nonoverlapping variance are essential for addressing these questions.

EFFECTIVE USE OF PARENT REPORT

Clearly there are legitimate concerns about the ability of parents to provide detailed and specific knowledge about their children's language. Many of the reservations that have been expressed, however, may have more to do with how parental experience is drawn upon rather than with the validity of that perspective in general. Parent report is most likely to be accurate under three general conditions:

• When assessment is limited to current behaviors
• When assessment is focused on emergent behaviors
• When a primarily recognition format is used

Each of these conditions acts to place fewer demands on the respondent's memory, relative to retrospective reports and/or "free-form" reports. The first condition reflects the fact that parents are better able to report on their child's present language abilities than on their child's past language abilities. The second condition reflects the fact that parents are better able to report on animal names in their child's vocabulary, for example, at the age at which their child is actively learning new animal words. Parents can track their child's receptive vocabulary to about 16–18 months, after which it is too large to monitor. Expressive vocabulary can be monitored until about 2½–3 years, after which it too becomes too large. The recognition strategy capitalizes on the greater ease of recognition as contrasted with recall. That is, it is better to ask parents to report on their child's vocabulary by selecting words from a comprehensive list rather than by having them write down all of the words that they can recall hearing their child use (or, even worse, asking whether the child "knows 50 words"). The recognition format also reduces the need for parents to make inferences about their child's ability relative to other children (e.g., "What do they mean by animal words?" or "What do they mean by 'lots' of animal words?").

There are, in fact, two uses of the recognition format for language assessment. In some cases, the language element of interest is a single form (e.g., a word such as *ball*). In such cases, the parent need only search his or her memory for one or more examples of the child producing that form. In other cases, typical of morphology and syntax, the linguistic element is a category. For example, does the child form plurals by adding the *-s* morpheme, or the progressive by adding *-ing*? No particular plural form is targeted; all examples of the category (*cats, dogs,* etc.) are appropriate. It would be difficult to explain English morphology to a linguistically untrained parent. In such cases, a recognition format can be used for the *contrast* rather than for the specific forms. In the MacArthur Communicative Development Inventories, parents read a series of sentence pairs, with the general instruction: "In each of the following pairs, please mark the one that sounds MOST like the way your child talks right now...." Among the pairs are *two shoe/two shoes* and *kitty sleep/kitty sleeping*. The contrast between the two sentences in each pair provides a concrete exemplification of the regular plural or the present progressive and thus serves as a basis for recognition.

EXAMPLES OF SUCCESSFUL PARENT REPORT MEASURES

In recent years, two types of parent report measures have been developed and extensively evaluated. The first type includes questionnaires or interviews that attempt to evaluate a broad range of ability domains including language (along with gross and fine motor skills, social abilities, and self-help skills), most often for screening purposes rather than for detailed diagnosis. It includes the Denver Developmental Screening Test (DDST) (Frankenburg & Dodds, 1969), the Minnesota Child Development Inventory (MCDI) (Ireton & Thwing, 1974; revised as the Child Development Inventory [Ireton, 1992]), and the Vineland Adaptive Behavior Scales (Sparrow, Balla, & Cicchetti, 1984). Both the DDST and the Vineland have been demonstrated to distinguish with some reliability and specificity the typically developing children from the children with developmental delays, though they are less effective as predictors of functioning within the typical range. Their limitations stem from the small number of items at each age focused on language and communication. The MCDI, for birth through age 6, is more comprehensive; its six subscales include a 64-item expressive language scale and a 67-item receptive language scale. The General Development Index computed from the MCDI has been observed to correlate significantly (correlations between .45 and .8) with standardized measures of intelligence such as the Bayley Scales of Infant Development (Bayley, 1969) and the McCarthy Scales of Children's Abilities (McCarthy, 1972). Both language scales of the MCDI correlate substantially with conventional language measures such as mean length of utterance (MLU) and the Sequenced Inventory of Communicative Development–Receptive (SICD–R) expressive scale (Tomblin, Schonrock, & Hardy, 1989). There still are relatively few items at each age level, however, and they are a mix of recognition-format items and more open-ended items (e.g., uses the word *not* in sentences, uses at least five words as names of familiar objects).

The second category of parent report includes measures developed specifically for language, again usually for screening purposes, reflecting a widespread belief that parent report is most appropriately used for screening rather than for detailed evaluation. It includes the Clinical Linguistic and Auditory Milestones Scale (CLAMS) (Capute et al., 1986) and the Receptive-Expressive Emergent Language Scale (REEL) (Bzoch & League, 1994). These measures also show some ability to separate typically developing children from those with delays but show limited effectiveness as measures across the full range of variability, again a result, in part, of the small number of items at each age. An additional limitation to their usefulness is the limited norms that have been obtained.

Rescorla's Language Development Survey (LDS) (Rescorla, 1989), although also designed as a relatively brief expressive language–screening instrument for children between 12 and 24 months, represents a different approach, more consistent with the three "design principles" for parent report discussed in the previous section. It contains a 309-word expressive vocabulary checklist, along with a section requesting that the parent write three of the child's longest recent sentences or phrases. The LDS demonstrates excellent reliability including internal consistency and validity as a screening device. Its usefulness as a screening device is greatly increased by the substantial norming data collected by Rescorla.

The most fully developed parent report measures for language (through 1996) are the MacArthur Communicative Development Inventories (Fenson et al., 1993). Unlike the screening measures just described, the primary purpose of which is to discriminate children at the lower percentile levels, the CDI questionnaires are designed to measure language development across the full range of ability levels. In addition, they evaluate dimensions of communicative development beyond expressive vocabulary.

The MacArthur inventories evolved from the work of Bates and her colleagues, during a period of 20 years, from relatively free-form interviews with parents through structured interviews to orally presented structured checklists to a self-administered checklist format, which in turn passed through several phases of revision. (See Fenson et al. [1994] for information on the earlier development of these measures.) Each phase of revision incorporated the results of previous studies; the revisions also represented a movement away from reliance on recall, elicited through open-ended questions, toward reliance on recognition memory. This continuing research effort was motivated by a series of findings that demonstrated the concurrent and predictive validity of parent report measures. For example, Bates et al. (1988) observed significant predictive correlations from a parent report vocabulary checklist at 20 months and both vocabulary ($r = .64$) and MLU ($r = .83$) measures obtained at 28 months.

The MacArthur inventories are a pair of measures: the MacArthur Communicative Development Inventories: Words and Gestures (MCDI:WG) for children at developmental levels between 8 and 16 months and the MacArthur Communicative Development Inventories: Words and Sentences (MCDI:WS) for children at developmental levels between 16 and 30 months. (The two forms originally were named CDI: Infants and CDI: Toddlers; because many professionals using the forms with older children with developmental delay found these titles to be awkward, the forms were renamed.) The major components of the MCDI:WG are a 396-item vocabulary checklist, organized into 19 semantic categories, and a 63-item list of actions and gestures, organized into five categories. For each word of the vocabulary checklist, parents are asked to check "understands," "understands and says," or "neither." The checklist of actions and gestures includes first communicative gestures (e.g., shakes head "no"), games and routines (e.g., plays pat-a-cake), actions with objects (e.g., blows to indicate something is hot), pretending to be a parent (e.g., feeds a doll or stuffed animal with a spoon), and imitating other adult actions (e.g., puts key in door or lock). These actions are hypothesized to represent important cognitive precursors to communicative development (Bates, Benigni, Bretherton, Camaioni, & Volterra, 1979) and to have diagnostic value for children who are late in developing expressive language (Thal & Tobias, 1994).

The major components of the MCDI:WS are a 680-item vocabulary checklist organized into 22 semantic categories, a 37-item list of forced-choice sentence pairs of the form discussed in the previous section (e.g., *that my truck* versus *that's my truck*), and, following Rescorla (1989), a request for the three longest sentences that the parent has heard recently. Both the MCDI:WG and the MCDI:WS contain a number of more minor sections focused on, for example, comprehension of familiar phrases in the MCDI:WG and production of irregular forms such as *flew, mans,* and *taked* in the MCDI:WS. These sections were included for specific research purposes; the discussion in this chapter is on the major components with the greatest demonstrated reliability and validity.

The norming study for the MacArthur inventories represents a uniquely large sample study of more than 1,800 children. A minimum of 30 males and 30 females were included at each age level (month). Children with serious health problems or extensive exposure to a language other than English were excluded from the study. The sample included a wide socioeconomic range, although it is heavily weighted toward the middle class. The study also included a second completion of the inventory approximately 6 weeks later for 500 children and approximately 6.5 weeks later for a different set of 503 children. The major measures listed previously have impressive internal consistency and test–retest reliability. One major substantive finding of the norming study was the enormous variability on virtually every measure of the inventories, a variability that was not substantially correlated with sex, birth order, or social class (see Fenson et al., 1994).

It is the concurrent *validity* of any particular parent report measure that will be of the greatest interest to most readers. Chapter IV of Fenson et al. (1994) summarizes numerous studies that have compared MCDI measures (and very similar measures from precursor versions of the MCDI) with either structured tests or measures derived from language samples. The MCDI expressive vocabulary measures correlate at levels between .40 and .80 with direct measures, with the highest correlations occurring for the two most valid and specific among the criterion measures: observed vocabulary and Expressive One-Word Picture Vocabulary Test (EOWPVT) (Gardner, 1979). Both MCDI grammatical measures (the 37-item forced-choice sentence pairs and the three longest sentence examples) are very highly correlated (r between .74 and .88) with language sample MLU. Fewer studies have been conducted on the validity of the gestures scale, but several studies have demonstrated that infants selected for high or low scores on total gestures are reliably different on laboratory measures of imitation, symbolic play, and vocabulary comprehension.

As Tomasello and Mervis (1993) have pointed out, for the youngest children, especially the 8- to 10-month-olds, the vocabulary comprehension scores reported by parents are surprisingly high, with a median of 15–25 and some scores much higher. Although these vocabulary scores do show good internal reliability and predictive validity and although children do appear to be increasing their understanding of language during this period, the actual numbers seem somewhat implausible. Tomasello and Mervis suggested that this is a result of a lack of clarity in the term "understands" on the part of parents of children at this young age, that caution be used in interpreting such comprehension scores in any absolute way, and that additional explanation of the term "understands" be given.

It should be noted that a major limitation in evaluating any new measure of language development for very young children is the absence of fully satisfactory criterion measures. Both structured tests and language sample measures have their own limitations of reliability and validity, which can depress validity correlations with the new parent report measures. For example, the reliability of MLU has been estimated to be approximately .80–.85 (Dale, 1991). That the validity correlations are in this range means that the parent report measure of grammatical development predicts *all* of the reliable variance in the language sample measure, and it is entirely possible that the parent report measure is *more* reliable and valid than the language sample measure. A similar argument is made in Dale (1991) concerning vocabulary measures. The EOWPVT is primarily a measure of concrete noun vocabulary, whereas the vocabulary observed in a relatively brief (e.g., 30-minute) language sample will be particularly sensitive to high-frequency words. Thus, each of these criterion measures may index only a portion of the child's semantic knowledge. The multiple correlation between these *two* criterion measures and children's vocabulary scores on the MCDI:WS was higher (.79) than either of the two simple correlations. A multiple regression analysis confirmed that each criterion measure was related to a distinct, significant portion of the variance in MCDI:WS vocabulary. The vocabulary checklist, then, appears to assess a broader vocabulary range than either the direct observation measure or the structured test, just as expected given that the checklist includes both types of words.

There is a second kind of evidence of the validity of parent report, even for such an apparently esoteric area as grammar. There is a remarkable consistency between the developmental trends in the parent report data and the results of research on child language development, which most parents are unlikely to have read. Parents, collectively, report that the progressive -*ing* and plural -*s* are produced before the past tense -*ed,* that overregularizations such as *comed* and *goed* do not occur until after common irregular forms such as *came* and *went,* and that certain word endings are learned before function words such as prepositions and auxiliaries. Furthermore, the ages at which various important milestones occur, such as combining words, generally are consistent with previous research.

As encouraging as the results just described are, the validity of parent report instruments, which were developed for assessing typically developing children, cannot simply be assumed to apply to children with developmental disabilities (Miller, Sedey, & Miolo, 1995). Can parents with children performing below typical levels provide equally valid information? Some disabilities such as Down syndrome are diagnosed shortly after birth; knowledge of this condition may limit parents' expectations of their children's development, which in turn may lead to underestimating the child. Conversely, both parental bias and a lack of experience with typically developing children might lead to overestimation. For other conditions, such as specific language impairment (SLI), which are not diagnosed until later, parents may find it difficult to acknowledge delays.

The available research on this question with respect to general developmental measures is highly inconsistent (Diamond & Squires, 1993), with perhaps a bit more evidence of overestimation of abilities than of the other possibilities (e.g., Hunt & Paraskevopoulos, 1980). The findings for the assessment of language, however, are much more encouraging. O'Hanlon and Thal (1991; summarized in Fenson et al., 1993) reported a correlation of .85 between vocabulary scores obtained on the CDI and EOWPVT scores for a sample of 20 children with language impairment between 39 and 49 months and a correlation of .62 between the sentence complexity measure from the CDI and MLU obtained in a 30-minute language sample. Miller et al. (1995) have reported both concurrent and predictive validity of the CDI for children with Down syndrome and for typically developing children at the mental age of approximately 18 months. Parent report vocabulary was highly correlated with both language sample vocabulary

(.82) and an expressive language subscale derived from the Bayley Scales of Infant Development (.77) for the children with Down syndrome. In fact, the correlations were slightly higher for the group with Down syndrome than for the typically developing comparison group (.75 and .70 for the two criterion measures, respectively). Similarly, there was a substantial predictive correlation for the children with Down syndrome between the first parent report and later laboratory measures obtained when the children were at the mental age of approximately 28 months; for language sample vocabulary and the expressive language measure derived from the Bayley, the correlations were .65 and .51, respectively. Although more research is greatly needed, especially with a wider variety of clinical populations, these results are highly encouraging. Also needed is research evaluating parent report of alternative communication modalities, such as sign and graphic symbol systems (Miller et al., 1995).

APPLICATIONS OF PARENT REPORT IN RESEARCH AND CLINICAL PRACTICE

Clinical Applications

The high validity of measures such as the MacArthur inventories is a *group* statistic. An individual parent may misunderstand the instructions or misperceive or misreport the child's language. Hence, it is essential that decisions concerning the diagnosis or treatment of a given child be corroborated by a home or clinic assessment. Conversely, the same caution is appropriate for home or clinic assessments; an independent confirmation is essential, given each child's unique response to observation, strange environments, and structured testing. A parent report measure is ideal for this purpose.

When adequate norms are available, a parent report measure can produce quantitatively defined profiles of different aspects of early language. These profiles have a number of different applications. One such application is screening for delayed language. Several research projects (e.g., Rescorla, 1989) have converged on a "rule of thumb" that children who are producing fewer than 50 words or who are not yet combining words at 24 months are at risk for language impairment. Both of these criteria represent the lowest 10% of the distribution, based on the norming sample for the MCDI:WS. Further research is needed to determine whether performance in the lowest 10% prior to 24 months also is diagnostic of impairment, but there is some evidence that a combination of low expressive vocabulary *and* a low gesture score does represent a higher risk for problems.

As the previous example demonstrates, comparing individual patterns of strengths and weaknesses may be especially revealing. Generally, the various measures in each of the MacArthur inventories are moderately correlated (see Fenson et al., 1994, for a detailed discussion of the significance of these correlations), but considerable variation frequently occurs and may be entirely typical.

Extreme discrepancies between vocabulary comprehension and production or between language and gesture, however, may identify a child as being at risk. It also may be useful to examine patterns of strengths and weaknesses across different aspects of communication while holding overall language level constant. For example, Bates et al. (1994) compared the composition of vocabulary among children at the same overall vocabulary size. This made it possible to characterize children as being especially high or low in nominals (they provide a table for this purpose). Similarly, it is possible to determine whether a given child is unusually high or low in comprehension and/or gesture and/or grammar compared with other children at the same level of expressive vocabulary. This information may have considerable predictive significance.

The development of individual profiles also can be useful in identifying aspects of a child's communicative skills to be targeted for intervention. These may include broad domains such as vocabulary production or more specific ones such as particular semantic or syntactic categories. Furthermore, as discussed previously, parent report measures are especially valuable in evaluating treatment effects, as they are based on a variety of contexts outside of the clinic or laboratory.

A long-standing concern in the use of parent report is the interpretation of discrepancies between parental information about their children and professional assessments. As noted previously, there has been a bias toward interpreting such discrepancies—especially when the parental report measure is higher than the direct measure—as evidence of the lack of validity of parent report. As thoughtful observers such as Diamond and Squires (1993) have noted, it is equally possible that professional assessments underestimate the capabilities of young children, particularly those with disabilities. Specific skills may not be demonstrated during the brief course of a language sample collected under unfamiliar circumstances or during a single administration of a structured test. In a study of specific infant behaviors, Hagekull, Bohlin, and Lindhagen (1984) found that parent–observer agreement was higher when the professional observer had the opportunity to observe the infant's behavior over a longer time period. In other words, the initial discrepancy (based on a shorter observational interval) reflected an underestimation of the infant on the part of the observer. It is probably true that cases of extreme discrepancy suggest a problem with one or both of the measures being compared. Moderate disagreement, however, may well serve to identify areas in which a skill is newly emerging, and the child can demonstrate it under certain conditions without yet being able to generalize the skill to a wide range of environments (Diamond & Squires, 1993).

Research Applications

The ease of use and substantial validity of parent report measures make possible a global assessment of language for larger samples of children than was previously possible. This capability has many research applications. One is the screening and preselection of children at different levels of development. Researchers often are interested in studying children who are at a specific point in the process of language acquisition. Rather than selecting a specific age and "hoping for the best," it is possible to use a parent report measure to screen a large number of children and select a sample that meets the desired criterion, such as a 50-word vocabulary but not yet combining words.

Similarly, parent report measures can be used to identify children with particular language characteristics or unusual profiles, for example, "late talkers" (Rescorla, 1989; Thal & Tobias, 1994), "linguistically precocious" children (Dale et al., 1989), children whose comprehension far exceeds their production (Bates, Dale, & Thal, 1995), children who are reported to gesture extensively despite language delays, or children who are surprisingly slow to produce word combinations despite their vocabulary level. These special categories of children often are highly relevant for studying specific hypotheses about the acquisition of language.

As discussed previously, the ability to assess the language of large samples of children makes it possible to examine the influence of a wide variety of other variables, such as family size, birth order, child-rearing practices, parental style, use of child care, and other factors that may be substantially intercorrelated among themselves. In addition, parent report measures may be highly useful in experimental designs. The power and validity of an experimental investigation of a specific environmental feature or intervention program is greatly increased when the groups initially are equivalent in communicative skills. Parent report measures can be used to ensure this equivalence prior to the treatment.

"BOUNDARY CONDITIONS" FOR USING PARENT REPORT

No single assessment instrument can be expected to be practical and valid under all conditions. This section considers factors that may make parent report more or less valid; that is, the possible "boundary conditions" for its effective use. Diamond and Squires (1993) provided a comprehensive review of family, child, and task characteristics that may influence parent report across a wide spectrum of developmental domains. This section focuses on parental, child, and cultural factors that may affect assessment of communication skills by parent report.

As Diamond and Squires (1993) pointed out, studies of the relationship between social class and the validity of parent report have produced inconsistent findings. Several studies (e.g., Eisert, Spector, Shankaran, Faigenbaum, & Szego, 1980) have obtained equally valid developmental information from parents of high and low socioeconomic status (SES). In Dale's (1991) evaluation of the validity of the MacArthur Communicative Development Inventories, there was no correlation between SES (assessed as maternal education) and the difference between parent report and laboratory measures of language development. In contrast, Frankenburg, Coons, and Ker (1982) obtained more reliable information from parents with a high school degree than from parents without a high school degree. It seems likely that there is a minimum level of interests and skills necessary for effective parent report, and a first estimate of this level may coincide with the distinction between completing versus not completing a high school education. It should be noted that university-based research projects, such as Dale's (1991), typically recruit few parents at the extreme low end of parental education, whereas field-based studies of high-risk children are more likely to do so. It remains an open question, however, whether any limitations that are observed are a result of less-accurate monitoring of children by low-education parents or of the difficulty of working with a printed questionnaire. A number of research projects have found that parent report questionnaires can be administered as interviews in person or by telephone with good results. For example, Toth (personal communication, February 1996) found that parents of children prenatally exposed to cocaine and other drugs provided, via a telephone interview when the children were 21 months old, information about their children's language that was highly correlated with laboratory measures of children at 24 months. These findings suggest that the knowledge base for valid parent report is available for the great majority of parents, although literacy issues may sometimes serve as a barrier.

A second potential source of boundary conditions is child characteristics, including age, gender, and developmental disability. Interestingly, there is some evidence (Diamond & Squires, 1993) that parental accuracy is higher during the preschool period than during either infancy or the school years. Such a finding, if reliably observed, is expected because the skills typically developed between 18 months and 5 years are more observable than are the perceptual and cognitive skills of infancy and are exhibited across more of the child's daily life than are the cognitive developments of the school years. Furthermore, the developments during this period include language, the most public of cognitive abilities; and even those skills that are not directly linguistic (e.g., memory skills) are exhibited through language. The possible influence of gender of child on parental reporting accuracy has yet to be investigated. As discussed in the section "Examples of Successful Parent Report Measures," in the domain of language development, parent report measures appear to be equally appropriate for children with disabilities such as Down syndrome and SLI as for typically developing children.

The greatest need for information, however, concerns the potential role of cultural differences in affecting parent report. This topic takes on a special significance in light of the changing demographics of American families. More than one third of the children born in the United States are born to linguistically and culturally diverse families, and it has been estimated that by the year 2000 more than one third of all children under 18 will be members of non-Caucasian or non-Anglo groups. Hanson, Lynch, and Wayman (1990) have provided a thoughtful and comprehensive review of the influences of cultural histories, values, and beliefs on parental participation in the assessment process. These include differences in views of children and child rearing, views of disabilities and their causes, and views of medicine and healing. Differences in language and communication styles also are widely known. They are not limited to formal, structural differences in language but include differences in the patterns of use in language, such as a preference for high-context communication in which situational cues and shared knowledge play a major role versus low-context cultures, which prefer direct messages and tend to rely more on what is said than on what is left unsaid. Similarly, in some cultures, asking questions is a sign of linguistic independence and self-expression, whereas in others it may be interpreted as a challenge of another person's knowledge and authority. How these differences might affect parental attending to and reporting on children's language is in much need of investigation, as is the development of culturally sensitive ways to use parental knowledge optimally. It is likely that an interview format will be useful in many situations in which a low-context printed questionnaire is not. In the meantime, the suggestions of Hanson et al. (1990) for early interventionists are well worth considering:

> First, they must clarify their own values and assumptions. Second, they must gather and analyze ethnographic information regarding the cultural community within which each family resides. Third, they must determine the degree to which the family operates transculturally [is comfortable in both cultures, in the mainstream culture only, or in the original culture only]; and finally, they must examine each family's orientation to specific childrearing issues. (p. 126)

PROMISING DIRECTIONS FOR PARENT REPORT MEASURES

The most highly developed parent report measures for language and communication have focused on vocabulary, grammar, and limited aspects of pragmatics. This section considers some promising directions for parent report measures for both research and clinical practice. Yet another advantage of parent report measures is that they do not require elaborate equipment or expertise for their development. Thus, researchers and practitioners can develop measures appropriate for their needs. Nevertheless, the challenges of developing such measures and the amount of effort required should not be underestimated. Several cycles of revision, piloting, and analysis are essential to produce a measure that is clear to parents; contains items that are appropriate for the domain of interest; and has appropriate psychometric properties of internal consistency, age and population discrimination, and concurrent validity. It is better to develop the first version or two on a small scale, seeking feedback from a modest number of parents and other professionals, before proceeding to a larger-scale norming study. Many of the suggestions in the next section for adapting measures for other languages are equally relevant for developing measures for new aspects of language and communication.

Adaptations for Other Languages

The validity and efficiency of the MacArthur Communicative Development Inventories have led several research groups to develop similar measures for other languages. Versions of the CDI have been developed, and normative data have been collected for Italian (Caselli, Casadio, & Sanders, 1993), Spanish (Jackson-Maldonado, Thal, Bates, Marchman, & Gutierrez-Clellen, 1993), Japanese (Ogura, Yamashita, Murase, & Dale, 1993), and American Sign Language (Reilly, Provine, & Bellugi, 1993). Adaptations are being developed in a number of other languages, including Hebrew, Chinese, Korean, Swedish, and Finnish. These adaptations are motivated by both clinical and research needs. The increasing number of Spanish-speaking children in the United States gives the Spanish adaptation a special clinical significance. The identification, diagnosis, and remediation of language disorders must rest on an accurate characterization of the range of typical variation. Investigating individual differences necessarily requires large samples of children; parent report is ideally suited for this purpose.

Cross-linguistic comparisons of language acquisition have constituted a particularly illuminating kind of research on the processes and mechanisms underlying language development. The extent to which the early phases of language development remain similar or diverge in languages with differing structure provides crucial evidence for the existence and nature of basic operating principles of language development (Slobin, 1985). Yet a comparison of two or three children acquiring one language with an equally small sample of children acquiring a different language can have only limited interpretability in the absence of information about variability among children acquiring those languages. An apparently large contrast between the two groups may simply reflect sampling fluctuation; alternatively, a genuine difference may be obscured by sampling variation in the opposite direction. The benefits of large samples and the utility of parent report are thus as important for research as for clinical issues.

It is important to note that each of these versions is an *adaptation* of the CDI, not just a simple translation (Dale, Fenson, & Thal, 1993). Languages and cultures differ substantially in both the form and the content of their communication systems, and there is every reason to believe that even in the earliest phases of development, differences in gestural communication, vocabulary, and grammar will be noticeable. For example, Ogura et al. (1993) included bowing as an early emerging gesture, while Jackson-Maldonado et al. (1993) included *tortillitas* (little tortillas), a variant of the pat-a-cake game that is played in Mexico.

As Dale et al. (1993) pointed out, it generally is most effective in developing a parent report tool to begin with a more open-ended format in which parents are invited to list additional words, gestures, and even sentences. In this way, a more inclusive list of potential items appropriate for the widest variety of young children in the linguistic community of interest can be generated. Feedback from parents can be used to clarify instructions and modify the instrument. Information from language samples also can be useful for identifying possible additions. Later in the development process, it is important to shift to the checklist (recognition) formation for the collection of norms in order to remove the variance that would otherwise be introduced by parental reporting style and recall abilities.

Semantic Development

Existing parent report measures of vocabulary ask only whether the word is in the child's expressive vocabulary or whether the child appears to understand the word. It is well-established that words may enter a child's vocabulary with meanings that are related but somewhat distinct from the meaning of the word in the adult language (e.g., the familiar phenomena of over- and underextension [Clark, 1987], confusion of related words [Bowerman, 1978]). Although structured experiments and tests based on a brief sample of the child's behavior often are useful, much of the most illuminating research on early semantic development has been conducted by parent-scientists such as Bowerman, who can draw on a rich store of linguistic experience.

Gopnik and Meltzoff (1993) have used a combination of recognition and recall techniques to investigate semantic development in a set of words hypothesized (and demonstrated) to be closely linked to specific aspects of cognition. Gopnik and Meltzoff hypothesized that different words would be used by children to express the same concept. Their "Early Language Questionnaire" (Gopnik & Meltzoff, n.d.) asks about 13 particular situations: when something disappears, when the child tries to do something and fails, when a child refuses suggestions, when the child wants more of something, and so forth. The parent is asked to supply the word and three examples of its use. The general instructions for the questionnaire are a model of clarity:

> Sometimes different children will use the same word in different ways. We have listed a variety of common ways that children use early words. We want to know whether your child uses a word consistently and spontaneously in any of these ways. Next to most of the uses is an example of a particular word that is often used in this way. For example, many children use "no" to refuse suggestions. But your child may use some other word. Please tell us which word in particular your child uses. We would like at least three specific examples of situations in which your child has used this word.

The general approach taken here—providing very specific examples of situations and contexts to communicate the general concept to parents and then requiring specific examples from the child being assessed for analysis—has considerable potential for many aspects of semantic development, such as the semantics of time, dimensionality, and evaluation. It is likely that such research would reveal that children with specific forms of language impairment have special difficulty in particular areas, along the lines of recent research that has demonstrated that children with autism have special difficulty with words that refer to mental state, such as *think* and *know,* consistent with a hypothesized cognitive limitation in "theory of mind" (Tager-Flusberg, 1992).

Prelinguistic Vocalizations

Accurately perceiving and analyzing speech is one of the most difficult skills even for professionals to acquire. For this reason, aspects of phonology—the sound system of language—rarely have been included in parent report measures. Even in this arena, parent report sometimes can play a role. In a longitudinal study of prelinguistic and early linguistic development, Stoel-Gammon (1989) wanted to record and analyze prelinguistic vocalizations at the beginning of the stage of "canonical babbling," which is characterized by alternating consonants and vowels integrated into syllables (e.g., [dada], [gugu]). The onset of canonical babbling has considerable age variability; therefore, parents were asked to watch for its emergence and to contact the researchers to schedule an appointment when it occurred. During a laboratory visit at 5 months, prior to this stage, parents were played a tape of some good examples of canonical babbling and asked to listen for "something similar." Later laboratory visits generally confirmed the accuracy of the parents' judgment that canonical babbling had begun.

Politeness Forms and Other Aspects of Pragmatics

As discussed previously, a major advantage of parent report is that it can overcome the pragmatic limitations of structured tests and naturalistic observation. The questions asked on a test have answers that are already known by the examiner; this fact generally is clear to the child being tested. These "public test questions" are thus pragmatically highly constrained, and performance on them may not be representative of spontaneous language in other settings. Although naturalistic observation is an improvement in this respect, the setting of mother–child free play in an unfamiliar setting also is unlikely to elicit a wide range of pragmatic intents. Nowhere is this constraint more of a problem than in the assessment of pragmatic abilities themselves, such as the use of politeness forms for specific speech acts, discourse maintenance skills, and interpersonal negotiating skills such as playing with a friend.

A few parent report items focused on pragmatic skills are included in available instruments (e.g., listens to a story for 5 minutes, delivers a simple message, says *please* when asking for something). This potentially is an area of great fruitfulness for developing measures. Can parents accurately report on their children's use of language for a variety of pragmatic functions such as announcing an impending action or denying the truth of another person's statement? What about the emergence of polite forms of requests (e.g., "Can I...?") or the ability to stay on topic in a conversation? The wording of these items will be crucial, as one major question is whether forms are used spontaneously, at least under certain circumstances, or only when prompted.

Metalinguistic Abilities and Emergent Literacy

Literacy skills are central to educational achievement. Research has convincingly demonstrated that the process that leads to effective reading and writing begins long before formal instruction in elementary school. Among the foundational skills for reading is the set of abilities known as *metalinguistic abilities,* or awareness, which includes the ability to recognize and manipulate words, syllables, and individual sounds as units. For example, a commonly used phonological awareness task is phoneme deletion: "Say *cat* without the [k]." Secret codes such as pig Latin require a high degree of phonological awareness. A second set of foundational skills is known as *concepts of print:* recognizing that it is the letters and not the pictures that tell the story, that letters proceed from left to right and from top to bottom, and so forth.

Questions about early reading and writing abilities sometimes are included in broad-range parent report measures. Following are some unpublished data from a longitudinal study of children selected for linguistic precocity at 20 months (Crain-Thoreson & Dale, 1992; Robinson, Dale, & Landesman, 1990). When the children were 4½ years of age, parents completed a questionnaire about their child's abilities and interests. A measure of the child's reading was obtained using a recognition-like format: recognizes most letters, reads at least three common signs, reads at least 10 words, tries to sound out new words, looks at book on own initiative, and reads on own initiative. A similar measure for writing was obtained using a list of three questions: prints or writes own name, prints or writes words on drawings, and prints or writes short notes or messages. The parental measure of early reading was significantly correlated ($r = .49$) with the child's score on the reading portion of the Peabody Individual Achievement Test (Dunn & Markwardt, 1970), whereas the parent measure of early writing was not significantly correlated. Both measures were significantly correlated ($r = .53$) with an invented spelling task, in which the child was asked to guess how the word might be spelled; partial credit was given for spellings that captured some of the word's pronunciation. Parental evaluation of their children's reading and writing abilities were not simply the reflection of a global assessment; neither rating was correlated with the Wechsler Preschool and Primary Scale of Intelligence–Revised (WPPSI–R) (Wechsler, 1989) Information subtest, a general measure of verbal intelligence.

Parents also appeared to be sensitive to some aspects of their child's developing metalinguistic abilities. The questionnaire included two open-ended questions about the child's language:

1. Do you feel your child's language is still exceptional? Can you describe particular abilities or incidents which typify his/her strongest language abilities?
2. Does your child show an interest in "playing" with language, for example, by making up or using secret codes (Pig Latin, etc.) or talking about words, or making jokes about words and their sounds?

Parents' responses to these questions were coded for mention of phonologically oriented activities such as rhyming, alliteration, and making up nonsense words by playing with sound and for mention of semantically oriented activities such as commenting on ambiguity and similarities of word meaning. (The two were not mutually exclusive.) Despite the informality of this technique and the use of recall rather than recognition, report of phonologically oriented activities was significantly related to a test of phoneme deletion and to invented spelling scores, whereas mention of semantically oriented activities was not related. These and other results suggest that effective parent report measures could be developed for aspects of emergent literacy, including metalinguistic awareness.

CONCLUSION

It is not the claim of this chapter that parent report is a panacea for the difficulties of assessing young children. Parent report is not effective for every family or for every aspect of language. Nevertheless, it is a tool that has been greatly undervalued in the past. With careful attention to the best way of drawing on the extensive experience of a parent with a child, it can be unsurpassed as a practical and effective source of information on individual children and for very large samples as well. For both clinical and research applications, it is a valuable complement to direct professional assessment.

Parent report instruments can translate the results of focused, small-sample research studies into a more widely usable assessment instrument. Conversely, the kind of normative information available from parent report can serve as a yardstick, a baseline that permits assessment of extreme variations from the mean and the variations that are associated with particular environmental conditions or biological facts. These quantitative frameworks can then facilitate identifying children with specific developmental profiles for further study with more traditional, intensive direct methods. For a truly adequate repertoire of assessment techniques, the whole should be greater than the sum of the parts. Parent report has the potential to play such a role.

REFERENCES

Bar-Adon, A., & Leopold, W.F. (Eds.). (1971). *Child language: A book of readings.* Englewood Cliffs, NJ: Prentice Hall.

Bates, E., Benigni, L., Bretherton, I., Camaioni, L., & Volterra, V. (1979). *The emergence of symbols: Cognition and communication in infancy.* New York: Academic Press.

Bates, E., Bretherton, I., & Snyder, L. (1988). *From first words to grammar: Individual differences and dissociable mechanisms.* New York: Cambridge University Press.

Bates, E., Dale, P.S., & Thal, D. (1995). Individual differences and their implications for theories of language development. In P. Fletcher & B. MacWhinney (Eds.), *Handbook of child language* (pp. 96–151). Oxford, England: Basil Blackwell.

Bates, E., Marchman, V., Thal, D., Fenson, L., Dale, P.S., Reznick, J.S., Reilly, J., & Hartung, J.P. (1994). Developmental and stylistic variation in the composition of early vocabulary. *Journal of Child Language, 21,* 85–124.

Bayley, N. (1969). *Bayley Scales of Infant Development.* New York: The Psychological Corporation.

Bowerman, M. (1978). Systematizing semantic knowledge: Changes over time in the child's organization of word meaning. *Child Development, 49,* 977–987.

Bzoch, K.R., & League, R. (1994). *Receptive-Expressive Emergent Language Scale* (2nd ed.). Austin, TX: PRO-ED.

Capute, A., Palmer, F., Shapiro, B., Wachtel, R., Schmidt, S., & Ross, A. (1986). Clinical Linguistic and Auditory Milestones Scale: Prediction of cognition in infancy. *Developmental Medicine and Child Neurology, 28,* 762–771.

Caselli, M.C., Casadio, P., & Sanders, L. (1993, July). *A parent report study of lexical and grammatical development in Italian.* Paper presented at the Sixth International Congress for the Study of Child Language, Trieste, Italy.

Clark, E. (1987). The principle of contrast: A constraint on language acquisition. In B. MacWhinney (Ed.), *Mechanisms of language acquisition* (pp. 1–33). Hillsdale, NJ: Lawrence Erlbaum Associates.

Crain-Thoreson, C., & Dale, P.S. (1992). Do early talkers become early readers? Linguistic precocity, preschool language, and emergent literacy. *Developmental Psychology, 28,* 421–429.

Dale, P.S. (1991). The validity of a parent report measure of vocabulary and syntax at 24 months. *Journal of Speech and Hearing Research, 34,* 565–571.

Dale, P.S., Bates, E., Reznick, J.S., & Morisset, C. (1989). The validity of a parent report instrument of child language at twenty months. *Journal of Child Language, 16,* 239–249.

Dale, P.S., Fenson, L., & Thal, D. (1993). *Some suggestions for the adaptation of the MacArthur Communicative Development Inventories to additional languages.* Unpublished manuscript, University of Washington, Seattle,

Diamond, K.E., & Squires, J. (1993). The role of parental report in the screening and assessment of young children. *Journal of Early Intervention, 17,* 107–115.

Dromi, E. (1987). *Early lexical development.* New York: Cambridge University Press.

Dunn, L., & Markwardt, F.C., Jr. (1970). *Peabody Individual Achievement Test.* Circle Pines, MN: American Guidance Service.

Education of the Handicapped Act Amendments of 1986, PL 99-457, 20 U.S.C. § 1400 *et seq.*

Eisert, D., Spector, S., Shankaran, S., Faigenbaum, D., & Szego, E. (1980). Mothers' reports of their low birth weight infants' subsequent development on the Minnesota Child Development Inventory. *Journal of Pediatric Psychology, 5,* 353–364.

Fenson, L., Dale, P.S., Reznick, J.S., Bates, E., Thal, D.J., & Pethick, S.J. (1994). Variability in early communicative development. *Monographs of the Society for Research in Child Development, 59* (5, Serial No. 242).

Fenson, L., Dale, P.S., Reznick, J.S., Thal, D., Bates, E., Hartung, J.P., Pethick, S., & Reilly, J.S. (1993). *MacArthur Communicative Development Inventories* (CDI). San Diego: Singular.

Frackowiak, R.S. (1994). Functional mapping of verbal memory and language. *Trends in Neurosciences, 17,* 109–115.

Frankenburg, W., Coons, C., & Ker, C. (1982). Screening infants and preschoolers to identify school learning problems. In E. Edgar, N. Haring, J. Jenkins, & C. Pious (Eds.), *Mentally handicapped children* (pp. 11–28). Baltimore: University Park Press.

Frankenburg, W.K., & Dodds, J.B. (1990). *The Denver Developmental Screening Test.* Denver: University of Colorado Medical Center.

Gardner, M.F. (1979). *Expressive One-Word Picture Vocabulary Test.* Novato, CA: Academic Therapy Publications.

Golinkoff, R., Hirsh-Pasek, K., Cauley, K., & Gordon, L. (1987). The eyes have it: Lexical and syntactic comprehension in a new paradigm. *Journal of Child Language, 14,* 23–45.

Gopnik, A., & Meltzoff, A. (1993). Words and thoughts in infancy: The specificity hypothesis and the development of categorization. In C. Rovee-Collier & L. Lipsitt (Eds.), *Advances in infancy research* (Vol. 8, pp. 217–249). Norwood, NJ: Ablex.

Gopnik, A., & Meltzoff, A. (n.d.). *Early language questionnaire*. Unpublished manuscript.

Hagekull, B., Bohlin, G., & Lindhagen, K. (1984). Validity of parent reports. *Infant Behavior and Development, 7*, 77–92.

Hanson, M.J., Lynch, E.W., & Wayman, K.I. (1990). Honoring the cultural diversity of families when gathering data. *Topics in Early Childhood Education, 10*, 112–131.

Hunt, J. McV., & Paraskevopoulos, J. (1980). Children's psychological development as a function of the inaccuracy of their mothers' knowledge of their abilities. *Journal of Genetic Psychology, 136*, 285–298.

Ireton, H. (1992). *Child Development Inventory Manual*. Minneapolis, MN: Behavior Science Systems.

Ireton, H., & Thwing, E. (1974). *The Minnesota Child Development Inventory*. Minneapolis: Behavior Science Systems.

Jackson-Maldonado, D., Thal, D., Bates, E., Marchman, V., & Gutierrez-Clellen, V. (1993). Early lexical development of Spanish-speaking infants and toddlers. *Journal of Child Language, 20*, 523–549.

MacWhinney, B. (1995). *The CHILDES Project: Tools for Analyzing Talk*. Hillsdale, NJ: Lawrence Erlbaum Associates.

McCarthy, D. (1972). *McCarthy Scales of Children's Abilities*. San Antonio, TX: The Psychological Corporation.

Miller, J.F., Sedey, A.L., & Miolo, G. (1995). Validity of parent report measures of vocabulary development for children with Down syndrome. *Journal of Speech and Hearing Research, 38*, 1037–1044.

Ogura, T., Yamashita, Y., Murase, T., & Dale, P.S. (1993, July). *Some preliminary findings from the Japanese Early Communicative Inventory*. Paper presented at the Sixth International Congress for the Study of Child Language, Trieste, Italy.

O'Hanlon, L., & Thal, D. (1991, November). *MacArthur Communicative Development Inventory: Toddlers—Validation for language impaired children*. Poster presented at the annual meeting of the American Speech-Language-Hearing Association, Atlanta, GA.

Osterhout, L., & Holcomb, P.J. (1995). Event-related potentials and language comprehension. In M.D. Rugg & M.G.H. Coles (Eds.), *Electrophysiology of mind: Event-related brain potentials and cognition* (pp. 171–216). Oxford, England: Oxford University Press.

Peterson, S., Fox, P.T., Posner, M.I., Mintun, M.A., & Raichle, M.E. (1988). Positron emission tomographic studies of the cortical anatomy of single word processing. *Nature, 331*, 585–589.

Reilly, J.S., Provine, K., & Bellugi, U. (1993, July). *Does modality affect lexical development: Parent report data on the emergence of American Sign Language*. Paper presented at the Sixth International Congress for the Study of Child Language, Trieste, Italy.

Rescorla, L. (1989). The Language Development Survey: A screening tool for delayed language in toddlers. *Journal of Speech and Hearing Disorders, 54*, 587–599.

Robinson, N.M., Dale, P.S., & Landesman, S. (1990). Validity of the Stanford-Binet IV with linguistically precocious toddlers. *Intelligence, 14*, 173–186.

Slobin, D.I. (1985). *The cross-linguistic study of language acquisition* (Vols. 1, 2). Hillsdale, NJ: Lawrence Erlbaum Associates.

Sparrow, S.S., Balla, D.A., & Cicchetti, D.V. (1984). *Vineland Adaptive Behavior Scales*. Circle Pines, MN: American Guidance Service.

Stoel-Gammon, C. (1989, May). *From babbling to speech: Some new evidence*. Paper presented at the Child Phonology Conference, Evanston, IL.

Tager-Flusberg, H. (1992). Autistic children's talk about psychological states: Deficits in the early acquisition of a theory of mind. *Child Development, 63,* 161–172.

Thal, D., & Tobias, S. (1994). Relationships between language and gesture in normally developing and late-talking toddlers. *Journal of Speech and Hearing Research, 37,* 157–170.

Tomasello, M. (1992). *First verbs: A case study of early grammatical development.* New York: Cambridge University Press.

Tomasello, M., & Mervis, C.B. (1994). Commentary: The instrument is great, but measuring comprehension is still a problem. *Monographs of the Society for Research in Child Development, 59* (5, Serial No. 242).

Tomblin, J.B., Schonrock, C., & Hardy, J. (1989). The concurrent validity of the Minnesota Child Development Inventory as a measure of young children's language development. *Journal of Speech and Hearing Disorders, 54,* 101–105.

Wechsler, D. (1989). *Wechsler Preschool and Primary Scale of Intelligence–Revised.* San Antonio, TX: The Psychological Corporation.

9

"Show Me X"
New Views of an Old Assessment Technique

Mabel L. Rice and Ruth V. Watkins

THE MOTHER OF A 3-YEAR-OLD girl holds her child in her lap as they look at a picture book together. The mother says to her daughter, "Show me the kitty. Where is the kitty?" When the child points to the picture of the kitty, the mother says, "That's right! You know the kitty, don't you?"

A psychologist wants to determine how intelligent children are. Knowing that an important kind of intelligence is the ability to learn new words and that this ability is evident in young children, the psychologist devises a test that consists of showing young children a set of pictures of everyday things. The child is instructed, for example, to "show me kitty." The number of correct responses shows how many words the child knows.

A behavioral scientist studies the ways in which young children come to know the meanings of words like "kitty." The scientist introduces 3-year-old children to novel things with novel names, like "blick." Then the scientist shows a child a set of three pictures—one is a "blick," and two are other novel things that differ from "blick" in carefully specified ways. The scientist says to the child, "Show me blick," and carefully records which picture the child chooses. The child's choice of pictures indicates the ways in which novel things can be interpreted and which novel things go together.

A speech-language pathologist evaluates a 3-year-old girl who does not yet talk very well. It is important to know how much the girl understands of the language she hears. The speech-language pathologist uses a test consisting of a book with four pictures per page and asks the girl, for example, to "show me kangaroo." The pathologist then calculates a test score that will determine whether the child's performance is within the range expected for children her age.

What these scenarios illustrate is that parents, psychologists, behavioral scientists, and speech-language pathologists all rely on the same simple proce-

Preparation of this chapter was supported in part by National Institutes of Health research grant #R01 DC01803 to the first author, #R03 DC02218 to the second author, and #R29 DC00485 to the first author for the studies supported herein.

dure for assessing young children's understanding of words. Binet and Simon, in 1916, advocated this procedure with their now-famous intelligence test:

> One of the best tests upon which to form a judgment [about the intelligence of individuals] is to ask them to designate in a picture the object which one names for them. The test is so much the more to be recommended because it has, for the normal child, the great attraction of curiosity. There is also a great advantage in asking him to point out the objects corresponding to the words which are said to him, rather than to make him name the objects which he himself sees, because of the defects of pronunciation which often prevent him from being understood. (p. 145)

Although "show me X" has long been considered a useful technique for assessing children's word comprehension, the contemporary literature introduces innovative ways of understanding lexical acquisition and language impairments. This chapter examines contemporary developments relevant to the third and fourth scenarios previously described; that is, using "show me X" to learn about the mechanisms and processes of lexical acquisition and to assess children with language impairments. In some ways, the available research is not fully in accordance with the conventional wisdom about this measure. In short, "show me X" has the advantage of ease and familiarity, but it also is a more subtle and complex assessment means than is self-evident.

BACKGROUND

"Show me X" methods for assessing vocabulary comprehension abilities have a long history, dating to at least 1900 (cf. Binet & Simon, 1916; Terman, 1916). Such vocabulary comprehension methods continue to be a component of several measures of intelligence (e.g., Stanford-Binet Intelligence Scale [Thorndike, Hagen, & Sattler, 1986], Kaufman Assessment Battery for Children [Kaufman & Kaufman, 1983]). Furthermore, the picture-identification method of evaluating vocabulary comprehension is a staple of conventional clinical assessment tools. The Peabody Picture Vocabulary Test–Revised (PPVT–R) (Dunn & Dunn, 1981) is the prototype vocabulary comprehension measure; the same basic task is used to assess vocabulary comprehension in a variety of other instruments, including the Receptive One-Word Picture Vocabulary Test (Gardner, 1985), as well as subtests of the Test of Language Development–P:2 (Newcomer & Hammill, 1991) and the Test for Auditory Comprehension of Language–Revised (Carrow-Woolfolk, 1985).

The motivations behind the widespread use of picture-identification methods of evaluating vocabulary comprehension are relatively straightforward. First, assessing vocabulary comprehension addresses the importance of lexical development. Children's comprehension of words is fundamental to children's emerging linguistic system. Understanding the meaning of words is a hallmark indicator of the beginnings of language. At very young ages, the ways in which children quickly learn new word meanings reveal much about the nature of their early lexical development and related cognitive abilities. Beyond the first stages, children's word comprehension serves as an indicator of lexical achievement that is interpretable as one important aspect of general intelligence and as a contributor to children's literacy.

Second, there are methodological advantages to the "show me X" method:

1. As noted by Binet and Simon (1916), the procedure capitalizes on children's inherent interest in looking and pointing; in short, children like to do this activity.
2. Young children often cannot or will not name objects; therefore, the pointing response is easier and probably more accurately elicited, especially for young children. It also is likely that comprehension of a particular word can be evident before a child may be able to say the word, presumably because the necessary phonetic representations for pronunciation may require greater experience with the words (cf. Bates, 1993).
3. Although the picture-identification procedure is suitable for and of interest to very young children, it also is appropriate for older children and adults. This makes it one of the few measures of language ability that can be employed across the life span.
4. Manipulating the foils can reveal much about the basis for a child's judgments about word meanings. Many studies in the contemporary literature have capitalized on this feature to increase what is known about early lexical development.
5. Such tasks can be used to identify children with language impairments, to study their lexical acquisition processes, to determine their relative growth in vocabulary as compared to their age-peers, and to plan for intervention.

This chapter addresses four specific issues: 1) the role of vocabulary comprehension tasks in revealing powerful processes and mechanisms of lexical acquisition; 2) using vocabulary comprehension tasks to detect lexical impairments and to reveal mechanisms of lexical development in children with specific language impairment (SLI); 3) using vocabulary comprehension as a predictor of developmental outcome for children with language impairments, as well as applying lexical comprehension measures to intervention efficacy studies; and 4) interpretive boundaries; that is, some surprising dissociations between vocabulary comprehension abilities and other linguistic skills, as well as limitations in the applicability of particular measures of lexical knowledge. The chapter concludes with a summary of issues in current and future applications of vocabulary comprehension measures in research and clinical contexts.

The main points are these: Just as hammers and screwdrivers are valuable tools in a carpenter's tool kit, so the "show me X" way of assessing vocabulary comprehension is a valuable tool in the armamentarium of researchers and practitioners. It is worthwhile, from time to time, to step back and reconsider the full range of usefulness of such procedures. The literature review and synthesis provided here is intended to yield that reconsideration. Just as hammers and screw-drivers cannot be applied indiscriminately to any woodworking problem, the "show me X" procedure is not without limitations. This chapter identifies some of those limitations and offers caveats where appropriate.

INSIGHTS FROM VOCABULARY COMPREHENSION TASKS ON LANGUAGE ACQUISITION AND IMPAIRMENT

Insights on Language Acquisition

A review of the available research on children's lexical acquisition reveals that vocabulary comprehension tasks play a central role in the study of processes of children's lexical learning. The use of vocabulary comprehension tasks has revealed much about young children's word-learning mechanisms. A large number of investigations have employed both picture-pointing and object-identification methods of measuring comprehension abilities, accompanied by a variety of verbal prompts such as "Where's X," "Find X," "Show me X," or "Point to X" (Carey & Bartlett, 1978; Dollaghan, 1985, 1987; Golinkoff, Mervis, & Hirsh-Pasek, 1994; Rice & Woodsmall, 1988). These studies have identified several powerful lexical acquisition capabilities including fast mapping, quick incidental learning, and mechanisms of word comprehension.

Fast Mapping Investigations of children's lexical comprehension demonstrate that young children can "fast map" new word meanings, forming initial (albeit somewhat sketchy) representations of a new word's meaning. This allows children to quickly build a lexicon of thousands of words by the time they enter school (Carey, 1982). Carey and Bartlett (1978; see also Carey, 1978, 1982) were among the first to document young children's impressive word-learning aptitudes. Carey and Bartlett used a relatively naturalistic vocabulary comprehension task to probe children's ability to learn new words. In this task, an adult presented children with two trays, one of a known color (e.g., red or blue) and the other of an unknown color (e.g., olive green). Children were then told, "Find the chromium tray. Not the red one, the chromium one." The phenomenon observed by Carey and Bartlett is widely recognized. Preschoolers were adept in fast mapping initial properties of a word's meaning from just one or two exposures to that word in a meaningful context; that is, young children were able to select the chromium tray without any explicit teaching of the novel word. A number of subsequent investigations confirmed children's aptitude for rapidly mapping new word meanings from limited experience with those words (Dickinson, 1984; Dollaghan, 1985; Heibeck & Markman, 1987; Rice & Woodsmall, 1988).

Quick Incidental Learning Vocabulary comprehension tasks have served as the vehicle for additional insights into children's word-learning mechanisms. For example, Rice and Woodsmall (1988) evaluated 3- and 5-year-old children's ability to map novel word meanings in a noninteractive context—video viewing. In this task, children were exposed to new object, action, attribute, and affective state words embedded in narration specifically developed to match a cartoon segment. Each novel word was used approximately five times during the course of the video cartoon. Children's comprehension of target words was assessed, pre- and post-video viewing, through a vocabulary comprehension task analogous to the PPVT–R; pictures taken from the video program were used in an array of four photographs with a "show me X" prompt. Rice and Woodsmall found that both 3- and 5-year-olds learned new words through video viewing, with greater learning demonstrated by the 5-year-old children.

The context for introducing novel words and evaluating children's learning was interactive in studies that preceded Rice and Woodsmall (1988) (cf. Carey & Bartlett, 1978; Dickinson, 1984; Dollaghan, 1985, 1987; Heibeck & Markman, 1987). In those investigations, novel words were presented in focused and presumably salient circumstances; an adult used the target word in a play-based activity, and the child was asked to demonstrate comprehension or knowledge of the new word in a similar manner using real objects (see Dollaghan, 1985, for example). The context for word exposure and the comprehension measure used by Rice and Woodsmall differed in fundamental ways from the majority of fast-mapping investigations. The Rice and Woodsmall study revealed that young children's word-learning mechanisms are robust enough to accomplish at least partial mappings of new word meanings through strictly incidental exposure to novel forms. Hence, Rice (1990, 1991) suggested, a quick incidental learning (QUIL) capability exists in children's word-acquisition competencies. This finding is important because it reveals that children can learn new words in indirect experiential contexts, such as television viewing, in addition to during highly focused interactions with an adult. Television's influence on word learning is well-documented (cf. Rice, Huston, Truglio, & Wright, 1990).

Mechanisms of Word Comprehension Evidence of children's powerful word-learning aptitudes and accomplishments has led scholars to consider mechanisms that may underlie and promote lexical achievements (Golinkoff et al., 1994). Specifically, investigators have proposed and evaluated particular principles or constraints thought to enable rapid word acquisition. The basic proposal is that these principles operate to reduce the amount of information that must be considered in determining a word's meaning (Baldwin & Markman, 1989; Clark, 1990; Golinkoff, Hirsh-Pasek, Bailey, & Wenger, 1992; Golinkoff et al., 1994; Markman & Wachtel, 1988; Merriman & Bowman, 1989; Mervis & Bertrand, 1993; Mervis, Golinkoff, & Bertrand, 1994; Waxman & Kosowski, 1990). For example, Golinkoff et al. (1994) summarized fundamental principles that direct children's lexical acquisition, principles such as *reference* (i.e., words are mapped onto representations of objects); *extendibility* (i.e., a word can refer to objects beyond a labeled exemplar); and *object scope,* or *whole object* (i.e., the first referent considered for a word is an entire object rather than its parts or attributes). These basic lexical principles are believed to be accessible to the young child at about 1 year of age. The principles focus the learner, constrain the hypotheses that the learner will entertain in attempting to infer the meanings of novel words, and, thus, narrow the scope and magnitude of the word-learning task.

A number of specific lexical principles have been proposed, some offering contradictory perspectives. Investigators continue to actively debate the status of such principles, accumulating evidence and negotiating the particulars of the various principles (cf. Markman, 1989; Mervis et al., 1994). One aspect of this debate, however, is abundantly clear: Vocabulary comprehension tasks, using either objects or pictures, have played a crucial role in understanding and evaluating proposed lexical principles. Research assessing two particular principles illustrates this point. Markman and her colleagues (Baldwin & Markman, 1989; Markman, 1989; Markman & Wachtel, 1988) proposed that a *mutual exclusivity* (ME) bias exists in young word learners, suggesting that children assume that an object will have only a single name. On this account, a novel label is attached to an unnamed object, and the children refrain from attaching a second label to an already named object. In situations in which a novel name occurs, and the surrounding context suggests that the novel name refers to a previously named object, Markman and her colleagues anticipated that ME will take precedence over the whole object principle described previously; that is, the child will assume that the novel name refers to a part or attribute of the object.

In contrast, Golinkoff et al. (1994; Mervis & Bertrand, 1993, 1994) suggested a lexical principle termed *novel name-nameless category* (N_3C). N_3C states simply that young children are able to associate novel terms and previously unnamed objects rapidly, presumably after one or two exposures in incidental or nonexplicit contexts. The onset of the principle is posited to be about 18 months—around the time the child begins to learn words at a brisk pace. Prior to that time, word acquisition typically proceeds at a relatively slow rate (cf. Golinkoff et al., 1994).

These components of N_3C are not in conflict with Markman's ME principle. In fact, in contexts in which a child encounters a novel word and an unnamed object, N_3C and ME both anticipate that the child will map the new term to the whole unnamed object. The two perspectives differ in situations in which the child hears a novel word in the presence of an already named object. Whereas ME suggests that the child will attach the new label to a salient attribute or component of the already named object, N_3C makes no specific predictions about likely word-referent pairings in a situation in which a named object receives a second label. Instead, Golinkoff et al. (1994) suggested that the child will evaluate candidate interpretations of the new term in accordance with available linguistic and nonlinguistic contextual information. For example, only if a child heard the novel word while viewing the manipulation of a part of an already named object would the child be likely to infer that the label referred to the object part (cf. Baldwin, 1993). Other plausible referents would be equally likely, as directed by salient contextual information. For example, if the object were a particularly unusual or previously unidentified color, the novel word might be hypothesized to be a color label. If reasonable candidate referents were not readily apparent, then the child would probably accept a second label for an already named object. Thus, a primary difference between the two lexical acquisition principles is that ME asserts that the child will automatically apply a competing label to a part or component of an already named object, whereas N₃C allows more degrees of freedom and contends that the child will consider a range of options, including a second label for an already named object. This learning is guided by the contextual information available as the child chooses a referent for the competing label.

Data obtained through the vocabulary comprehension paradigm (i.e., "show me X") have helped tease out the relative merits of the ME and N₃C perspectives. For example, Markman and Wachtel (1988) tested the predictions of the ME account by assessing children's willingness to apply a novel name when they heard the new term paired with a known or identified object. In about half of the comprehension trials, Markman and Wachtel found that 3-year-olds selected object components or attributes, and about half of the time they selected the object itself. Because the children were willing to accept a second label in many of the trials used by Markman and Wachtel, Golinkoff et al. (1994) interpreted these findings as inconsistent with the ME principle.

Additional data support the predictions of N₃C versus ME. Specifically, Mervis et al. (1994) conducted an experiment similar to Markman and Wachtel's, again evaluating young children's comprehension of novel words when the terms were used in the presence of an already named object. Following exposure to novel terms, the children were willing to apply both known and novel words to the same object (i.e., children who knew the word "truck" were willing and able to select a truck when both "show me truck" and "show me lorry" were probed in comprehension). These findings conflict with the expectations of the ME lexical principle.

In summary, accounts of early word acquisition have underscored the role of lexical principles in simplifying the child's task and explaining rapid learning curves. Key insights into these impressive word-acquisition mechanisms have been obtained through measures of language comprehension. Vocabulary comprehension tasks have uncovered the boundaries of initial word mapping, the process of QUIL, and the existence of lexical principles that expedite word acquisition by focusing children on particular candidate referents for novel word meanings.

Insights on Language Impairment

It is well-documented that children with SLI demonstrate difficulties in lexical acquisition (Leonard, 1988; Rice, 1991). The typical profile of a child with SLI is a pattern of late appearance of first words, followed by slower-than-expected lexical acquisition through the preschool and early school years (Crystal, 1987). Parallel impairments in vocabulary comprehension also may be a frequent component of the SLI profile (Johnston, 1988; Leonard, 1988; Rice, 1991).

Because many young children with language-learning difficulties evidence vocabulary comprehension impairments, researchers and clinicians use vocabulary comprehension measures as a diagnostic marker of the impairment. Many scholars in the field use below-average PPVT–R standard scores as a criterion in SLI identification and/or rely on the PPVT–R as a key index for subject description (e.g., Craig & Evans, 1993; Craig & Washington, 1993; Kelly & Rice, 1994; Masterson, 1993; Oetting & Rice, 1993; Rice, Buhr, & Nemeth, 1990; Rice, Buhr, & Oetting, 1992; Rice, Oetting, Marquis, Bode, & Pae, 1994; Rice, Wexler, & Cleave, 1995; Tomblin, Freese, & Records, 1992; Watkins, Buhr, & Davis, 1993; Watkins, Kelly, Harbers, & Hollis, 1995; Watkins & Rice, 1991; Weismer, 1991; Weismer & Hesketh, 1993).

Research addressing word learning in children with SLI has revealed not only delays in lexical acquisition but also apparent differences in the mechanisms driving development. Rice and her colleagues (Rice, Buhr, et al., 1990; Rice et al., 1992; Rice et al., 1994) have extended the QUIL paradigm to the SLI population as a means to understand processes of impaired lexical development. Again, vocabulary comprehension tasks have played a central role in revealing breakdown in word-learning mechanisms. Rice, Buhr, et al. (1990) replicated the videotape task developed in Rice and Woodsmall (1988) with 5-year-old children with SLI. Results revealed that children with SLI learned fewer words, as measured in a vocabulary comprehension format, than did either language- or age-equivalent peers with typical language development. Children with SLI did demonstrate some QUIL abilities but at a reduced level relative to typical counterparts (i.e., the children with SLI comprehended an average of 1.5 new words, of 20 possible, after the video-viewing activity; language-equivalent peers learned 2.3 new words, and age-equivalent peers learned 4.2 new forms). Rice, Buhr, et al. evaluated plausible sources of the limited ability of children with SLI to quickly comprehend new words; candidate explanations involved restrictions in processing and/or segmenting abilities whereby children with SLI may be unable to identify novel words in the incoming stream of verbalization. This limitation, in turn, could be tied to particular syntactic difficulties, such as impairments in grammatical morphology.

In subsequent investigations, Rice and her colleagues systematically evaluated potential sources of the restricted QUIL aptitudes of children with SLI. These studies extended the use of the vocabulary comprehension format developed by Rice and Woodsmall (1988). Rice et al. (1992) increased the salience of target words in a video-viewing QUIL task by presenting the target words in sentence-final position and adding a brief pause immediately before presentation of the target word. The general aim of this project was to evaluate whether manipulations of target-word salience would enhance the QUIL abilities of children with SLI. Results revealed no advantage for children with SLI or for their typically developing counterparts in the enhanced salience condition. In general, these findings suggest that the restricted QUIL capabilities of children with SLI are not likely to be tied to an inability to segment novel words within the context of the language stream.

Next, Rice et al. (1994) assessed the influence of varied input frequencies and word types on the QUIL abilities of children with SLI and age- and language-equivalent counterparts. Both initial comprehension and later retention of new words were examined. Several intriguing findings were revealed. First, given more instances of target words, children with SLI demonstrated robust QUIL abilities; with 10 exposures to target words, children with SLI showed posttest comprehension gains that were comparable to their age-equivalent peers. Second, contrasts of nouns and verbs in QUIL revealed a surprising pattern of verb learning and loss in children with SLI. During posttesting in the high input frequency condition (10 exposures), children with SLI performed as well on comprehension of novel verbs as did their age-equivalent peers; however, the children with SLI subsequently displayed a sharp loss of verb forms in the retention condition (verb comprehension measured 1 week later). Thus, Rice et al. suggested that increased frequency is necessary to promote lexical comprehension for children with SLI. At the same time, increased input alone is not likely to be sufficient to ensure retention of new word forms. Rice et al. hypothesized that verb learning, specifically long-term storage of verbs in semantic networks, may be influenced by the grammatical markings associated with verb forms (e.g., the inflections associated with them and the grammatical frames in which they appear). In this study, available grammatical markings may not have been particularly helpful in mapping new words. Target verbs were modeled in the video presentation in limited grammatical contexts that consisted predominantly of uninflected forms and forms with past-tense markings. Because the children with SLI and the language-equivalent peers who participated in this study lacked mastery of the regular past-tense inflection, the verb presentation may not have been informative enough to ensure adequate storage for long-term retention.

Finally, Rice, Cleave, Oetting, and Pae (1993) evaluated young children's ability to use grammatical devices that cue differences in novel mass versus count noun forms. In a QUIL word-learning task, presented via videotape and evaluated in a picture-pointing comprehension format, children with SLI and age- and language-equivalent peers were required to differentiate between novel mass and count nouns, as specified by different determiner cues presented with novel objects and substances (e.g., "a keelwug," "some blick"). Findings revealed that children with SLI were less capable than were their age-equivalent counterparts in distinguishing mass versus count nouns, making errors in the association between novel label and novel substance or object. In contrast, typically developing 5-year-olds (age-equivalent peers) made use of grammatical cues in achieving links between novel labels and substances or objects. These findings suggest an interaction between morphosyntactic difficulties and lexical development in children with SLI, insofar as learning new words is constrained by challenges in recognizing grammatical cues to particular word classes.

In summary, measures of vocabulary comprehension are fundamental to the study of child language disorders, serving as a diagnostic indicator of SLI. The PPVT–R is the measure most commonly used for this purpose. Furthermore, within the context of QUIL investigations, measures of vocabulary comprehension that emulate the PPVT–R format have revealed that 1) children with SLI are less able than are their peers to map initial word meanings, at least in contexts in which incidental, nonsalient exposure to novel forms is provided; 2) such impairments are not likely to be attributable to problems with segmenting language input; 3) with enhancement of input frequency, children with SLI demonstrate QUIL capabilities roughly commensurate with their peers, but they may experience additional difficulties in long-term retention of new forms; and 4) children with SLI are less facile in using grammatical devices to cue particular distinctions in novel word form class when presented in a QUIL context. In brief, these investigations and the vocabulary comprehension format central to them have revealed much about the nature and character of SLI, including insight into the mechanisms of acquisition operative for children with language limitations.

One caution about using the PPVT–R as a diagnostic marker of SLI warrants mention. A high proportion of the items on the PPVT–R are nouns. Given that children with SLI display unique problems in retaining verb forms (cf. Rice et al., 1994; see also Rice & Bode, 1993; Watkins, Rice, & Moltz, 1993), the PPVT–R may, in fact, underestimate the lexical difficulties of children with SLI.

VOCABULARY COMPREHENSION: DEVELOPMENTAL OUTCOMES, RELATED DOMAINS, AND INTERVENTION STUDIES

The use of vocabulary comprehension measures has not been limited to the study of typical and atypical lexical development. Vocabulary comprehension measures have been utilized in a considerable number of investigations with a range of aims (Arnold, Lonigan, Whitehurst, & Epstein, 1994; Butler, Marsh, Sheppard, & Sheppard, 1985; Chaney, 1994; Crain-Thoreson & Dale, 1992; Dunning, Mason, & Stewart, 1994; Karweit, 1989; Lonigan, 1994; Rice, Huston, et al., 1990; Scarborough & Dobrich, 1994; Schleicker, White, & Jacobs, 1991; Tunmer, Herriman, & Nesdale, 1988; Walker, Greenwood, Hart, & Carta, 1994; Whitehurst et al., 1988; Whitehurst et al., 1994). Key applications of vocabulary comprehension measures include 1) predicting developmental trajectories (Bishop & Edmundson, 1987; Rice & Hadley, 1995; Thal & Tobias, 1992; Thal, Tobias, & Morrison, 1991); 2) assessing associations between language skills and other developmental areas, such as social competence, literacy experiences, reading development, and academic achievement (Anderson & Freebody, 1981; Chaney, 1994; Gertner, Rice, & Hadley, 1994; Walker et al., 1994); and 3) evaluating the outcomes of specific and general intervention programs (Arnold et al., 1994; Brody, Stoneman, & McCoy, 1994; Karweit, 1989; Rice & Hadley, 1995; Whitehurst et al., 1988; Whitehurst et al., 1994). In these various investigations, vocabulary comprehension measures have served a number of functions, most often acting as either a variable predicting status in other domains or as an index of developmental outcome.

The widespread use of vocabulary comprehension measures can undoubtedly be attributed to many of the reasons cited at the beginning of the chapter (e.g., they can be used with young children and across the life span, they place minimal demand on the individual tested). The PPVT–R in particular has two additional attributes that make it an appealing choice in large-scale research endeavors that employ multiple measures: It is easy to administer, and it is brief (i.e., the PPVT–R does not require extensive training or practice and typically is completed in 10–15 minutes). Beyond these functional benefits, however, measures of vocabulary comprehension appear to be powerful indices of language ability that have predictive and concurrent associations with multiple other dimensions of developmental competence. Key findings related to three specific applications of vocabulary comprehension measures are highlighted: 1) prediction of continued language impairment and intervention outcomes, 2) concurrent relations between vocabulary comprehension and social competence, and 3) use in intervention studies.

Developmental Outcomes

Investigations of early language development have revealed that a substantial number of children demonstrate delayed onset of lexical acquisition and slow word-learning patterns. These children have been identified in the research and clinical literature as "late talkers" (Paul, 1991; Paul & Alforde, 1993; Paul, Spangle-Looney, & Dahm, 1991; Rescorla, 1993; Rescorla & Schwartz, 1990; Thal et al., 1991; Thal & Tobias, 1992, 1994). Furthermore, studies suggest that approximately half of the children who experience such delays at 18–24 months of age continue to have language-learning problems in the late preschool years (Fischel, Whitehurst, Caulfield, & DeBaryshe, 1988; Paul, 1991; Paul & Alforde, 1993; Rescorla, 1993; Thal et al., 1991; Thal & Tobias, 1992). A central issue then becomes specifying factors that predict persistent versus transient language difficulties (i.e., that provide prognostic information about language outcomes).

Predicting outcome also is pertinent in language intervention. More specific, it is beneficial to know which profiles of language impairment are likely to be most responsive to intervention and in what ways. This information is important to families that are working toward understanding language impairment and striving to make future plans for their children, as well as for clinicians who are seeking to develop optimal intervention plans for the present and future needs of the children that they serve.

Research findings suggest that measures of vocabulary comprehension may be useful prognostic indices in terms of both predicting developmental trajectory and estimating intervention outcomes. First, in differentiating the overall population of late talkers into those with persistent versus transient delays, Thal et al. (1991) found that two measures of language comprehension are strong predictors of developmental outcome. In this project, 10 late talkers were identified at roughly 2 years of age and evaluated again 1 year later. At the 1-year follow-up evaluation, four of the children still experienced delays (true delays), whereas six demonstrated age-appropriate language skills (late bloomers). Examining data from the first visit, Thal et al. found that all of the children with true delays experienced delays in language comprehension, as measured by the number of words understood in the Language and Gesture Inventory (cf. Thal & Bates, 1988) and by a two-way forced-choice picture-identification test. In contrast, the language comprehension skills of the late-bloomer group at the initial visit were equivalent to those of an age-matched control group.

Second, Rice and Hadley (1995) reported language outcomes of children enrolled in a preschool classroom–based intervention program (Language Acquisition Preschool [LAP], Rice & Wilcox, 1995). Thirty-six children with SLI were enrolled in the intervention program for either 1 or 2 academic years. The protocol used to monitor progress and evaluate intervention efficacy included the PPVT–R, the Reynell Developmental Language Scales (Reynell & Gruber, 1990), and mean length of utterance (MLU). Overall, children with SLI gained an average of 9–11 standard score points on the language measures following enrollment in the intervention program. These standard score gains indicate that the children with SLI were learning new language skills at a rate that exceeded typical developmental expectations.

Of interest here are the observed profiles of language impairment among the children studied and their associations with outcome measures. Rice and Hadley (1995) found that children with an expressive disability profile at the outset of intervention programming (i.e., delays in expressive language and speech but age-appropriate receptive language, of which PPVT–R was a key component) made dramatic gains in expressive language skills during intervention (i.e., increases of 14–18 standard score points) and demonstrated average-range abilities on all language measures at preschool exit. Children with global language disabilities at the time of enrollment in the program (receptive, expressive, and speech delays) displayed standard score gains of 5–12 points but remained below the average range on all language measures except the PPVT–R at preschool exit. In addition, 79% of the children with global language impairments continued to receive intervention services through kindergarten and early elementary grades. In contrast, 56% of the expressive group were enrolled in language intervention in kindergarten; enrollment declined to 33% by the end of second grade. In summary, Rice and Hadley (1995) reported that for children with SLI enrolled in the LAP intervention program, intact receptive language abilities were associated with substantive gains in expressive language abilities and a reduced rate of future enrollment in intervention programming, relative to children with global disabilities.

Research findings in these two areas converge to suggest a predictive capacity for measures of vocabulary comprehension. Relatively little is known about the overall strength or confines of relations between early vocabulary comprehension and long-term language development status and/or responsiveness to early intervention. Important issues are whether vocabulary knowledge is the most robust predictor of future linguistic competence and the extent to which productive language difficulties are linked to later outcomes. In an investigation similar to that of Thal and her colleagues (Thal et al., 1991), Paul et al. (1991) did not find a pattern of greater risk for continued delay among children with concomitant receptive and expressive impairments. The discrepancy between studies may be attributed to differences in the particular measures of language competence that were used; Thal et al. (1991) specifically measured vocabulary comprehension, whereas Paul et al. (1991) measured general receptive and expressive language skills through the Vineland Adaptive Behavior Scales (Sparrow, Balla, & Cicchetti, 1984). Additional investigation is needed to sort out the particulars of links between early vocabulary knowledge and later language outcomes. (See Chapter 1 for further discussion.)

Related Domains

Research has revealed that children with language disabilities are at risk for difficulties in social interaction and acceptance and may be vulnerable to negative social bias (cf. Craig & Washington, 1993; Fujiki & Brinton, 1994; Hadley & Rice, 1991; Rice, 1993; Rice, Hadley, & Alexander, 1993; Rice, Sell, & Hadley, 1991; Windsor, 1995). An investigation by Gertner et al. (1994) assessed positive and negative peer nominations among three groups of preschoolers who attended a classroom-based language intervention program: children with typically developing language skills, children with speech and/or language impairments (S/LI), and children learning English as a second language. The peer nomination task asked children to "point to the picture of who you like to play with" and "point to the picture of who you do not like to play with," with three positive and three negative nominations obtained from each child.

Multiple regression analyses revealed that 1) PPVT–R standard scores were the single best predictor of positive peer nominations, and 2) age and IQ did not significantly add to the variance in positive peer nominations accounted for by language measures (PPVT–R, Reynell Developmental Language Scales). Furthermore, examination of the patterns of peers' nominations for individual children with S/LI revealed that language comprehension skills (as measured by performance on the PPVT–R and Reynell Receptive Scale) were a key factor in social acceptance. Children with S/LI whose receptive language skills were age appropriate received fewer-than-average negative nominations. In contrast, children whose S/LI profile included receptive language impairments tended to receive more negative peer nominations.

Intervention Studies

Measures of vocabulary comprehension also have played a central role in numerous treatment efficacy studies. The Rice and Hadley (1995) investigation of children's PPVT–R standard score gains following enrollment in the Language Acquisition Preschool is an example of this use of the measure. Standardized measures can be optimal tools for assessing generalized treatment outcomes. Bearing in mind restrictions on the frequency of administering standardized tests, using vocabulary comprehension indices as treatment outcome measures enables the evaluation of global language change, supplementing the more common and circumscribed focus on specified treatment targets. Furthermore, using standard scores permits evaluation of whether language change exceeds that anticipated on the basis of maturation alone.

Research evaluating the influence of enhancing parental book-reading skills on children's rate of language learning is one line of inquiry that has heavily used standardized vocabulary tests such as the PPVT–R as intervention outcome measures. In a series of studies, Whitehurst and his colleagues (Arnold et al., 1994; Whitehurst et al., 1988; Whitehurst et al., 1994) trained parents to use interactive strategies likely to enhance parent–child book reading; that is, strategies that provide optimal language models for children and encourage child participation in book-reading events (e.g., asking open-ended rather than yes–no questions, positively acknowledging child comments and questions, expanding on child comments). In these studies, the children had not been identified as having language impairment. In general, the design involves both experimental (parents learn about book-reading strategies) and control groups (no parent training occurs). The basic design also includes 1) a set of pretest measures of child language competence, 2) training parents in book-reading strategies and allowing a brief intervention period (roughly 6 weeks), and 3) readministering the measures of child language competence as a posttest. Pretest and posttest measures included the PPVT–R, as well as other standardized tests, such as the Expressive One-Word Picture Vocabulary Test–Revised (EOWPVT–R) (Gardner, 1990) and particular subtests of the Illinois Test of Psycholinguistic Abilities (ITPA) (Kirk, McCarthy, & Kirk, 1968). In some of the studies, nonstandardized measures such as MLU and a specific test of expressive vocabulary designed by the investigators also were used as pretest and posttest measures of child language skill (cf. Whitehurst et al., 1994).

Findings of these investigations generally revealed positive influences of enhancing parental book-reading styles on the rate of children's language acquisition, specifically in expressive language areas, and, to a lesser extent, in vocabulary comprehension (as measured by the PPVT–R). For example, Whitehurst et al. (1988) found that children in the experimental group scored significantly higher at posttest on the EOWPVT–R, the ITPA verbal expressive subtest, and MLU than did the control-group children (groups were equated at the outset of intervention). Posttest scores on the PPVT–R did not differ between groups. Valdez-Menchaca and Whitehurst (1992) implemented the basic design, outlined previously, in the context of Mexican child care; the experimental group scored significantly higher than did the control group at posttest on Spanish versions of the PPVT–R, the EOWPVT–R, and the ITPA. Arnold et al. (1994) contrasted a control group and two experimental groups, one in which parents received book-reading training through a videotape format and one in which parents received training in a typical passive instruction format. Posttest results revealed significant differences in PPVT–R standard scores between children whose parents received book-reading training in the videotape format versus children in the control and typical instruction groups.

In summary, measures of vocabulary comprehension have played a significant role in evaluating the effectiveness of various intervention programs and, more specific, have made a contribution to understanding how environmental manipulations in parental book-reading strategy and style can enhance the rate of children's language development. Although expressive vocabulary skills appear more amenable to change, the Arnold et al. (1994) and Valdez-Menchaca and Whitehurst (1992) studies suggest that vocabulary comprehension abilities also can be enhanced through book-reading interventions. It is important to remember that the participants in these investigations are children with a full set of language-learning resources who are growing up in low-income environments. It may be the case that comprehension abilities are less easily promoted by brief enriching experiences, whereas production abilities, when language comprehension skills are intact, are more readily enhanced. An additional point of interest is the extent to which these changes are durable. Arnold et al. (1994) reported that investigations of the long-term consequences of such interventions for oral language development and emerging literacy development are under way. Researchers anticipate that measures of vocabulary comprehension will constitute a central component of the research protocol in addressing these issues.

INTERPRETIVE BOUNDARIES:
LIMITATIONS OF VOCABULARY COMPREHENSION MEASURES

The findings reviewed in the previous section point to the ubiquity of measures of vocabulary comprehension, particularly the PPVT–R. Furthermore, measures of vocabulary comprehension clearly are informative indices of linguistic ability and language change across a range of purposes and contexts. Recent studies, however, also have uncovered some surprising dissociations between vocabulary comprehension and other linguistic abilities. In addition, limitations in the populations for whom particular measures of vocabulary comprehension are appropriate have become apparent.

Dissociations Between Initial and Full Mapping of Words

Several investigations have demonstrated that existing lexical knowledge (as measured by the PPVT–R) is not a powerful predictor of fast-mapping aptitude or QUIL abilities (cf. Rice, Buhr, et al., 1990; Rice et al., 1992). On the contrary, Rice and her colleagues have found little association between children's past lexical accomplishments (i.e., their accumulated lexicons) and their aptitude for gaining new words in comprehension during fast-mapping tasks. Initial-word mappings are only a tentative first step in the process of full mastery of lexical items. Although fast mapping is a very useful ability and one that almost certainly plays a central role in learning new words, the partial, or perhaps even superficial, word knowledge that begins in fast mapping must undergo substantial refinement before the novel lexical item is "acquired" in any complete sense. For example, a new form introduced through fast mapping must be associated with the existing lexicon and appropriately placed within the network of semantically related forms, the boundaries of the new word's meaning must be identified (i.e., the range of exemplars to which the word applies will need to be specified), and the grammatical function and role of the new form must be recognized. At best, competence in fully working through these steps seems to be indirectly, rather than directly, linked to initial–word-mapping aptitude (Rice, Buhr, et al., 1990; Rice et al., 1992).

Predicting Early Reading Success

Although vocabulary comprehension abilities are associated with literacy accomplishments (i.e., PPVT–R scores are significantly correlated with phonological, print, and metalinguistic awareness abilities [cf. Chaney, 1994; Tunmer et al., 1988]), vocabulary knowledge is only one contributor in a complex interaction of variables that influence reading achievement. For example, Mason (1992) identified multiple factors that influence reading acquisition, including home literary experiences, language understanding and expression, and early decoding and print-labeling skills. Mason developed an intricate model to depict the interdependence of such factors in directing reading outcomes. These findings are substantiated by numerous investigations (see Dunning et al., 1994; Lonigan, 1994; Scarborough & Dobrich, 1994, for reviews).

Furthermore, vocabulary comprehension ability does not appear to be the most powerful predictor of the basic decoding abilities that are crucial for early reading achievement. In a longitudinal investigation of associations between spoken language development and reading acquisition, Catts (1993) and his colleagues (Catts, Hu, Larrivee, & Swank, 1994) assessed the oral language skills of preschoolers with and without language impairments, using both standardized measures of language skill (including the PPVT–R) and informal measures of phonological awareness (e.g., segmentation and blending tasks, rapid-naming measures). Results of multiple regression analyses revealed that the best predictors of early reading achievement were the phonological awareness measures. In a study of precocious language learners, Crain-Thoreson and Dale (1992) found that children with advanced linguistic and vocabulary abilities were not particularly facile early readers. In general, these findings concur with a number of other investigations demonstrating that performance on phonological awareness tasks is highly predictive of early reading achievement—more predictive than vocabulary abilities (Adams, 1990; Menyuk et al., 1990; Wagner & Torgesen, 1987).

Limitations with Diverse Populations

A significant issue in language assessment is identifying and developing measures that are appropriate for the diverse population of children whose language skills are evaluated. The widespread use of vocabulary comprehension measures such as the PPVT–R does not ensure that the measures are appropriate for the racially, ethnically, and economically diverse children who need appropriate assessment and intervention services or who may participate in research activities.

In fact, research findings suggest that, in particular circumstances, frequently used standardized measures are not appropriate. For example, Washington and Craig (1992) examined the performance on the PPVT–R of 105 urban, African American children from low-income backgrounds. The children were 4- to 6-year-olds enrolled in preschool or kindergarten programs at the time of the study. The mean standard score equivalent achieved on the PPVT–R was 79.7; nearly all children in this sample scored below the mean, and 65% scored below −1.00 standard deviation. A follow-up analysis revealed largely random error patterns, suggesting general bias in the overall test rather than specific content bias in a limited number of individual test items. Washington and Craig concluded that the PPVT–R is an inappropriate measure of vocabulary comprehension for African American children from urban, low-income environments. In brief, the measure provided limited information about individual abilities in vocabulary comprehension. The overall vocabulary tested by the PPVT–R and that known by the children appeared to be mismatched. In addition to potential bias present in the PPVT–R, the test context itself may have been alien to the children. Overall, the PPVT–R failed to provide useful information about the vocabulary knowledge of these participants. Other investigators also have suggested that the PPVT–R is an inappropriate measure for speakers of African American dialect (cf. Kreschek & Nicolosi, 1973).

Limitations with Very Young Children

As mentioned previously, one of the attractive features of vocabulary comprehension measures is their applicability across a broad age range; however, this advantage does not robustly apply to very young children. Standardized measures, such as the PPVT–R, generally require a reasonable amount of attention, ability to scan several pictures, and impulse control in selecting the frame named by the examiner. Very young children frequently find these task demands excessive. Norms for the PPVT–R begin at 2;6. Many children between the ages of 2;6 and 3;0 are capable of the task demands required by the PPVT–R, yet certainly some are not; few children below age 2;6 can complete a PPVT–R or other structured vocabulary comprehension tasks. Clearly, for children below age 3, standardized measures of vocabulary comprehension should be used with caution and interpreted in light of the child's interest in and attention to the task. With early identification and intervention services extending to the birth-to-3 period, the need for accurate and appropriate measures of language proficiency in this population is particularly pressing. However, measures of vocabulary comprehension in the picture-identification "show me X" format appear to be best-suited to children ages 2;6–3;0 and above. (See Chapter 8 for a discussion of using parent report in assessing vocabulary in young children.)

In summary, much of this chapter has been devoted to the insights gained from measures of vocabulary comprehension. This discussion would be both incomplete and inaccurate without acknowledging interpretive boundaries for measures of vocabulary comprehension, which include areas of dissociations between vocabulary knowledge and other developmental areas and limitations in the application of particular vocabulary comprehension measures.

CONCLUSION

Overall, one of the most striking aspects of the familiar "show me X" vocabulary comprehension task is that it is relatively unique among the multitude of available assessment tools and approaches in both the scope of uses to which it has been applied and the shared research and clinical insight it offers. Assessing vocabulary knowledge appears to tap some fundamental aspect of linguistic skill near the core of language capabilities. Perhaps the most convincing support for this conclusion comes from the literature on children with limitations in vocabulary knowledge. Insofar as restricted understanding of vocabulary is closely associated with negative social status among peers, it seems to strike at the very center of what it means to be an individual with less-than-typical linguistic abilities. Similarly, as variations in vocabulary knowledge relate to different developmental trajectories and varied outcomes of language intervention, the integral contribution of lexical skills to overall linguistic aptitude and knowledge is revealed.

The literature reviewed in this chapter indicates that a fair amount of what is known about the mechanisms and processes of both typical and atypical lexical development has come about through measures of vocabulary comprehension. Available literature suggests a fundamental clinical role for measures of vocabulary knowledge, with potential applications to clinical decision making and intervention planning, yet vocabulary knowledge also dissociates in some surprising ways from other linguistic competencies; existing vocabulary does not accurately predict how readily new words can be mapped and does not provide direct insight into probable reading achievement. Furthermore, measures of vocabulary comprehension, particularly standardized instruments such as the PPVT–R, appear vulnerable to cultural bias and must be used cautiously with individuals who differ from normative populations. Another population for which caution is warranted is that of very young children, in the age range of 2;6–3;0 and below, who may not successfully manage the task demands.

Despite the insights gained from measures of vocabulary comprehension, a number of issues have yet to be resolved. Of particular importance are issues that arise regarding clinical concerns. For example, additional information on the role of vocabulary and/or general comprehension abilities in differentiating children with persistent versus transient language difficulties is needed, as is more study delineating the contribution of intact versus impaired comprehension abilities to outcomes of language intervention. In both of these areas, longitudinal analyses of children with varied language comprehension and production profiles, including assessment of performance in specifically linguistic and related domains (i.e., reading and academic achievement), would be highly informative. Available research offers relatively broad clinical "hints" for anticipating outcomes (cf. Rice & Hadley, 1995; Thal et al., 1991); additional studies are needed to specify the particulars of clinical decision making and prognosis that seek to make use of vocabulary comprehension profiles.

In the general context of available means and methods of language assessment, this chapter conveys a relatively positive theme: Straightforward, brief, and widely used measures of vocabulary comprehension can be highly informative in research and clinical endeavors. Vocabulary comprehension tasks of the "show me X" type have contributed substantially to the knowledge base in child language development, disorders, and assessment.

REFERENCES

Adams, M. (1990). *Beginning to read: Thinking and learning about print.* Cambridge: MIT Press.

Anderson, R.C., & Freebody, P. (1981). Vocabulary knowledge. In J.T. Guthrie (Ed.), *Comprehension and teaching: Research reviews* (pp. 77–117). Newark, DE: International Reading Association.

Arnold, D.H., Lonigan, C.J., Whitehurst, G.J., & Epstein, J.N. (1994). Accelerating language development through picture book reading: Replication and extension to a videotape training format. *Developmental Psychology, 86,* 235–243.

Baldwin, D. (1993). Infants' ability to consult the speaker for clues to word reference. *Journal of Child Language, 20,* 377–394.

Baldwin, D.A., & Markman, E.M. (1989). Establishing word–object relations: A first step. *Child Development, 60,* 381–389.

Bates, E. (1993). Comprehension and production in early language development. Commentary on E.S. Savage-Rumbaugh, J. Murphy, R. Sevcik, K. Brakke, & S. Williams, Language comprehension in ape and child. *Monographs of the Society for Research in Child Development, 58*(3–4), 222–242.

Binet, A., & Simon, T. (1916). *The development of intelligence in children.* Vineland, NJ: The Training School.

Bishop, D.V.M., & Edmundson, A. (1987). Language-impaired 4-year-olds: Distinguishing transient from persistent impairment. *Journal of Speech and Hearing Disorders, 52,* 156–173.

Brody, G.H., Stoneman, Z., & McCoy, J.K. (1994). Contributions of protective and risk factors to literacy and socioemotional competency in former Head Start children attending kindergarten. *Early Childhood Research Quarterly, 9,* 407–425.

Butler, S., Marsh, H.W., Sheppard, M.J., & Sheppard, J.L. (1985). Seven-year longitudinal study of the early prediction of reading achievement. *Journal of Educational Psychology, 77,* 349–361.

Carey, S. (1978). The child as word learner. In M. Halle, G. Miller, & J. Bresnan (Eds.), *Linguistic theory and psychological reality* (pp. 264–293). Cambridge: MIT Press.

Carey, S. (1982). Semantic development: The state of the art. In E. Wanner & L.R. Gleitman (Eds.), *Language acquisition: The state of the art* (pp. 347–389). Cambridge, England: Cambridge University Press.

Carey, S., & Bartlett, E. (1978). Acquiring a single new word. *Papers and Reports on Child Language Development* (Stanford University), *15,* 17–29.

Carrow-Woolfolk, E. (1985). *Test for Auditory Comprehension of Language–Revised.* Allen, TX: DLM Teaching Resources.

Catts, H.W. (1993). The relationship between speech-language impairments and reading disabilities. *Journal of Speech and Hearing Research, 36,* 948–958.

Catts, H.W., Hu, C., Larrivee, L., & Swank, L. (1994). Early identification of reading disabilities in children with speech-language impairments. In R.V. Watkins & M.L. Rice (Eds.), *Communication and language intervention series: Vol. 4. Specific language impairments in children* (pp. 145–160). Baltimore: Paul H. Brookes Publishing Co.

Chaney, C. (1994). Language development, metalinguistic awareness, and emergent literacy skills of 3-year-old children in relation to social class. *Applied Psycholinguistics, 15,* 371–394.

Clark, E.V. (1990). On the pragmatics of contrast. *Journal of Child Language, 17,* 417–431.

Craig, H.K., & Evans, J.L. (1993). Pragmatics and SLI: Within-group variations in discourse behaviors. *Journal of Speech and Hearing Research, 36,* 777–789.

Craig, H.K., & Washington, J. (1993). Access behaviors of children with specific language impairment. *Journal of Speech and Hearing Research, 36,* 322–337.

Crain-Thoreson, C., & Dale, P.S. (1992). Do early talkers become early readers? Linguistic precocity, preschool language, and emergent literacy. *Developmental Psychology, 28,* 421–429.

Crystal, D. (1987). Teaching vocabulary: The case for a semantic curriculum. *Child Language Teaching and Therapy, 3,* 40–56.

Dickinson, D.K. (1984). First impressions: Children's knowledge of words gained from a single experience. *Applied Psycholinguistics, 5,* 359–374

Dollaghan, C. (1985). Child meets words: "Fast mapping" in preschool children. *Journal of Speech and Hearing Research, 28,* 449–454.

Dollaghan, C. (1987). Fast mapping in normal and language-impaired children. *Journal of Speech and Hearing Disorders, 52,* 218–222.

Dunn, L.M., & Dunn, L.M. (1981). *Peabody Picture Vocabulary Test–Revised.* Circle Pines, MN: American Guidance Service.

Dunning, D.B., Mason, J.M., & Stewart, J.P. (1994). Reading to preschoolers: A response to Scarborough and Dobrich (1994) and recommendations for future research. *Developmental Review, 14,* 324–339.

Fischel, J., Whitehurst, G., Caulfield, M., & DeBaryshe, B. (1988). Language growth in children with expressive language delay. *Pediatrics, 82,* 218–227.

Fujiki, M., & Brinton, B. (1994). Social competence and language impairment in children. In R.V. Watkins & M.L. Rice (Eds.), *Communication and language intervention series: Vol. 4. Specific language impairments in children* (pp. 123–143). Baltimore: Paul H. Brookes Publishing Co.

Gardner, M. (1985). *Receptive One-Word Picture Vocabulary Test.* Austin, TX: PRO-ED.

Gardner, M. (1990). *Expressive One-Word Picture Vocabulary Test–Revised.* Austin, TX: PRO-ED.

Gertner, B., Rice, M.L., & Hadley, P.A. (1994). Influence of communicative competence on peer preferences in a preschool classroom. *Journal of Speech and Hearing Research, 37,* 913–923.

Golinkoff, R.M., Hirsh-Pasek, K., Bailey, L.M., & Wenger, R.N. (1992). Young children and adults use lexical principles to learn new nouns. *Developmental Psychology, 28,* 99–108.

Golinkoff, R.M., Mervis, C.B., & Hirsh-Pasek, K. (1994). Early object labels: The case for a developmental lexical principles framework. *Journal of Child Language, 21,* 125–155.

Hadley, P.A., & Rice, M.L. (1991). Conversational responsiveness of speech- and language-impaired preschoolers. *Journal of Speech and Hearing Research, 34,* 1308–1317.

Heibeck, T., & Markman, E.M. (1987). Word learning in children: An examination of fast mapping. *Child Development, 58,* 1021–1034.

Johnston, J.R. (1988). Specific language disorders in the child. In N. Lass, J. Northern, L. McReynolds, & D. Yoder (Eds.), *Handbook of speech-language pathology and audiology* (pp. 685–715). Philadelphia: B.C. Decker.

Karweit, N. (1989). The effects of a story-reading program on the vocabulary and story comprehension skills of disadvantaged prekindergarten and kindergarten students. *Early Education and Development, 1,* 105–114.

Kaufman, A.S., & Kaufman, N.L. (1983). *Kaufman Assessment Battery for Children.* Circle Pines, MN: American Guidance Service.

Kelly, D.J., & Rice, M.L. (1994). Preferences for verb interpretation in children with specific language impairment. *Journal of Speech and Hearing Research, 37,* 182–192.

Kirk, S.A., McCarthy, J.J., & Kirk, W.D. (1968). *Illinois Test of Psycholinguistic Abilities.* Urbana: University of Illinois Press.

Kreschek, J., & Nicolosi, L. (1973). A comparison of black and white children's scores on the Peabody Picture Vocabulary Test. *Language, Speech, and Hearing Services in Schools, 4,* 37–40.

Leonard, L.B. (1988). Lexical development and processing in specific language impairment. In R.L. Schiefelbusch & L.L. Lloyd (Eds.), *Language perspectives: Acquisition, retardation, and intervention* (2nd ed., pp. 69–87). Austin, TX: PRO-ED.

Lonigan, C. (1994). Reading to preschoolers exposed: Is the emperor really naked? *Developmental Review, 14,* 303–323.

Markman, E.M. (1989). *Categorization and naming in children.* Cambridge: MIT Press.

Markman, E.M., & Wachtel, G.F. (1988). Children's use of mutual exclusivity to constrain the meaning of words. *Cognitive Psychology, 20,* 121–157.

Mason, J.M. (1992). Reading stories to preliterate children: A proposed connection to reading. In P. Gough, L. Ehri, & R. Treiman (Eds.), *Reading acquisition* (pp. 215–242). Hillsdale, NJ: Lawrence Erlbaum Associates.

Masterson, J.J. (1993). The performance of children with language-learning disabilities on two types of cognitive tasks. *Journal of Speech and Hearing Research, 36,* 1026–1036.

Menyuk, P., Chesnick, M., Liebergott, J., Korngold, B., D'Agostino, R., & Belanger, A. (1990). Predicting reading problems in at-risk children. *Journal of Speech and Hearing Research, 34,* 893–903.

Merriman, W.E., & Bowman, L. (1989). The mutual exclusivity bias in children's word learning. *Monographs of the Society for Research in Child Development, 54.*

Mervis, C.B., & Bertrand, J. (1993). Acquisition of early object labels: The roles of operating principles and input. In A.P. Kaiser & D.B. Gray (Eds.), *Communication and language intervention series: Vol. 2. Enhancing children's communication: Research foundations for intervention* (pp. 287–316). Baltimore: Paul H. Brookes Publishing Co.

Mervis, C.B., & Bertrand, J. (1994). Acquisition of the novel name-nameless category (N₃C) principle. *Child Development, 65,* 1646–1662.

Mervis, C.B., Golinkoff, R.M., & Bertrand, J. (1994). Two-year-olds readily learn multiple labels for the same basic level category. *Child Development, 65,* 1163–1177.

Newcomer, P.L., & Hammill, D.D. (1991). *Test of Language Development–P:2.* Austin, TX: PRO-ED.

Oetting, J.B., & Rice, M.L. (1993). Plural acquisition in children with specific language impairments. *Journal of Speech and Hearing Research, 36,* 1236–1248.

Paul, R. (1991). Toddlers with slow expressive language development. *Topics in Language Disorders, 11,* 11–13.

Paul, R., & Alforde, S. (1993). Grammatical morpheme acquisition in 4-year-olds with normal, impaired, and late-developing language. *Journal of Speech and Hearing Research, 36,* 1271–1275.

Paul, R., Spangle-Looney, S., & Dahm, P. (1991). Communication and socialization skills at ages two and three in "late-talking" young children. *Journal of Speech and Hearing Research. 34,* 858–865.

Rescorla, L. (1993, March). *Outcome of toddlers with specific expressive language delay at three, four, five, and six.* Paper presented at the biennial meeting of the Society for Research in Child Development, New Orleans.

Rescorla, L., & Schwartz, E. (1990). Outcome of toddlers with specific expressive language delay. *Applied Psycholinguistics, 11,* 393–408.

Reynell, J.K., & Gruber, C.P. (1990). *Reynell Developmental Language Scales–U.S. Edition.* Los Angeles: Western Psychological Corporation.

Rice, M.L. (1990). Preschoolers' QUIL: Quick incidental learning of words. In G. Conti-Ramsden & C. Snow (Eds.), *Children's language* (Vol. 7, pp. 171–195). Hillsdale, NJ: Lawrence Erlbaum Associates.

Rice, M.L. (1991). Children with specific language impairment: Toward a model of teachability. In N.A. Krasnegor, D.M. Rumbaugh, R.L. Schiefelbusch, & M. Studdert-Kennedy (Eds.), *Biological and behavioral determinants of language development* (pp. 447–480). Hillsdale, NJ: Lawrence Erlbaum Associates.

Rice, M.L. (1993). "Don't talk to him; he's weird": A social consequences account of language and social interactions. In A.P. Kaiser & D.B. Gray (Eds.), *Communication and language intervention series: Vol. 2. Enhancing children's communication: Research foundations for intervention* (pp. 139–158). Baltimore: Paul H. Brookes Publishing Co.

Rice, M.L., & Bode, J.V. (1993). Gaps in the verb lexicons of children with specific language impairment. *First Language, 13,* 113–131.

Rice, M.L., Buhr, J.C., & Nemeth, M. (1990). Fast mapping word learning abilities of language-delayed preschoolers. *Journal of Speech and Hearing Research, 55,* 33–42.

Rice, M.L., Buhr, J.C., & Oetting, J.B. (1992). Specific-language-impaired children's quick incidental learning of words: The effect of a pause. *Journal of Speech and Hearing Research, 35,* 1040–1048.

Rice, M.L., Cleave, P.L., Oetting, J.B., & Pae, S. (1993, November). *SLI children's use of syntactic cues in lexical acquisition.* Poster presentation at the American Speech-Language-Hearing Association National Convention, Anaheim, CA.

Rice, M.L., & Hadley, P.A. (1995). Language outcomes of the language-focused curriculum. In M.L. Rice & K.A. Wilcox (Eds.), *Building a language-focused curriculum for the preschool classroom: Vol. I. A foundation for lifelong communication* (pp. 155–169). Baltimore: Paul H. Brookes Publishing Co.

Rice, M.L., Hadley, P.A., & Alexander, A. (1993). Social biases toward children with speech and language impairments: A correlative causal model of language limitations. *Applied Psycholinguistics, 14,* 443–471.

Rice, M.L., Huston, A.C., Truglio, R., & Wright, J. (1990). Words from "Sesame Street": Learning vocabulary when viewing. *Developmental Psychology, 26,* 421–428.

Rice, M.L., Oetting, J.B., Marquis, J., Bode, J., & Pae, S. (1994). Frequency of input effects on word comprehension of children with specific language impairment. *Journal of Speech and Hearing Research, 37,* 106–122.

Rice, M.L., Sell, M.A., & Hadley, P.A. (1991). Social interactions of speech- and language-impaired children. *Journal of Speech and Hearing Research, 34,* 1299–1307.

Rice, M.L., Wexler, K., & Cleave, P. (1995). Specific language impairment as a period of extended optional infinitive. *Journal of Speech and Hearing Research, 38,* 850–863.

Rice, M.L., & Wilcox, K.A. (Eds.). (1995). *Building a language-focused curriculum for the preschool classroom: Vol. I. A foundation for lifelong communication.* Baltimore: Paul H. Brookes Publishing Co.

Rice, M.L., & Woodsmall, L. (1988). Lessons from television: Children's word learning when viewing. *Child Development, 59,* 420–429.

Scarborough, H.S., & Dobrich, W. (1994). On the efficacy of reading to preschoolers. *Developmental Review, 14,* 245–302.

Schleicker, E., White, D.R., & Jacobs, E. (1991). The role of day care quality in the prediction of children's vocabulary. *Canadian Journal of Behavioural Science, 23*(1), 12–24.

Sparrow, S.S., Balla, D.A., & Cicchetti, D.V. (1984). *Vineland Adaptive Behavior Scales.* Circle Pines, MN: American Guidance Service.

Terman, L.M. (1916). *The measurement of intelligence.* Boston: Houghton Mifflin.

Thal, D., & Bates, E. (1988). Language and gesture in late talkers. *Journal of Speech and Hearing Research, 31,* 115–123.

Thal, D., & Tobias, S. (1992). Communicative gestures in children with delayed onset of expressive vocabulary. *Journal of Speech and Hearing Research, 35,* 1281–1289.

Thal, D., & Tobias, S. (1994). Relationships between language and gesture in normally developing and late-talking toddlers. *Journal of Speech and Hearing Research, 37,* 157–170.

Thal, D. Tobias, S., & Morrison, D. (1991). Language and gesture in late talkers: A 1-year follow-up. *Journal of Speech and Hearing Research, 34,* 604–612.

Thorndike, R.L., Hagen, E.P., & Sattler, J.M. (1986). *Stanford-Binet Intelligence Scale* (4th ed.). Chicago: Riverside.

Tomblin, J.B., Freese, P.R., & Records, N.L. (1992). Diagnosing specific language impairment in adults for the purpose of pedigree analysis. *Journal of Speech and Hearing Research, 35,* 832–843.

Tunmer, W.E., Herriman, M.L., & Nesdale, A.R. (1988). Metalinguistic abilities and beginning reading. *Reading Research Quarterly, 23,* 134–158.

Valdez-Menchaca, M.C., & Whitehurst, G.J. (1992). Accelerating language development through picture book reading: A systematic extension to Mexican day care. *Developmental Psychology, 28,* 1106–1114.

Wagner, R., & Torgesen, J. (1987). The nature of phonological processing and its causal role in the acquisition of reading skills. *Psychological Bulletin, 101,* 192–212.

Walker, D., Greenwood, C., Hart, B., & Carta, J. (1994). Prediction of school outcomes based on early language production and socioeconomic factors. *Child Development, 65,* 606–621.

Washington, J., & Craig, H.K. (1992). Performance of low-income, African American, preschool and kindergarten children on the Peabody Picture Vocabulary Test–Revised. *Language, Speech, and Hearing Services in Schools, 23,* 329–333.

Watkins, R.V., Buhr, J.C., & Davis, C. (1993, June). *Production of one derivational morpheme by children with SLI.* Paper presented at the Symposium for Research in Child Language Disorders, Madison, WI.

Watkins, R.V., Kelly, D.J., Harbers, H.M., & Hollis, W. (1995). Measuring children's lexical diversity: Differentiating typical and atypical language learners. *Journal of Speech and Hearing Research, 38,* 1349–1355.

Watkins, R.V., & Rice, M.L. (1991). Verb particle and preposition acquisition in children with specific language impairment. *Journal of Speech and Hearing Research, 34,* 1134–1141.

Watkins, R.V., Rice, M.L., & Moltz, C.C. (1993). Verb use by language-impaired and normally developing children. *First Language, 13,* 133–143.

Waxman, S.R., & Kosowski, T.D. (1990). Nouns mark category relations: Toddlers' and preschoolers' word-learning biases. *Child Development, 61,* 1461–1470.

Weismer, S.E. (1991). Hypothesis-testing abilities of language-impaired children. *Journal of Speech and Hearing Research, 34,* 1329–1338.

Weismer, S.E., & Hesketh, L. (1993). The influence of prosodic and gestural cues on novel word acquisition by children with specific language impairment. *Journal of Speech and Hearing Research, 36,* 1013–1025.

Whitehurst, G.J., Arnold, D.S., Epstein, J.N., Angell, A.L., Smith, M., & Fischel, J.E. (1994). A picture book reading intervention in day care and home for children from low-income families. *Developmental Psychology, 30,* 679–689.

Whitehurst, G.J., Falco, F.L., Lonigan, C.J., Fischel, J.E., DeBaryshe, B.D., Valdez-Menchaca, M.C., & Caulfield, M. (1988). Accelerating language development through picture book reading. *Developmental Psychology, 24,* 552–559.

Windsor, J. (1995). Language impairment and social competence. In M.E. Fey, J. Windsor, & S.F. Warren (Eds.), *Communication and language intervention series: Vol. 5. Language intervention: Preschool through the elementary years* (pp. 213–238). Baltimore: Paul H. Brookes Publishing Co.

10

Plotting the Complexities
of Language Sample Analysis
Linear and Nonlinear
Dynamical Models of Assessment

Julia L. Evans

THE ANALYSIS OF A SPONTANEOUS language sample is the cornerstone of any clinical assessment protocol. Unfortunately, the range of indices included in the analysis, the methods employed in collecting a sample, and even the definition of a language disorder have continued to change since the 1950s, coinciding with theory shifts in the fields of psychology and linguistics. Traditionally, models of language disorders have been derived from models of typical language development. As a result, the changes in the theoretical assumptions regarding the mechanisms of typical language development have profoundly influenced the conceptualization of children's language disorders, resulting in the parallel shifts in theories of disorder.

These theoretical shifts, however, are characteristic of the nature of research in general. Scientific inquiry is not an orderly process whereby information is accumulated in a steady, step-by-step manner, with each discovery being added to an evergrowing body of knowledge. The process of scientific inquiry is characterized either by periods of stability, or "normal" science, which are marked by the presence of a clear, overriding theory or research paradigm; or by the sudden and drastic dissolution of a given paradigm in favor of an alternative theory (Kuhn, 1970). The "shared" paradigm that characterizes periods of normal science is a symbolic construction employed to interpret, criticize, or unify a set of laws or assumptions. The implicit agreement on this rigid set of assumptions enables a research community to function effectively by providing a meaningful context by which the relevancy of research hypotheses or experimental results can be judged. In addition to determining the significance of specific research questions, a given paradigm also imposes a strict set of definitions regarding acceptable experimental methodology and instrumentation. Thus, the underlying assumptions of a research paradigm function continuously, driving the entire process of inquiry, guiding the search for data, and defining the laws that encompass this search.

The process of scientific inquiry, however, is not characterized solely by these stable periods of normal science. Often, sudden and drastic shifts in theoretical orientation, or "scientific revolutions," occur that radically alter the direction of inquiry within a given field. Ironically, it is the very process of normal science that is the catalyst for this sudden dissolution of a particular theoretical domain. The goal of normal science is to test the prediction of a given theory. This process, however, invariably yields data that cannot be accounted for by the very theory driving the research. During periods of normal science, the research community will defend the existing theory by repeatedly overlooking findings that are inconsistent with its predictions. Initially, these inconsistencies are viewed as "noise" in the data, or irrelevant to the specified research goal. Over time, however, researchers attempt to account for the anomalous findings by expanding and altering their theory. It is this extension of the theory that ultimately results in the shift to an alternative theoretical orientation.

Three major paradigm shifts in child language have occurred since the early 1950s. These are defined broadly as 1) the behaviorist learning paradigm; 2) the formalist competence-based paradigm, which includes generative syntax, generative semantics, and a narrow interpretation of pragmatics; and 3) the functionalist performance-based paradigm. Each of these theoretical orientations is clearly marked by a distinct set of assumptions regarding the mechanism involved in the process of language acquisition and the definition of the critical unit of analysis.

Craig (1983) clearly showed that the study of children's language disorders has shifted in conjunction with each of these paradigm shifts in child language. Given that models of disorder are derived from models of normal language acquisition, the assumptions from each of the three major paradigms have profoundly influenced the study of children with disorders. As a result, each paradigm shift in child language has altered clinical researchers' definitions of disorder, methods of assessment, and the development of assessment indices.

To understand the vast array of indices available for assessing children with language disorders, an understanding of the impact of each of the theories of language acquisition on models of disorder is needed. The goals of this chapter, therefore, are to 1) outline the underlying theoretical assumptions of each of the three paradigms, identifying the anomalies confronting them and exploring the impact of these paradigms on the nature of assessing populations with disorders; and 2) propose a model of dynamical complex systems as an alternative account of the anomalies that confront assessment models in the mid-1990s.

BEHAVIORISM

Theoretical Assumptions

The prominent paradigm in child language during the 1940s and 1950s has been referred to collectively as behaviorism (United States), or operant learning theory (Great Britain). The single-stage stimulus–response models of classical conditioning (Pavlovian), the operant models of Skinner (1954, 1957), and the representational mediation models of Mowrer (1954) and Osgood (1963) can be considered part of this broad theoretical orientation. Despite individual differences in the models, these learning theories all worked from the assumption that behavior was determined exclusively by the environment (Skinner, 1957). Language, within the behaviorist paradigm, was considered a verbal behavior analogous to other behaviors and, therefore, was subject to the same governing laws and principles. Given this orientation, verbal behavior was assumed to be independent of any central processes or internal cognitive mechanisms (Mowrer, 1954; Skinner, 1954).

Unit of Analysis

The critical unit of analysis within the behaviorist paradigm was the verbal operant, broadly defined as an environmental stimulus and a verbal response (Osgood, 1963; Skinner, 1957). When conceptualized as a behavior, language becomes a continuous phenomenon. As such, an operational definition of this continuous verbal behavior had to be formalized. Thus, a verbal operant was defined as the largest meaningful segment of language that was "highly redundant, frequent in occurrence, of relatively short duration and defined so as to maintain an internal integrity and interdependence among response elements" (Osgood, 1963, p. 744). Researchers focused, therefore, on identifying a unit of analysis that could be perceived and that was functionally related to other verbal forms (Skinner, 1957). Based on this operational definition, the *word* became the primary unit of analysis.

The relationship between an environmental stimulus and a verbal response was believed to be causal. In particular, it was assumed that the production of a verbal response was an immediate reaction to the presence of a specific environmental stimulus or stimulus complex. This relationship between the environmental stimulus and the verbal response was believed to be learned, not predetermined (Skinner, 1954). In addition to the initial *discriminative* stimulus, which was considered to be responsible for eliciting the verbal behavior, a second *reinforcer* stimulus, which occurred after the verbal response, was believed to increase the likelihood that a particular verbal behavior would occur again under the same circumstances (Bandura, 1977; Johnson, 1965; Pollio, 1968). It was assumed that principles of classical conditioning were involved in connecting meaning responses to words and that higher-ordered operant conditioning was involved in the transfer of meaning responses from one word to another. Investigations, therefore, focused on the process by which word meanings were conditioned from one word to another when they occurred in a sentence or on the specific manner in which individual words came to elicit specific connotative meaning responses (Mowrer, 1954; Osgood, 1957).

Implications for Language Learning

Extending the behaviorist paradigm to account for the process of language acquisition required identifying the specific manner in which the child acquired individual verbal response units and identifying the secondary process by which these response units subsequently were related, or "chained," to one another to form larger response units (e.g., sentences). It was believed that the child started with a repertoire of unpatterned vocalizations that were shaped into words through selective reinforcements in the environment (Skinner, 1954). The parents were viewed as the source of external reinforcement that modified the child's verbal behavior, and the child's verbal productions were viewed as incorrect attempts at the adult's verbal model. Thus, it was assumed that the child selected speech models from the environment, and the relative strength of competing stimuli reinforced those productions that were closest to the adult verbal models (Skinner, 1957). By definition, therefore, the child's role in the process of language acquisition was believed to be passive (Mowrer, 1952). For example, a child presented with a cookie might respond with the verbal behavior "cookie." This verbal response may have been elicited by a complex group of stimuli, including the presence of the cookie, the smell of the cookie, and the sound of the opening of the cookie jar; the reinforcer stimulus might have been the child's eating the cookie.

Learning was believed to occur through a well-prescribed sequence of external events; the relationship between the stimulus, the response, the time interval between behaviors, and the relative strength of the response behaviors was considered critical to the characterization of the verbal behavior in question (Skinner, 1954). Chaining—a process whereby each segment of verbal behavior was reinforced in such a way that it served as the stimulus for the next response behavior—and shaping—a process whereby verbal behavior was gradually altered through selective reinforcement of closer and closer approximations to a final verbal form—were proposed as accounts of the acquisition of the more complex verbal behaviors characteristic of adult language.

Language-Sampling Techniques

Calculating the probability of the production of a specific verbal response was the crucial test of a behaviorist account for both language production and comprehension. The primary research goal, therefore, was discovering the precise relationship between a verbal response unit and its external stimulus conditions (Shanon & Weaver, 1949; Sloane & MacAulay, 1968). Language sampling and data analysis consisted of frequency counts of different verbal behaviors, such as the occurrence of different words, different parts of speech, or the length of individual sentences (Johnson, 1965; McCarthy, 1954; Smith, 1933a, 1933b; Templin, 1957); and calculating the frequency with which these units were paired with one another (Pollio, 1968). Given that verbal behaviors were considered equivalent, linguistic classifications such as pronouns, verb tenses, and questions were not relevant tests of the theory.

Assessing Children with Language Disorders

The behaviorist paradigm had a profound impact on theories of disorder with respect to both the mechanism believed to be responsible for the disorder and the indices developed to assess verbal behavior. Because verbal behavior was believed to be determined exclusively by the environment, a language disorder, by definition, had to be the result of either an incorrect relationship between the child's verbal behavior and environmental reinforcement or limitations in the size or organization of the child's verbal response units. The principles of secondary reinforcement as outlined in operant learning theory were believed to be the cause of language disorders in children. For example, Mowrer (1952) argued that a positive relationship between the child and the adult was critical to the child's acquisition of language. Specifically, if the child's initial neutral sounds were associated with positive reinforcements based on the nature of the adult's behavior, then a nonverbal child must be the result of a negative environment created by the parent; intervention, accordingly, would focus on modifying the parent's verbal style.

Given that the mechanism underlying verbal behavior was believed to reside in the environment and that complex behavior was the result of chaining of smaller response units, assessment focused on identifying the critical discriminating stimulus in the environment assumed to be responsible for the disorder. In addition, frequency counts of different verbal behaviors such as the number of phonemes or lexical response units present in the child's response repertoire were compared with developmental norms (e.g., vocabulary size) (Darley & Moll, 1960; Dunn, 1959; Johnson, Darley, & Spriestersbach, 1952; Schiefelbusch, 1963).

Normed tests developed at the time reflected these behaviorist assumptions, providing quantitative measures of different verbal behaviors. For example, the Type-Token Ratio (TTR) (Templin, 1957) measured the diversity in the child's lexical response units, whereas the Peabody Picture Vocabulary Test (Dunn, 1959; revised, Dunn & Dunn, 1981) measured the actual size of a child's vocabulary. The Templin-Darley Test of Articulation (Templin & Darley, 1960) quantitatively measured the actual size of the child's verbal response units at the phonological level. Language tests, such as the Illinois Test of Psycholinguistic Abilities (ITPA) (Kirk & McCarthy, 1961), were developed directly from the operant principles derived from Osgood's (1957) Associations branch of operant learning. The ITPA differentiated assessment of stimulus parameters such as visual and auditory reception from internal mediational stimuli such as visual and auditory associations and response behaviors such as visual and manual output.

The Anomaly

As noted previously, theory shifts are the result of a research community's attempts to account for anomalous findings that, on the surface, appear to be solvable by the known rules and procedures outlined in the existing theory but that resist attempts at explanation. Two issues became problematic for a behaviorist account of language acquisition. First, it was assumed that the acquisition of verbal forms relied on the child's attempts to imitate the adult models that were subsequently reinforced. Unfortunately, characterizations of the adult's language—the model that the child was supposed to imitate—revealed that the adult rarely directly reinforced the child's verbal behavior and, moreover, that the adult's verbal behavior was full of false starts, dysfluencies, and breaks in speech flow instead of being a clean verbal model (Brown & Hanlon, 1970; Chomsky, 1957a, 1957b; McNeill, 1971).

Second, investigation of children's error patterns revealed the presence of novel forms that never occurred in the adult verbal models and that resisted adult corrections. The classic examples of these types of verbal behaviors produced by the child include overregularizations of past tense -ed, as in "I goed" or "I eated" (Berko, 1958; Brown, 1973; Brown & Bellugi, 1964).

Ongoing research in unrelated fields often provides a means of accounting for problems confronting a given group of researchers (Kuhn, 1970). The difficulty with the incomplete language models and the seemingly rule-governed forms in the child's language suggested that some internal processes might be involved in the acquisition of language. Unfortunately, the behaviorist accounts provided no framework to address the prospect of underlying cognitive aspects of language acquisition. Work in the field of linguistics at the time (Chomsky, 1957a, 1957b, 1965) seemed to provide psychologists with an alternative framework to account for these anomalies in children's verbal behavior. Abandoning a research paradigm in acceptance of another results in drastic changes in the research community (Kuhn, 1970). Prior theoretical conceptualizations must be reconstructed, fundamental assumptions must be altered, "traditional" experimental procedures must be reevaluated, and new and rigid definitions of critical research questions must be generated. This is precisely what occurred during the early 1960s as researchers abandoned behaviorism in exchange for a linguistic theory of language acquisition.

FORMALISM

Competence-Based Theories

The prevailing paradigm governing the study of child language since the 1960s has been a modular, competence-based account of language. An underlying assumption of this paradigm is that there is a stable set of cognitive structures, or linguistic competencies, that a hypothetical speaker-listener possesses that are independent of the demands of the ongoing processes of real-time language production or comprehension. This linguistic competence is the abstract knowledge that an ideal speaker-listener possesses about language. This competence-based paradigm encompasses Chomsky's (1957a, 1957b) theory of generative syntax, generative semantics (Fillmore, 1968; Schlesinger, 1974), and narrow pragmatics models (Dore, 1975; Halliday, 1975).

These theories are modular in that each level of the linguistic hierarchy—phonology, morphology, syntax, and semantics—is believed to be a distinct, rule-governed system that can be identified and studied in isolation (Berwick & Weinberg, 1984; Bresnan, 1982; Chomsky, 1957a, 1957b; Dore, 1975; Pinker, 1984; Schlesinger, 1973). These systems are believed to be generative in that the internal set of finite rules for each linguistic system generates an infinite set of structures (Chomsky, 1957a, 1957b; Dore, 1974; Lakoff, 1972; Schlesinger, 1973). Thus, it is believed that there is a direct one-to-one mapping between underlying linguistic rules and their manifestation in the surface form of an utterance (Brown, 1973; Chomsky, 1963; McNeill, 1971). Linguistic competence is believed to be autonomous of aspects of the environment and independent of the variations in the surface form of language production or comprehension resulting from actual communication demands (Chomsky, 1957a, 1957b; Fodor, Bever, & Garrett, 1974).

Generative Syntax　Chomsky's theory of transformational grammar was not developed to address the anomalies confronting psychologists in the late 1950s but was, instead, a response to a different set of problems confronting linguists (Chomsky, 1957a, 1957b, 1964). Chomsky's theory of transformational grammar was a purely mathematical approach to writing grammars. Instead of writing a grammar for a single language in isolation, Chomsky argued that the strongest test of a grammar was its ability to mark grammatical sentences from nongrammatical sentences produced by an ideal speaker-listener in any language. Thus, according to Chomsky, a finite set of universal linguistic rules should be able to generate an infinite set of sentences for any language; the ultimate goal for linguists, therefore, was to discover these linguistic universals.

Theoretical Assumptions　Researchers' acceptance of a new theoretical paradigm results in a profound and qualitative restructuring of relevant questions, with previously considered key evidence suddenly becoming irrelevant background facts. In contrast to behaviorism, the fundamental assumption of linguistic theories is that languages are rule governed and are generated by an internal set of competencies, not derived from the environment. Scientific inquiry focuses on identifying regularities in a language, with the goal being to construct an explicit grammar or set of rules to account for these regularities. The test of a grammar is the goodness of fit between the sentences generated by the grammar and the naturally occurring forms of the language in question (Gleason, 1961; Hockett, 1960).

Specifically, Chomsky's model of transformational grammar divided sentences into *deep structures* and *surface structures*. Deep structures are meaning-free, formal constituents, such as noun phrase and verb phrase, mapped in a hierarchical relationship. The final surface structure of a sentence is generated by deleting or rearranging deep structures into lexical strings through a series of transformations. These transformations result in the direct mapping of deep structures onto the final surface structures. According to Chomsky, these deep structures are the same as mathematical objects that are manipulated through the application of the transformations. Chomsky argued that for a grammar to generate all of the sentences of a language, these syntactic constituents had to be independent of and unconstrained by meanings.

Implications for Language Learning   Within the behaviorist paradigm, language acquisition was believed to be the result of a complex interaction among a stimulus, the child's verbal behavior, and a subsequent environmental reinforcement. Chomsky's generative theory of syntax stated that language was generated from a set of underlying rules that resulted in a one-to-one mapping between rules and the surface forms they generated. This posed a critical problem for the psychologist. If deep structures and transformations were internal, symbolic, rule-governed events, then they could never be present in the environment and, therefore, could never be observed by the child. If, according to Chomsky, language no longer was derived from the environment, then researchers would have to alter their assumptions regarding language acquisition. This fundamental shift in orientation was clearly revealed in McNeill's (1971) critique of behaviorism:

> In acquiring the transformations that define language, what children learn is how to relate deep structures and surface structures. But the deep structures of sentences are never displayed in the form of examples, stimulus, responses or anything else in the environment. They are abstract and for one who does not already know the language, inaccessible. It is this simple linguistic fact which every child faces and overcomes that eliminates Stimulus–Response theory as a serious explanation of language acquisition. There is no form of this S–R theory that can account for the emergence of a relation, one half of which is never manifested. The most fundamental ground rule of behavioral analysis—that a phenomenon can be analyzed into responses paired with a stimulus—is contradicted. Moreover, there is no conceivable elaboration of S–R theory, short of abandonment, that can apply to the acquisition of linguistic abstractions. (p. 18)

If the child could not observe the deep structures and transformations in the environment, then clearly some internal mechanism had to be involved in the process of language acquisition. Thus, by accepting Chomsky's theory, psychologists were forced to assume that the child's acquisition of language was the result of an interaction between some internal process or innate linguistic capacity and linguistic experience (McNeill, 1971). Because the generative syntax theory implied that language development consisted of the acquisition of underlying deep structures and transformations, researchers shifting from behaviorism were forced to restructure their thinking and start from the premise that the child began with clues about the nature of language and that language acquisition was the active search for underlying linguistic structures (Braine, 1973; Brown, Cazden, & Bellugi, 1973; Chomsky, 1963; McNeill, 1966).

Unit of Analysis Because the research goal for psychologists shifted to identifying deep structures, which were believed to generate the surface forms observed in a child's sentences, the concept of the verbal behavioral unit no longer was useful. Instead of frequency counts of verbal behavior, the unit of analysis became the *sentence*—a very specific form of verbal output that was believed to be a direct manifestation of the child's internal linguistic knowledge. Researchers restricted their efforts solely to the investigation of the linguistic structure of children's sentences independent of cognitive, perceptual, or social context.

Language-Sampling Techniques The critical test of Chomsky's theory was determining whether children's language acquisition was, in fact, rule governed. Language analysis, therefore, focused on the emergence of specific syntactic constituents. In contrast to behaviorism, in which emphasis was placed on predicting the probability of the occurrence of different response units, psychologists attempted to identify the structures that generated children's sentences. The first instances in which syntactic structures could be identified were the child's earliest two-word constructions (Braine, 1973; Brown et al., 1973; McNeill, 1966). Thus, children's productions were analyzed with respect to the form and distribution of specific syntactic elements and were classified on the basis of the privilege of co-occurrence of particular syntactic constituents, such as noun or verb phrases, or on the emergence of different transformations, such as negatives, interrogatives, or passives (Braine, 1973; Brown et al., 1973; McNeill, 1966). Studies at this time were characterized by a large amount of data collected from a small number of children beginning around 20–24 months of age when the child began to produce two-word utterances—the point at which it was believed that children's earliest instances of grammatical knowledge were revealed.

The findings from these studies revealed regularities in children's two-word utterances that were consistent with the theory's predictions. Children's earliest sentences appeared to be rule governed, consisting primarily of a small class of words occurring frequently in relatively fixed positions, and a larger class of words occurring less frequently. These two classes of words were referred to respectively as pivot and open classes by Braine (1963), functor and contentive classes by Brown and Bellugi (1964), and operators and nonoperators by Miller and Ervin (1964).

Assessing Children with Language Disorders With respect to models of disorder, the consequence of shifting to a generative model is evident in changes in assessment protocols, development of new tests, and shifts in the beliefs regarding the underlying etiology of language disorders. Parallel with psychologists' reinterpretation of language acquisition from a syntactic framework, the child with language disorders also was reconceptualized. If, as predicted by the generative syntax model, the child was born with the innate capacity to learn language, and the process of language acquisition consisted of the active formation of hypotheses regarding the regularities in a language, then the problems exhibited by children with language disorders, by logical extension, had to be the result of impairments in the child's innate linguistic competence either at the level of the deep structures or in the acquisition of the transformations necessary for generating the final surface structures.

By accepting a competence-based model, language disorders no longer could be interpreted as deficits in the size or organization of verbal response units or as incorrect relationships between the verbal behavior and its stimulus or reinforcer. By definition, a language disorder had to be, instead, the result of impairments in the child's underlying linguistic competence or innate linguistic abilities (Adams & Pace, 1969; Menyuk, 1964). This shift to a competence-based model of disorders drastically altered the critical unit of analysis. Clinical researchers now had to assess the underlying syntactic competence in attempts to identify the gaps or missing features in the child's linguistic competencies. Models of disorder attempted to determine whether the child was missing phrase structures, transformations, or morphological features (Johnson & Schery, 1976; Lee, 1966; Lee & Cantor, 1971; Leonard, 1972; Menyuk, 1964; Menyuk & Looney, 1972; Morehead & Ingram, 1973).

Given that the child's language impairments were now interpreted as a manifestation of an impaired rule-governed system, in contrast to the previous presumption of an incorrect approximation of the adult's verbal model, assessment of children's spontaneous language was compared with child models instead of adult language models (Bloom & Lahey, 1978; Lee, 1971, 1974). The earliest stages of language development were believed to represent experimentation with grammatical forms, such as noun phrase and verb phrase constructions, as a means of understanding the subject–predicate relationships essential to later adult English syntax (Dale, 1976). The child learning language typically was believed to progress through clearly marked stages in the acquisition of these different syntactic structures. As a result, the syntactic constructions observed for the child with a language disorder were compared with typically developing children at different stages in linguistic development (Johnson & Schery, 1976; Lee, 1966; Lee & Cantor, 1971; Leonard, 1972; Menyuk, 1964; Menyuk & Looney, 1972; Morehead & Ingram, 1973).

Both formal assessment indices and spontaneous language protocols developed at this time reflected the shift from a model of disorders defined by the environment to one predicated on innate internal mechanisms. Standardized tests such as the Reynell Expressive Developmental Language Scale (Reynell, 1969), Berko's (1958) assessment of morphological structures, Carrow Elicited Language Inventory (CELI) (Carrow, 1974), and the Northwestern Syntax

Screening Test (NSST) (Lee, 1971) all were developed to determine the state of a child's internal linguistic competence.

Assessment protocols of spontaneous language worked from the assumption that the state of the child's underlying competence was revealed in the surface form of the child's utterances. Thus, protocols such as Developmental Sentence Analysis (DSS and DST) (Lee, 1966; Lee & Koenigsknecht, 1974); Language Sampling, Analysis, and Training (Tyack & Gottsleben, 1974); and the Language Assessment Remediation and Screening Procedure (LARSP) (Crystal, 1974; Crystal, Fletcher, & Garman, 1989) focused exclusively on the syntactic structure of the child's language productions as a window to the state of the child's underlying grammar.

Because it was believed that the syntactic form of an utterance was a manifestation of direct one-to-one mapping between underlying linguistic rules and surface forms, the structure of the child's utterances was believed to be a direct window to the child's linguistic knowledge. Errors in the surface form of sentences were assessed, therefore, as a direct reflection of impairments in the state of the child's underlying linguistic competence. Unfortunately, Chomsky (1963) stated explicitly that linguistic theories had *nothing* to say about actual speaker performance, arguing that a strict distinction had to be maintained between a speaker's competence (i.e., the individual's knowledge of his or her language) and a speaker's actual performance (i.e., the real-time use of language in communicative situations) if linguists were to identify the linguistic universals of languages. Chomsky claimed that the traditional method of writing grammars from a corpus of spontaneous speech prevented linguists from identifying the underlying grammar of a language because of variations in the spontaneous speech produced by any individual speaker. These variations resulted from an infinite set of variables such as memory limitations, speaker distractions, shifts in attention, and interest and formulation errors.

Chomsky (1964) argued that linguists should study only the *ideal* speaker-listener in an ideal speech-community, who knows the language perfectly and is unaffected by the characteristic constraints of real-time language processing. As a result, only under idealized conditions could a speaker's actual performance ever be a direct reflection of linguistic knowledge. Given that these conditions never exist, Chomsky maintained that spontaneous language production could *never* be used as a map of underlying linguistic competence (Chomsky, 1964).

Maintaining the distinction between speaker competence and real-time language performance posed a particular problem for researchers investigating children's acquisition of linguistic rules. The only data available for psychologists to test the predictions of the generative theory—that children had innate internal linguistic knowledge—was to infer the existence of this knowledge from the syntactic structure of the utterances children actually produced (Braine, 1963; Brown & Bellugi, 1964; Miller & Ervin, 1964). Thus, directly counter to Chomsky, researchers interpreted the presence or absence of linguistic structures in the surface form of children's spontaneous verbal performance as direct evidence of internal rules.

This subtle shift in the methodology had a profound impact on clinical researchers' attempts to characterize the innate knowledge states of children with disorders. Consistent with psychologists, researchers investigating children's language impairments also began to interpret the surface structures of children's spontaneous productions as direct reflections of underlying linguistic competence (Lee, 1966; Lee & Koenigsknecht, 1974). For example, Lee (1974) argued that her Developmental Sentence Scoring (DSS) was developed to evaluate verbal *performance*—the child's use of grammatical rules in spontaneous speech—as a measure of the child's internal knowledge. Accordingly, the DSS system does not consider a particular linguistic structure to be present in the child's linguistic repertoire until all of the required syntactic and morphological rules are observed in spontaneous speech. A child who demonstrates consistent accuracy in the *use* of a particular syntactic structure is assumed to have generalized that rule into his or her deep structures.

Chomsky's separation of the study of innate linguistic competence and actual speaker performance was an attempt to control or filter out variability in real-time performance resulting from memory limitations, attention, or even speaker distractions. Using performance as a window to underlying competence, however, made obtaining a representative sample a serious problem for clinical researchers. Because it was assumed that structures present in a child's spontaneous language provided clues to the missing structures or rules in the child's underlying linguistic competence, obtaining evidence for the existence of these structures in spontaneous speech became critical to characterizing a child with a language disorder (Bloom & Lahey, 1978; Lee, 1966; Lee & Koenigsknecht, 1974). Suddenly, a range of variables affecting the child's production of grammatical forms, including variations resulting from different sampling contexts (e.g., "optimal," "typical," "best"), the effect of different materials such as pictures versus toys, even the effect of conversational style of the speaking partner, now had to be controlled in an attempt to collect a representative sample (Dailey & Boxx, 1979; Darley & Moll, 1960; Johnson, Darley, & Spriestersbach, 1963; Kramer, James, & Saxman, 1979).

The Anomaly In contrast to the behaviorist paradigm in which sentence meanings were believed to be attached to words through a series of associations (Pollio, 1968), semantics had no place in the generative theory of syntax (Chomsky, 1957a, 1957b, 1964). Semantics was a separate component of the grammar, containing lexical rules that interpreted abstract syntactic structures into semantic notions in the last step of formalizing the final surface form of the sentence. That syntactic constituents such as subjects or verbs often were occupied by semantic roles such as "agent" or "action" was believed to be purely coincidental (Bolinger, 1975). Researchers believed that the formal study of semantics could benefit from a precise definition of underlying syntactic structures but that the reverse was not true. Meanings expressed by the speaker and contextual information from the environment were considered irrelevant to writing grammars for any language (Chomsky, 1965).

This strict exclusion of meaning became problematic both for psychologists studying children's acquisition of grammar and for the field of linguistics as a whole. In attempting to write the rules for English, linguists discovered that certain kinds of meanings were not independent of the syntactic transformations that they were trying to identify. For example, the semantic content of the sentence *John hit the ball* remains the same after being subjected to the passive transformation resulting in the sentence *The ball was hit by John.* This was not the case for grammatical structures such as pronouns, negation, and reflexives, nor for passive transformations such as *All women kiss some men* to *Some men are kissed by all women,* which results in a radically different meaning (Fillmore, 1968; McCawley, 1968; Ross, 1970).

Psychologists also were confronted with the problem of the meanings inherent in children's expressions. To write the earliest grammars for children's language, the meanings evident in surface forms of children's sentences had to be included. If the semantic interpretations of children's sentences were not taken into account in the surface structures, then differences in underlying deep structures could not be captured (Bloom, 1970; Bowerman, 1976). For example, the sentence *Mommy sock* was produced by Kathryn at 21 months in two separate contexts—while picking up her mother's sock and while Kathryn's mother was putting Kathryn's sock on Kathryn's foot (Bloom, 1970). To an investigator working within Chomsky's transformational theory, both of these sentences were examples of Pivot + x-word constructions. However, this level of interpretation did not capture the semantic–syntax relations between "Mommy" and "sock." In the first utterance, "Mommy" is the attribute of "sock"; in the second utterance, "Mommy" is the agent-actor. These two utterances clearly were the result of different underlying deep structures.

Taken within the context of a semantic, or "rich," interpretation, the child's expression of two distinctly different meanings with the same surface structure suggested that the child had a far greater awareness of the relationship between linguistic elements. A strict syntactic account based solely on "privilege of occurrence" of linguistic constituents in the surface form of the sentence could not capture this relationship. By including semantics in the analysis, children's earliest two-word constructions no longer appeared to represent the mapping of the child's innate abstract syntactic structures onto surface forms void of meaning; rather, they seemed to reflect underlying semantic knowledge. When semantic intentions were included in the interpretations of children's two-word constructions, pivot-open-type grammars only captured children's underlying language competence in a superficial way (Bloom, 1970).

That the meanings expressed in a speaker's sentences persistently appeared to have some role in the final syntactic surface form kept intruding on researchers' attempts to write the grammars for children's language. The child's intuitive knowledge of linguistic code obviously involved more than was captured by the purely linguistic descriptions of the surface form of the child's utterances. Ignoring that the child's induction of underlying syntactic structures seemed to be intimately tied to the underlying semantic intentions that the child was expressing became increasingly more difficult.

Generative Semantics   In their attempts to fit newly discovered "facts" regarding semantic intentions into the existing accounts of language, psychologists and linguists both modified Chomsky's generative theory of syntax to include semantics. This extension of the generative syntactic theory has been referred to as the generative semantic account (Craig, 1983; Lakoff & Ross, 1967; Lund & Duchan, 1983, 1988; Postal, 1972; Schlesinger, 1971).

Theoretical Assumptions   One example of this extension of the generative model is Schlesinger's (1971) model, which replaced subject and verb constituents from Chomsky's original theory with agent-action, or receiver of action, notions that were mapped directly into a string of lexical items without passing through a separate syntactic level of subject–verb entities. Schlesinger maintained the deep structure constructs but redefined them from a semantic perspective by replacing syntactic phrase markers with semantic intention markers instead. Thus, the fundamental framework of the generative paradigm was maintained and merely extended to include semantic information. Because the basic assumptions were maintained, researchers continued to view language as a rule-governed system with a direct link between these underlying rules and surface forms. These underlying symbolic rules still were presumed to be generative, but a finite set of semantic intentions, which could generate an infinite set of meanings expressed in the surface form of the speaker's sentences, were added (Antinucci & Parisi, 1973; Bloom, 1970; Fillmore, 1968; Lakoff, 1973).

Implications for Language Learning   This shift to a generative semantic model did not alter the existing assumptions of the competence-based paradigm, but researchers had to redefine the critical unit of analysis. No longer were syntactic constituents and their mapping onto surface structures the unit of analysis; instead, semantic intentions and their mapping onto surface forms became the unit of investigation (Schlesinger, 1971; Sinclair, 1971). In response to this shift, psychologists began to focus on the meanings contained in children's utterances in an attempt to identify these new semantic structures and subsequently to capture the underlying semantic deep structures for all of the meanings signaled in the final surface form of children's utterances.

The early semantic intentions expressed by children became the focus of investigations, and the same two-word utterances that previously had been interpreted as a representation of underlying subject–verb relationships were reinterpreted from a semantic framework. The critical issue no longer was whether children's earliest utterances reflected the existence of syntax; it was whether their utterances suggested the existence of underlying semantic structures such as agent-vehicle/action rules. Emphasis was placed on identifying these semantic universals (Bach & Harms, 1968; Bowerman, 1974; Brown, 1973; Chafe, 1970; Ingram, 1972; Lakoff, 1971; Slobin, 1970). The results of these studies revealed that children expressed a similar set of meaning structures across a range of different languages (Johnston & Slobin, 1979). This high degree of overlap in the earliest semantic intentions expressed by children learning different languages was interpreted as an indication that the earliest stages in language acquisition had to be tied to cognitive development (Miller, Chapman, Branston, & Reichle, 1980). That the early meanings expressed by children seemed to parallel stages in cognitive development as predicted by Piaget therefore came as no surprise (Edwards, 1973; Sinclair, 1971).

Language-Sampling Techniques Given that the basic tenets of the generative paradigm were still operative, only slight modifications in language sampling techniques and definitions of data resulted from the shift to investigations of children's early semantic intentions. In spite of Chomsky's separation of competence and performance, researchers continued to view the patterns observed in spontaneous verbal performance as a window to underlying linguistic competence. During the generative syntax era, investigations of children's language acquisition began at 20–24 months—the point at which two-word constructions begin to emerge in children's spontaneous speech. The goal at the time was to write the rules for the relationship between syntactic constituents. Two-word utterances were the earliest instances of grammar in children's language and were considered the critical test of the theory (Braine, 1973; Brown et al., 1973; McNeill, 1966). Because the earliest stages of language acquisition appeared to be semantic instead, researchers began to focus on the first instances in which meaning could be conveyed by the child—the production of one-word utterances. Thus, data collection began at the point at which single words appeared, around 10–12 months of age, instead.

In addition to characterizing the range of meanings expressed at the single-word level, the relationship between these meanings and the child's stage of cognitive development also became the focus of investigations (Antinucci & Parisi, 1973; Bowerman, 1973; Brown, 1973; Greenfield & Smith, 1976; Ingram, 1971). These early one-word utterances were viewed either as static semantic features that were present or absent for a given word (Clark, 1973) or as meaning acts manifested as actions within meaningful communicative context (Antinucci & Parisi, 1973; Greenfield & Smith, 1976).

Reconceptualizing language development as the acquisition of semantic deep structures reflected researchers' attempts to capture these new data by extending the existing theoretical framework and maintaining the fundamental assumptions of the original linguistic theory. For example, by recalculating the length of children's utterances in morphemes reflecting the smallest unit of meaning instead of in syntactic constituents (i.e., nouns, verbs), Brown (1973) showed a relationship between the actual length of children's utterances in morphemes and underlying semantic and syntactic knowledge. Brown (1973) identified five distinct stages in language development that, he argued, captured the transition from the expression of early semantic notions to later syntactic constructions. When compared by age and rate of development of syntactic milestones, children appeared to differ substantially; however, when compared by the mean length of their utterances in morphemes, distinct stages in language development appeared to emerge.

According to Brown (1973), Stage I (mean length of utterance [MLU] 1.0–2.0) reflected the child's emphasis on the merging of syntactic and semantic influences and was characterized by the child's acquisition of semantic roles and early syntactic relations. Stage II (MLU 2.0–2.5) was characterized primarily by the child's acquisition of grammatical morphology and modulation of meanings. Stage III (MLU 2.5–3.25) captured the child's development of modalities of simple sentences. Stage IV (MLU 3.25–3.75) reflected the child's acquisition of embedded structures. Last, Stage V (MLU 3.75–4.0) reflected the presence of the coordination of phrase-level constructions necessary for the production of complete syntax.

Assessing Children with Language Disorders   Extending the existing generative model to incorporate semantic constituents also was incorporated into models of language impairments (Freedman & Carpenter, 1976; Inhelder, 1976; Leonard, Bolders, & Miller, 1976; Morehead & Ingram, 1973; Snyder, 1975). For example, Morehead and Ingram (1973) completed a complex transformational analysis of utterances produced by children with language disorders that was designed to represent the five linguistic levels outlined by Brown (1973). They argued that to effectively capture the relationship between the deep structure and surface forms, the linguistic competence of the child with language disorders had to be investigated from a rich interpretation. Because it was readily apparent that two or more semantic interpretations might be necessary for an accurate grammatical analysis of the linguistic competence of the child with language disorder, semantic information was considered critical in the analysis of the child's verbal productions.

Normal models again were employed in the development of these assessment indices, which were designed explicitly to document the underlying semantic competence of children with impairments. The relational semantic models of Fillmore (1968) and Schlesinger (1974), which provided a generative framework for early agent-action and locative relationships observed in children's early utterances, were incorporated into language assessment models to evaluate the range of relational meanings expressed by the child with impairments (Chapman, 1981; Retherford, Schwartz, & Chapman, 1982). In addition, the lexical semantic models of Ingram (1972) and Peach (1977) were employed as measures of the diversity of meanings in the child's repertoire (Freedman & Carpenter, 1976; Leonard et al., 1976).

Formal assessment protocols also were derived from Fillmore's (1968) case grammar, which provided profiles of the relational meanings used by children with language disorders. Bloom and Lahey's (1978) assessment profile was an example of the extension of the existing generative syntax constructions and attempted to capture the early semantic–syntactic notions expressed by a child.

Standardized tests developed at the time clearly reflected the shift in emphasis to assessment of the underlying semantic competence of the child with language disorder. Tests, including the Environmental Language Inventory (ELI) (MacDonald, 1978), were based upon Schlesinger's (1971) transformational semantic rules and Brown's (1973) early semantic categories. Assessment of lexical meanings expressed in the child's spontaneous speech samples included using the TTR, recommended as an overall measure of lexical diversity (Chapman, 1981), and documenting the range of different lexical meanings expressed by the individual child (Lund & Duchan, 1983).

The belief that the impairments of a child with language disorder were a direct reflection of the state of the child's underlying linguistic competence was still maintained. Because children's earliest utterances were being interpreted as reflections of early sensorimotor cognitive development (Bates, Camaioni, & Volterra, 1975; Bowerman, 1974; Clark, 1974; Morehead & Morehead, 1974), researchers assumed that the impairments observed for children with language disorders were a reflection of underlying cognitive deficits (Cromer, 1976; de Ajuriaguerra et al., 1976; Inhelder, 1976; Johnston & Ramstad, 1978; Morehead & Ingram, 1973). Studies investigating children's underlying cognitive impairments and language impairments focused on the symbolic play skills of children with language disorders (Brown, Redmond, Bass, Leibergott, & Swope, 1975), their use of figurative and operational thought (Inhelder, 1976; Johnston & Ramstadt, 1978), and the relationship between the child's verbal skills and nonverbal cognitive skills (Snyder, 1975). Formal assessment measures developed at the time, such as the Boehm Test of Basic Concepts (Boehm, 1971), reflected the assumption that the meanings expressed by the child were representations of underlying cognitive development.

The discovery that the linguistic complexity of the utterances produced by children appeared to be related to their acquisition of underlying roles for typical children (Brown, 1973; Brown & Hanlon, 1970) suggested that the length and complexity of the utterances of the child with language impairment also could be used as a direct index of the underlying semantic–syntactic competence of the child with language disorder. As a result, the use of MLU was incorporated into assessment protocols as a means of identifying the linguistic level of the child with language disorder and has become the cornerstone of spontaneous language assessments (Miller, 1981).

The Anomaly In the same way that researchers had to employ a rich semantic interpretation of children's language to write the grammars for two-word utterances, psychologists in the late 1970s were having to rely on a rich interpretation of children's one-word utterances. Specifically, coding semantic intentions required extensive reference to the verbal and nonverbal communicative context associated with the language event in question. Thus, researchers had to rely heavily on the child's communicative intent to accurately code semantic intentions in children's earliest expressions (Bates et al., 1975; Carter, 1974; Lakoff, 1972; Lock, 1972).

For example, prior to determining the underlying meaning constituents in an utterance such as *Those cookies were great,* investigators had to determine whether the speaker's intended meaning was a simple declarative statement or under a different set of contextual conditions—an indirect request. Even something as simple as different intonation patterns clearly distinguished the compliment *Gee, you look great* from sarcasm. In the same way that using a rich semantic interpretation of children's two-word utterances to write early grammars ultimately revealed that children's earliest expressions were in fact semantic in nature, including a rich communicative interpretation to write the semantic grammars for children's one-word utterances began to reveal that children's earliest utterances were highly communicative (Bates et al., 1975; Carter, 1974; Lakoff, 1972; Lock, 1972).

Again, instead of rejecting the formalist competence-based theory, researchers extended the existing paradigm, adding a set of competencies designed to capture this underlying communicative knowledge in the same manner that semantic information had been incorporated into the existing syntactic models during the late 1960s (Fillmore, 1968; Schlesinger, 1971). Thus, in the same way that the paradigm had been extended to include the additional set of semantic deep structures, which were distinct from syntactic deep structures but which maintained the same conceptual model, the generative theory once again was extended to include a distinct set of underlying language-use competencies. The modularity of the paradigm still was maintained, and it was assumed that these conversational competencies could be studied independent of the syntactic and semantic systems (Gordon & Lakoff, 1971; Grice, 1968; Kiefer, 1973; Morris, 1946).

This extension was clearly revealed in Lakoff's (1973) suggestion that the early pragmatic presuppositions expressed by children could be reduced to traditional semantics if they were conceptualized as an additional part of the semantic tree structure underlying individual sentences. However, studies of children's earliest one-word utterances suggested that the intentions expressed by children were not simply the result of a set of combined symbolic deep meaning tree structures (Bates, 1976; Greenfield & Smith, 1976). It appeared, therefore, that in the same way that a purely syntactic analysis had not captured the child's underlying semantic knowledge evident in utterances such as *Mommy sock* used in different contexts, the communicative intentions of one-word expressions such as *bye-bye* could not be captured by a purely semantic referential model.

Closer inspection of the verbal and nonverbal communicative intentions of children's one-word utterances such as *doggy,* occurring with a certain set of gestures and eye contact, appeared to suggest two levels of meaning. The first was the primary aspect of the context *dog* as the intended referent, and the second was the communicative force of the utterance such as *Look at the dog!* while pointing to a dog in the park. Children's single-word constructions, when viewed as communicative acts, revealed underlying communicative intentions that could not be captured by a purely semantic referential analysis (Antinucci & Parisi, 1973; Dore, 1974; Greenfield & Smith, 1976). Within the context of a richer interpretation, most of children's earliest utterances, instead of expressing semantic notions, suddenly appeared to be pragmatic, performing communicative acts in and of themselves (Bates et al., 1975).

Narrow Pragmatics   Relying on early communicative intentions to study the emergence of semantic knowledge resulted in a third extension of the existing competence-based paradigm, which has been referred to as a narrow interpretation of pragmatics (Craig, 1983, 1995). Several different definitions of pragmatics evolved at this time, resulting in distinct lines of research for both typical language learners and children with language impairments (Austin, 1962; Bates, 1978; Craig, 1983, 1995; McTear & Conti-Ramsden, 1992; Prutting & Kirchner, 1983; Searle, 1969).

Theoretical Assumptions   The narrow interpretation of pragmatics maintained the fundamental theoretical assumptions of the generative paradigm. It was tacitly believed, therefore, that an additional set of generative rules governed the relationship between conversational entities in the same way that syntactic and semantic structures governed the relationship between syntactic or semantic constituents. As a result, the generative paradigm was extended once again to incorporate an additional set of communicative competencies in such a way that children's earliest pragmatic intentions could later become "grammaticalized" as semantic and syntactic structures instead (Dore, 1975; Lakoff, 1973). Researchers' attempts to explicitly maintain the fundamental assumptions of the existing paradigm are evident in Dore's (1975) argument that there had to be an analogous set of pragmatic universals that were distinct from semantic and syntactic universals but that functioned in the same manner. Thus, researchers simply extended the generative paradigm to include children's earliest communicative expressions and attempted to write the rules for the communicative functions evident in children's one-word utterances, such as declarative and imperative acts, in the same way that they had written the rules for children's combining of semantic or syntactic constituents (Antinucci & Parisi, 1973).

Within this narrow interpretation of pragmatics, researchers focused primarily on 1) the child's knowledge of communicative intents, 2) the child's understanding of the concept of a shared speaker knowledge, and 3) the child's knowledge of the rules governing communicative interactions. The study of the intentional aspects of communication was grounded in the speech act theory (Austin, 1962; Searle, 1969), which focused on language as a social act. Within this speech act theory, researchers attempted to document the developmental progression of the child's acquisition of communicative intentions and the impact of communicative intentions on the listener (Dore, 1974; Halliday, 1975). Researchers also attempted to characterize the child's presuppositional knowledge—knowledge not contained in the sentence itself but the result of the shared speaker–listener understanding of the communicated meaning (Kiefer, 1973; Levison, 1983). Researchers focused on the meanings that children expressed that could not be captured by the traditional generative semantic model. For example, the correct interpretation of the response *It's not your birthday* to the question *Can I wear this sweater?* had to go beyond the literal meaning of the utterance and include the shared knowledge of both the speaker and the listener (Bates, 1978; Greenfield & Westerman, 1978). In addition, researchers focused on children's awareness of the subtle meanings conveyed by the rules governing discourse or conversational postulates (Bloom, Rocissano, & Hood, 1976; Garvey, 1975; Grice, 1968; Sacks, Schegloff, & Jefferson, 1974).

Language-Sampling Techniques   To investigate the intentional aspects of children's communication, the analysis of spontaneous language samples had to be substantially modified from the traditional structural analysis of individual utterances in isolation to a richer analysis of the child's utterances within the larger context of the communicative interaction. To correctly interpret the intended force of a child's utterances or to accurately determine a child's underlying knowledge of discourse functions, a whole new level of information from the language samples had to be included in the transcriptions themselves (Ochs, 1979). Detailed documentation of the nonverbal communication behaviors such as gaze and gestures (Craig & Gallagher, 1983; Ochs, 1979) and microanalysis of turn management behaviors such as speaker overlaps or speaker response times now had to be included in the spontaneous language samples (Craig & Gallagher, 1983; Gallagher & Craig, 1982; Garvey & Hogan, 1973; Keenan, 1974).

With this major reconceptualization of language as a communicative act, a richer analysis of children's communication revealed not only that children expressed a range of communicative acts in their earliest utterances, which were highly intentional (Dore, 1975; Garvey, 1975; Greenfield & Smith, 1976; Gruber, 1973; Halliday, 1973; Ingram, 1971), but also that children appeared to have underlying communicative competence as revealed by the wide range of conversational postulates such as indirect requests and politeness markers used by children in their earliest dyadic interactions (Bates, 1976; Garvey & Hogan, 1973; Lakoff, 1972). In addition, it appeared that children clearly understood the fundamental discourse management rules necessary to participate in two- and three-party interactions (Craig & Gallagher, 1983).

Assessing Children with Language Disorders   The most profound implication of the studies of children's early communicative attempts was that there was an additional set of underlying competencies—the rules governing the use of language within context—that needed to be identified and assessed for children with language disorders. As a result, the pragmatic skills of children with language disorders became the focus of clinical investigations in the early 1980s. It had to be determined whether the child with language disorder had impaired underlying communicative competence governing the use of language in context in addition to having impaired syntactic and semantic competence (Brinton, Fujiki, Froem-Loeb, & Winkler, 1986; Craig & Evans, 1989; Gallagher, 1981; Gallagher & Craig, 1984; Prutting & Kirchner, 1983; van Kleeck & Frankel, 1981).

Because pragmatics was viewed as an additional set of rules underlying the use of language, new language assessment protocols were developed to identify possible impairments in this additional set of competencies. The range of speech acts expressed by children with impairments was compared with children developing language typically to provide some measure of a child's conversational knowledge (Brinton et al., 1986; Gallagher & Craig, 1984; Leonard, Camarata, Rowan, & Chapman, 1982; van Kleeck & Frankel, 1981). The presence or absence of individual speech acts was viewed as a measure of the child's underlying pragmatic competence. The studies investigating the presuppositional knowledge of the child with language impairment focused on the child's ability to prioritize new information while maintaining old information in background discourse (Leonard, Chapman, Rowan, & Weiss, 1983; Skarakis & Greenfield, 1982) and his or her ability to manipulate episodes and cohesive devices within narrative and discourse contexts (Craig & Evans, 1993; Liles, 1985).

Preliminary investigations of the underlying knowledge of conversational postulates produced by children with language impairment and their ability to employ the rules of discourse focused on turn-taking abilities in dyads and multiparty interactions. These studies included detailed analysis of children's abilities to manage the turn exchange, to use both verbal and nonverbal cues (Craig & Evans, 1989), to produce conversational interruptions (Craig & Evans, 1993), and to gain access to ongoing discourse (Craig & Washington, 1993).

Given that the child's pragmatic skills were revealed only during ongoing verbal interactions, formal pragmatic profiles, which were based on the spontaneous speech sample (Penn, 1988; Prutting & Kirchner, 1983; Roth & Spekman, 1984), had to be developed to evaluate the child's verbal and nonverbal communicative competence. In addition to these pragmatic profiles, a few formal test measures were developed, including the Test of Pragmatic Skills–Revised (Shulman, 1986) and the Interpersonal Language Skills Assessment (Blagden & McConnell, 1985).

Competence-Based Paradigm

Assessing Children with Language Disorders As noted previously, the fundamental tenets of the paradigm restrict the research community's definition of relevant research questions, acceptable research methods, and critical units of analysis. As a competence-based model of language, the formalist paradigm is predicated on the assumption that the final surface form of any utterance is a direct manifestation of its direct relationship to underlying rules or structures (Chomsky, 1957a, 1957b). By logical extension, these linguistic structures have been assumed to be the underlying source of children's acquisition of language and the mechanisms responsible for disorder.

Characterizing these underlying competencies at each linguistic level (e.g., phonology, morphology, syntax, semantics, pragmatics) has been the focus of investigations since the mid-1960s. Starting with Chomsky's stark division of syntax and semantics, a fundamental tenet of the formalist paradigm has been that the underlying rules for each of these linguistic levels are distinct and should be studied as independent systems that subsequently can be recombined in an additive manner for a complete account of the state of the child's language competence at any given time.

The impact of the extensions of this competence-based paradigm on the assessment of children with language disorders has been monumental (Craig, 1995; McTear & Conti-Ramsden, 1992; Prutting & Kirchner, 1983). Given that each linguistic system consists of a separate set of underlying rules within the competence-based paradigm and that language disorders are a direct reflection of the missing features in each underlying morphological, syntactic, semantic, or pragmatic system, the state of each of these systems must be assessed independently and then added to the states of other linguistic systems to provide an overall impairment profile. By definition, therefore, within the competence-based paradigm the child with language disorders is the sum of the state of his or her impairments and abilities in each area of competence. The child with a language disorder, from this perspective, is a static knowledge state minus specific structures—the underlying mechanism responsible for the missing features in surface form. Thus, a complete account of the entire disorder profile for a child is the sum of the impaired underlying features (Kirchner & Skarakis-Doyle, 1983; Prutting & Kirchner, 1983; Rice, 1995).

Unfortunately, this implies that all assessment indices developed since the 1950s are still relevant to evaluating the child with language disorders. This orientation is reflected both in protocols that contain detailed outlines for assessing syntactic, semantic, and pragmatic indices as distinct linguistic systems (Bloom & Lahey, 1978; Lund & Duchan, 1983, 1988; Miller, 1981) and in recent theoretical work conceptualizing the nature of the impairments for children with language disorders (Fletcher & MacWhinney, 1995; McTear & Conti-Ramsden, 1992; Watkins & Rice, 1995). For example, Crystal, Fletcher, and Garman (1990), in the most recent edition of their book *Grammatical Analysis of Language Disabilities,* continued to argue that a fundamental understanding of language disorders must come from a syntactic framework that is independent of semantic analysis. They suggested, therefore, that

> while the study of language disorders can benefit from the occasional insights of the semantic approaches currently being developed, we are of the opinion that there is no chance of a theoretical or descriptive framework capable of application in a therapeutic or remedial context being evolved in the foreseeable future. (p. 6)

This view of the child as the sum of the underlying state of his or her abilities and disabilities across a range of linguistic competencies is maintained at the theoretical level as well. The recent theoretical works outlining advances in the study of children with language impairments continue to conceptualize the phonological, morphological, semantic, pragmatic, and social impairments of children with language disorders as distinct systems (Fletcher & MacWhinney, 1995; Watkins & Rice, 1995).

Technological Advances This shift toward profile analysis reflects researchers' attempts to capture the final state of impairments for children with language disorders with larger models that include detailed assessment information across all language domains. This attempt to sum the findings of analysis across individual subsystems (e.g., phonological, morphological, lexical) is a result, in part, of advances in microcomputer technology. With these advances, researchers are able to rapidly code and analyze large amounts of data. This goal of including multiple indices across language subsystems, however, also reflects an underlying attitude consistent with 20th-century science in general—to discover order and regularity in the world. Specifically, the implicit goal of research in child language disorders has been to break down language systems into the smallest units of analysis that will obey a governing set of rules resulting in predictability of verbal performance. This view is consistent with traditional Newtonian physics, which holds that the world can be unfolded along a deterministic path that is rule-bound like the planets in a linear, deterministic manner (Hayles, 1991; Kaplan, 1963; Kuhn, 1970; Vallacher & Nowark, 1994).

A specific characteristic of linear models, relevant to the study of child language, is their modularity. Linear models can be taken apart and put back together, and the relationship between the individual parts is additive. With linear models, small changes in the input of the system result in similarly small effects on the output of the system. In keeping with this viewpoint, research in child language has emphasized discovering order and regularity in language, with the test of the goodness of fit of any set of rules being the degree to which verbal performance is predicted by these rules. In addition, within this framework, measurements are never believed to be perfect; yet given an approximate knowledge of the initial conditions, it has been assumed that one can predict the overall behavior of the child while ignoring the fluctuations in performance.

The development of the computer has fueled the myth that order and regularity can be discovered; researchers tacitly have assumed that, given a large enough computer, all of the individual rules of any complex system can be written down and subsequently added back together to ultimately capture the behavior of the entire system (Gleick, 1987; von Neumann, 1950). The development of language analysis software reveals that this assumption also is operating in the study of children's language. The language analysis programs that have been developed fall into two broad categories: 1) those that are reimplementations of existing assessment indices such as Developmental Sentence Scoring (Hughes & Low, 1989); Automated LARSP (Bishop, 1985); mean length of analysis calculated by Lingquest (Mordacai, Palin, & Palmer, 1985); computerized profile analysis (Long & Fey, 1988), which includes LARSP, DSS, PRISM (lexical analysis), PROPH (phonological analysis), and APRON (semantic analysis); and 2) those that start from the premise that the structure of the child's linguistic competence can be captured in an infinite degree of detail. These programs are designed to provide researchers with the tools to code and analyze language at infinite levels of detail, resulting in profiles at any level of analysis for an individual speaker, as measured by aggregated counts of the frequency of occurrence of the range of linguistic behaviors in question.

The two most notable examples of software developed to generate language profiles are the Systematic Analysis of Language Transcripts (SALT) (Miller & Chapman, 1983) and the Child Language Analysis Programs (CLAN) (MacWhinney, 1991, 1993). Each of these programs has been designed to provide the individual researcher with an infinite degree of freedom to code and analyze any level of linguistic performance. Given unlimited time and computer memory, a transcript theoretically can be analyzed to any degree of detail at the phonological, morphological, syntactic, semantic, and discourse level, resulting in an overall profile of verbal performance. Emphasis has been placed on creating a transcription system that allows an infinite amount of information to be coded and analyzed. Thus, the advent of the personal computer has provided researchers with the power to break language into its smallest analyzable units.

The Anomaly The shifts in theoretical orientation in the field of child language since the 1950s are the result of researchers' attempts to account for findings that were inconsistent with prior models. Two problems confront the formalist account. First, if language is composed of autonomous, encapsulated subsystems that have their own set of rules but that are highly interactive at the level of verbal performance (Fodor & Crain, 1987; Pinker, 1989), then it is unclear how these individual subsystems are combined to result in a whole model of language competence, and it is unclear exactly how the subsystems of language competence are manifested as an integrated whole during the process of real-time language performance (MacWhinney & Bates, 1989; Thelen & Smith, 1994).

This is particularly relevant for assessing children with language impairments. In spite of the advent of the personal computer and ostensibly having the power to assess everything that might possibly be impaired for the child with language disorders, every linguistic structure that could possibly pertain to an account of the disorder is now equally relevant without some overriding account of the interaction between the impairments in the separate linguistic systems (Miller, 1991; Prutting & Kirchner, 1983). As Kuhn (1970) noted, "In the absence of a unifying theory, facts simply become miscellaneous observations which have no significance in and of themselves and which are indistinguishable from the plethora of facts from which they have been selected" (p. 15). A formalist competence-based assessment of the child with language disorders merely provides a list of impaired competencies or missing structures without a unifying account of the interaction between these linguistic levels.

If linguistic competence is defined as a set of internal structures, then the goal for assessment is to identify these underlying rules. If it is assumed that there is a linear relationship between these underlying rules or features and observed verbal performance and that these features are stable and predictable, then, given the correct model, the language impairments of the child should be predictable. Unfortunately, this means that if each linguistic system functions in an independent linear manner, then effective assessment of a child with language disorders is contingent upon the microanalysis of *all* aspects of language.

The second major anomaly confronting a formalist account of language competence is the variability evident in individual language performance both moment to moment and developmentally over time. Researchers studying both typical and impaired language development have worked from the belief that the structure of children's language is a direct reflection of underlying knowledge. They maintained the belief that the form of a child's utterance is generated from an underlying set of linguistic structures and that the critical test of the competence-based paradigm is the discovery of the innate underlying linguistic universals that could account for these regularities at the syntactic, semantic, or pragmatic level. However, in his original theory, Chomsky (1957a, 1957b) clearly and explicitly stated that a speaker's actual performance could not be used as a window to underlying linguistic competence. He argued that the spontaneous speech produced by any individual speaker is a reflection of the interaction between linguistic competence and an infinite set of environmental and individual processing constraints that would result in such a range of variability in performance that the underlying structures could not be identified.

Unfortunately, children acquire language in radically different ways, particularly in the early stages of language development (Bates, Bretherton, & Snyder, 1988; Bates, Dale, & Thal, 1995; Bloom, Lightbown, & Hood, 1975; Bretherton, McNew, Snyder, & Bates, 1983; Nelson, 1973, 1981). This individual variation in language development clearly is a distinct characteristic of the children themselves, not a result of differences in linguistic input or other environmental factors (Furrow & Nelson, 1984; Goldfield & Snow, 1985; Nelson, 1973). Thus, a great deal of individual variability is evident in children's language acquisition within the context of larger patterns of stable language universals (Bates & MacWhinney, 1987).

In attempting to identify the global regularities, or linguistic universals, predicted by the competence-based account of children's language, a clear research style evolved that focused exclusively on identifying the similarities in the structure across children's language because it was the regularities in children's language that were considered proof of underlying linguistic universals.

As a result, individual differences in language performance, developmentally or moment to moment, were either 1) ignored in a classic "Kuhnian" sense and interpreted as noise in the data collection or 2) accounted for by the creation of ad hoc performance accounts that were developed in conjunction with the structural accounts of underlying linguistic competence (Thelen & Smith, 1994).

For clinical researchers, the goal has been to determine the extent to which linguistic competencies are either absent or impaired for children with disorders. In the same way that psychologists focused on the global similarities in the structure of children's language during acquisition, clinical researchers focused on identifying stable deficit profiles across groups of children. However, variability in language performance for children with disorders also has been a consistent source of frustration (Gallagher, 1991).

Variability in impairment profiles consistently has been observed both developmentally (Whitehurst, Fischel, Arnold, & Lonigan, 1992) and across language-sampling contexts (Evans & Craig, 1992; Fujiki & Brinton, 1983, 1987; Johnson, Miller, Curtiss, & Tallal, 1993; Klee, 1992; Miller, 1981; Prutting, Gallagher, & Mulac, 1975). For example, studies of differences in MLU for children with language disorder have shown variability across different contexts including type of conversational partner (Fey, Leonard, & Wilcox, 1981; Kramer et al., 1979; Olswang & Carpenter, 1978; Scott & Taylor, 1978; van Kleeck & Frankel, 1981), different conversational context (Evans & Craig, 1991; Longhurst & File, 1977; Stalnaker & Craighead, 1982), and discourse style of the conversational partner (Johnson et al., 1993). From the traditional formalist account in which verbal performance is considered a window to underlying linguistic competence, this variability in verbal performance inherent in the child with language disorder is problematic.

Unfortunately, a formalist model of language competence cannot account for the variability in the actual form of utterances produced by children with impairments because, according to a competence-based account, the underlying state of the child's linguistic system (i.e., the presence or absence of linguistic features or structures) is static and does not change over time. If verbal performance (be it syntactic, semantic, or pragmatic) is a manifestation of this underlying language competence, then the variability inherent in real-time language performance cannot be accounted for within a competence-based theory and becomes a confound in researchers' attempts to diagnostically capture this knowledge for the child with language disorders.

FUNCTIONALISM

Theoretical Assumptions

In contrast to the competence-based formalist paradigm, functionalist theories focus on changes in the form of a speaker's utterances during actual verbal performance (Bates & MacWhinney, 1989). The fundamental assumption of a functionalist performance-based paradigm is that similarities and differences are *expected* across individuals in the actual process of language use. Cross-linguistic studies have revealed that at a global level exists a core set of communicative functions that are present in all languages. Yet closer inspection reveals a wide range of variability in the form in which these communicative devices are constructed moment to moment for any given individual. (See Bates & MacWhinney, 1989, for a complete review.) Studies reveal that any communicative function can be expressed by a range of different linguistic devices; alternatively, a single linguistic device can capture a range of different communicative functions (MacWhinney & Bates, 1989). In contrast to the formalist account in which the mapping between linguistic devices and language forms was presumed to be a linear one-to-one relationship, the mapping between underlying linguistic structures and communicative function clearly is one to many or many to one instead (Bates & MacWhinney, 1982; MacWhinney, Bates, & Kliegel, 1984).

Competence-based models focus exclusively on the abstract linguistic knowledge of an ideal speaker-listener (Chomsky, 1957a, 1957b), whereas the emphasis of performance-based models is the actual process of real-time language use by real speakers in real communicative interactions. Specifically, performance-based models start from the premise that "the forms of natural languages are created, governed, constrained, acquired, and used in the service of communicative functions" (Bates & MacWhinney, 1989, p. 3). The critical question from a functionalist performance-based perspective is not, "What are the underlying linguistic structures?" but is instead, "What is the relationship between the various language forms and communicative functions?"

Grammar, within a functionalist perspective, is viewed as the final state of the system or the solution to the problem of mapping nonlinear meanings onto a highly constrained linear production system whose only devices include word order, lexical items, morphology, and suprasegmentals (Bates & MacWhinney, 1982; MacWhinney et al., 1984). All sources of information are presumed to be integrated equally in the process of real-time verbal performance. As a result, all underlying meanings, presuppositions, beliefs, case-role relationships, and communicative intentions must compete for access to these four surface forms (Bates & MacWhinney, 1979).

Unit of Analysis

The critical unit of analysis within a functionalist theory is not the stable rule-governed state of a speaker's linguistic competence but the moment-to-moment changes in a speaker's verbal performance during the process of communicating—the very data for which the formalist paradigm cannot account. A functionalist account assumes that the variability in speaker performance is simply the final solution to the interaction among the internal state of a complex system (i.e., the underlying speaker competence), the structure of the system (e.g., word order, lexical items, morphology, suprasegmentals), and the impact of external constraints such as real-time language processing demands. As Bates et al. (1995) argued, an understanding of the quantitative and qualitative variations both within and across all components of language performance is *critical* to any account of the possible mechanisms underlying both typical and impaired language learning.

Assessing Children with Language Disorders

It seemed initially that the traditional account of pragmatics could solve the problem of the variability in the performance of children with language disorders. Given that pragmatics was defined as the rules governing the use of language in context, it appeared that if all of the contributing contextual factors were identified and controlled, then the variability in children's performance could be accounted for, and the stable underlying linguistic competence of the child with disorder ultimately could be diagnosed. Thus, once all of the contextual factors accounting for changes in verbal behavior were identified, the variability in performance of individual linguistic systems could be documented, and the impairments in individual competencies could be combined for a total diagnostic profile. However, in an evaluation of the success of pragmatics as a model for assessment, Brinton (1990), Craig (1990), and Skarakis-Doyle (1990) argued that this approach to language assessment can neither characterize the language skills of children in real-time nor address the interaction between multiple linguistic levels during ongoing discourse.

Craig (1995) has argued for a broader account of language disorders in which language is not viewed as a static entity that is assessed across multiple contexts but in which the child's language performance is assessed as a dynamic, integral part of the communicative contexts themselves. If verbal performance is defined as the final solution to the interplay between contextual demands and underlying linguistic knowledge, then the goal for assessment is not to determine the child's linguistic competence but is to develop an account of the child's performance as it changes during ongoing language processing. A functionalist account is based on the assumption that variability in verbal performance is the critical unit of analysis. By this account, the verbal performance of the child with language disorder no longer is a window to linguistic competence but is a manifestation of a complex system that may or may not be in a stable state at any given point in time.

Unfortunately, investigations of language performance have employed only formal experimental techniques whereby different linguistic cues are manipulated in an effort to study moment-to-moment language processing (Bates, Friederici, & Wulfeck, 1987; Bates, Wulfeck, & MacWhinney, 1991; Evans & MacWhinney, 1995). The results of these studies have been effective in illuminating individual patterns in language processing at a microanalysis level; however, they do not provide a means of capturing both variability and stability in a child's verbal performance in real time.

DYNAMIC COMPLEX SYSTEMS

Advances in the study of dynamic complex systems suggest a possible solution to the problems inherent in attempting to capture both the stability and the variability in children's spontaneous language productions. Dynamic systems theory provides a set of assumptions regarding the organization of the behavior of complex systems, how systems' behavior changes over time, and methods to empirically unlock these processes (Arnold, 1983; Devany, 1989; Glass & Mackey, 1988; Kelso, Holt, Kugler, & Turvey, 1980; Nicolis & Prigogine, 1989; Parker & Chua, 1989; Vallacher & Nowark, 1994). Principles of dynamic systems have been employed to model the behavior of a wide range of complex systems including thermal convection (Haken, 1978; Nicolis & Prigogine, 1989), weather patterns (Lorenz, 1963), biological phenomena (Glass & Mackey, 1988), the physiology of motor development (Kelso, Ding, & Schöner, 1993; Robertson, Cohen, & Meyers-Kress, 1993), and development issues in cognition and language acquisition (Bates & Carnevale, 1993; Buder, 1991; Thelen & Smith, 1994; van Geert, 1991).

The study of dynamic systems is predicated on the assumption that a complex interdependency among *all* of the individual components of a system exists and that the interaction between these components under different conditions will result in the emergence of different global patterns of behavior without the role of the individual components being specified or controlled (Devany, 1989; Feignbaum, 1980; Nicolis & Prigogine, 1989; Parker & Chua, 1989). Dynamic systems change and evolve over time, exhibiting both stable and variable patterns of behavior. These systems are *dynamic* in that the state of the system at any given time is a reflection of the prior state of the system and the interaction between the system's present state and external constraints on the system. Dynamic systems are highly sensitive to slight variations in external conditions, also known as control parameters (Kelso et al., 1993; Robertson et al., 1993), which can result in dramatic and instant qualitative changes in the behavior exhibited by the system.

Most dynamic systems can be conceptualized as either discrete or continuous. Discrete dynamic systems are systems whose behavior evolves in distinct time steps. Thus, the state of the system at time t is part of what determines the state of the system at time $t + 1$. Discrete dynamic systems are modeled with difference equations (e.g., measures of populations year to year, fluctuations in stock market prices). Continuous dynamic systems evolve in a continuous fashion whereby the rate of change of the system is expressed as a function of the state of the system. Continuous dynamic systems are expressed with differential equations. A simple example of a continuous dynamic system is the oscillating movement of a pendulum over time.

The goal in constructing a model of a dynamic system is to capture the time-based history of the system by characterizing the *state* of the system at any point in time (Nicolis & Prigogine, 1989; Robertson et al., 1993). Complex systems can exhibit behavior that appears highly variable when observed moment to moment but that appears regular and stable when observed over a longer time frame. Thus, emphasis is placed on capturing these changes in the behavior of the system as it changes over time (Nicolis & Prigogine, 1989; Robertson et al., 1993). The study of dynamic systems uses both mathematical models (Glass & Mackey, 1988; Parker & Chua, 1989) and visual plots of the changes in the state of a system over time (Abraham & Shaw, 1982; Mandelbrot, 1983; Peitgen & Richter, 1986; Robertson et al., 1993). The dynamic properties of a system and the system's evolution over time are captured by plotting the changes in the behavior of the system—changes in the state of specific variables called *state variables*. Given knowledge of the state variables of a system, a plot can be constructed where the state of the system is represented as its position in a multi-dimensional state space. This final plot of the system as it moves through its state space over time is called the *phase portrait* of that system.

Dynamic systems often settle or stay in localized portions of the state space. The area where the system tends to converge is called an *attractor*. There are several different types of attractors. The simplest type of attractor conceptually is known as a *fixed-point attractor*. Imagine a pendulum swinging back and forth. As the pendulum slows, both the amplitude and the velocity of its movement—the state of the system as it comes to a stop—change over time. The pendulum is "attracted" to its final resting point. The phase portrait of the behavior of the pendulum as it settles to a fixed-point attractor is shown in Figure 1, plotted as a con-

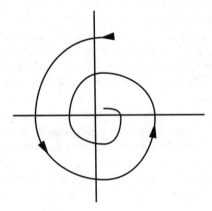

Figure 1.   Fixed-point attractor.

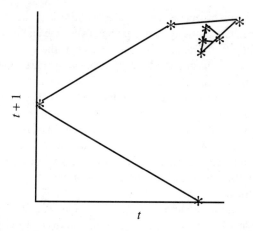

Figure 2.   Discrete fixed-point attractor.

tinuous system. A system that has settled to a fixed-point attractor is most often in a highly stable state. An example of a fixed-point attractor for a discrete system is shown in Figure 2. Each point of the plot represents the position of the pendulum as measured in discrete time steps, and the phase portrait of the pendulum in the state space is plotted for each set of coordinates $(t; t+1)$ as the pendulum converges to a fixed point. A different type of attractor, called a *limit-cycle attractor,* captures the portrait of a system that is oscillating continuously over time without losing energy. The phase portrait of a pendulum in this self-excitatory state is plotted as a continuous system in Figure 3. Thus, an attractor is the subset of the system's state space where the system may converge under certain conditions and that often represents the preferred state, or range of behaviors, of the system.

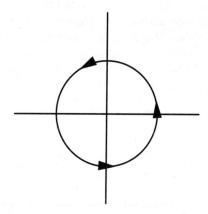

Figure 3.   Limit-cycle attractor.

The moment-to-moment behavior of a dynamic system may be highly variable, yet when the state of the system is plotted over time and is represented by its phase portrait, general regularities can be seen as the system moves away from and then returns to its preferred state. Related to the idea of attractors is the concept of attractor basins. The basin of an attractor refers to the region of the state space where almost all conditions of the system will converge. A system may have several different basins of attractors, which coexist. As Kelso et al. (1993) pointed out, a system that has several attractor basins, or states, is said to have multistability—an essential characteristic of all biological systems. Changes in the values of external control parameters will cause the system to move back and forth across these multiple attractor basins, as represented conceptually in Figure 4.

Thus, according to dynamic systems principles, a complex system can exhibit both stable and variable behavior as it moves from one attractor state to another because of changes in external conditions. But what does this really mean? A simple example of the interaction between external conditions and the resulting changes in the behavior of a complex system is the model of the heat convection originally proposed in the 1900s by the physicist Bernard and presented in detail in Nicolis and Prigogine (1989). Imagine a layer of water between two horizontal plates. The temperature of the top plate is represented by T1 and the temperature of the bottom plate is represented by T2. When there is no difference between the temperature of the two plates, the system is said to be in a stable state of equilibrium because the temperature throughout the system is the same. In this state, if the temperature of the system were plotted either continuously or discretely as T1 against T2, then the phase portrait of the system would reveal a fixed-point attractor.

If, however, the system is in a state of equilibrium but is at a temperature slightly lower than body temperature and someone briefly were to touch one of the plates, then that area would warm slightly, and the system would shift out of that attractor state. Once cooled back to ambient temperature, the system returns to its original attractor state (Figure 5). This external incident, which occurred locally in the system but which had no long-term influence on the system, is called a *perturbation*. Because there was no long-term effect on the temperature

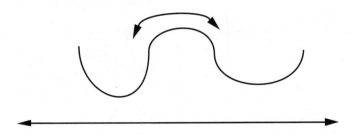

Figure 4.   Movement across multiple attractor basins with changes in external conditions.

of the system as a result of this perturbation, the system is said to be asymptotically stable, and the behavior of the system as a whole is stable. The phase portrait of the temperature of the system would show a shift out of its attractor state and then its return as represented in the hypothetical plot shown in Figure 5.

The behavior of a system can be changed qualitatively, however, if the external conditions change enough. By applying constant heat to the bottom plate (T2), instead of merely touching it, the temperature of the bottom plate becomes greater than the temperature of the top plate, and the conditions of equilibrium will be violated because the temperature of T1 no longer is the same as T2. The important point here is that by changing an *external constraint* (e.g., applying heat to the bottom plate), the state of the system is altered, and the *behavior* of the system changes. If the amount of heat applied to the system is small, and the difference between T1 and T2 stays within a certain range, then the system will be able to adapt to a second different stable state in which the heat will be transported from the lower to the upper plate and then transferred through the top plate as it cools. The only difference in the system from its prior state of equilibrium is that the temperature throughout the system no longer is uniform. The temperature changes from warmer at the bottom to colder at the top in a linear additive fashion and can be modeled as such. In this state, as a result of small changes in the external constraints placed on the system, the system has adapted to a simple yet unique state in response to these constraints, and the behavior of the system again appears stable and predictable but is now in a different attractor basin. This second attractor basin would not be a fixed-point attractor because there is ongoing yet stable *change* in the movement of the molecules.

The system can be moved farther and farther from its state of equilibrium by continuing to change the external constraints on the system. Increasing the difference between T1 and T2 by applying more heat to the bottom plate will

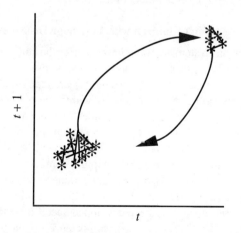

Figure 5.   External perturbation of a stable system.

cause a qualitative shift in the behavior of the system at a certain critical value of the difference between the temperature of T2 and T1. The heat, instead of rising in layers in a linear, additive manner through the system, suddenly will cause the system to "boil," and the movement of the molecules suddenly will shift to "bulk" movement, known as Bernard cells. The molecules in the system, instead of rising in the previous linear fashion, will begin to move in a circular, rolling fashion rising in the center, splitting at the top, and moving back down the outside edges. Thus, by continuing to change the value of the *same* external parameter, the behavior of the system will change qualitatively to a third type of attractor state that has no resemblance to either of its previous behavior states. What is important about this example is that as the value of the same external condition moves into a different range (e.g., increasing its temperature), the system's behavior will change suddenly as it shifts to a different state. Thus, what emerges is "organized complexity out of the interplay between the disordered thermal motion of the individual molecules and the nonequilibrium constraints" (Nicolis & Prigogine, 1989, p. 13).

A biological example of how changes in external conditions can modify the state of a system is presented by Thelen and Smith (1994). Imagine the hypothetical "fitness space" of the range of heart rates and blood pressure levels for an individual. This individual will have a "preferred" range of values that, if plotted in their state space, will show that these values tend to stay within a certain attractor basin as revealed by the system's phase portrait. However, with changes in external conditions such as increased stress from the environment or exercise, the "fitness state" of the person shifts out of the preferred attractor basin to a second, less stable, attractor space. Once the external constraint has been removed, the individual's system will return to its preferred fitness space in the phase portrait. With changes such as continuous exercise or aging, this attractor state can shift over time and become either more or less stable.

Implications for Assessing Children with Language Disorders

What does a dynamic systems account have to offer the study of children with language disorders? A research paradigm provides researchers with a set of assumptions about an area of interest, specific research questions, definitions of the unit of analysis, and a methodology by which these questions might be answered. A dynamic systems account provides 1) a theoretical framework to conceptualize the variability in the performance of the child with language impairment, which accounts for patterns of both correct and incorrect language performance over time; 2) a possible conceptual approach to formalizing the interaction across language levels; and 3) implications for intervention.

As evidenced throughout this chapter, the traditional models of spontaneous language assessment have been developed specifically to document the stable state of the child's internal linguistic competence. As such, the structure of the child's language production has been used as a map of this knowledge. Traditional assessment indices have been developed to provide an aggregated summary measure of a particular linguistic structure as measured by the structure's occurrence in a spontaneous speech sample such as MLU (Miller, 1981), TTR, Index of Productive Syntax (IPSyn) (Scarborough, 1990), or DSS.

But as Craig and Evans (1993) have cautioned, traditional assessment indices provide single summary measures of a specific feature or structure in the child's language, which subsequently is interpreted as impaired competence. These summary measures are not sensitive to qualitative differences in children's use of language. They do not lend themselves to real-time analysis nor to the assessment of qualitatively unique adaptive behavior often exhibited by children with impairments. Even the profiles generated by computer analysis provide single summary statistics for the particular linguistic structure in question. But as Rice (1995) noted, computer-generated calculations of mean-percentage correct use of a particular structure can be misleading and can obscure individual differences in children's use of these structures.

Researchers studying verbal performance in children with language disorders are confronted with the same issues as are scientists attempting to characterize the dynamics of any complex system (Kugler, Kelso, & Turvey, 1982; Thelen, Kelso, & Fogel, 1987). These issues include the degrees of freedom for a given system, the indeterminacy of the subcomponents of the system, and the interplay between the state of the system at any given time and external constraints that can affect the behavior, or performance, of the system. The problem of degrees of freedom is directly related to Bates and MacWhinney's (1987) argument that there are an infinite number of meanings and ideas that a speaker may want to communicate, yet there are only four channels by which this infinite range of meanings can be expressed—word order, morphology, lexicon, and paralinguistic cues.

A dynamic systems account would predict that because the phonological, morphological, syntactic, semantic, and pragmatic components of language are all linked together, and because the moment-to-moment interplay among all of these components is continuously changing, the state of the child's linguistic behavior during the processing of language is dynamic—changing moment to moment over time. From a dynamic systems framework, the interaction between the child's state of linguistic knowledge and the external constraints on the child's system should result in evolving and adaptive verbal behavior that will be stable under certain conditions yet suddenly highly variable under other conditions. As Farmer and Packer (in Gleick, 1987) noted,

> Adaptive behavior is an emergent property which spontaneously arises through the interaction of simple components. Whether these components are neurons, amino acids, ants, or bit strings, adaptation can only occur if the collective behavior as a whole is qualitatively different from that of the sum of the individual parts. (p. 339)

But how does this change the way that children's language is assessed? From a dynamic systems account, the goal in assessing children with language disorders is not to focus exclusively on the stable presence of specific linguistic features in the child's speech. The goal is twofold: 1) to capture both periods of stability and the sudden dissolution of this stability; thus, the shift from stable usage of a particular form to the sudden omission of the same form during ongoing language processing must be accounted for without invoking ad hoc accounts of the presence or absence of internal constraints; and 2) to understand the interaction between external control parameters (i.e., contextual variables) and the internal state of the child's language processing over time. The critical distinction between this approach and prior attempts to assess the child's language across multiple contexts is that prior attempts aimed to identify only the percentage of occurrence of the structure in the child's language while controlling or factoring out the variability (i.e., standard deviation) in the rate of occurrence of these structures across contexts.

A dynamic systems account, by contrast, would focus both on correct forms and on the dissolution of these forms. A key feature of dynamic systems is that the behavior of a high-dimensional complex system can be described by low-dimensional space if critical control parameters can be identified. A dynamic systems account would predict that the form of the child's behavior should change qualitatively and suddenly as external contextual parameters are altered. For example, if the child were viewed as a complex system, then there should be a set of external conditions that when decreased should result in one type of verbal behavior (e.g., absence of morphological errors). Yet the model would predict that if these same external conditions were increased, then the child's verbal behavior would become unstable and would suddenly shift to a qualitatively different state of behavior.

The contextual constraints within which the child is communicating are continually changing; from a dynamic systems account, the child's verbal performance is *always* a manifestation of the *interaction* between the child's internal state and external contextual parameters. The change in the state of the child's system cannot be captured by traditional approaches that represent language as the sum of a set of linguistic competencies captured by single summary statistics (Craig, 1995; Miller, 1991; Rice, 1995). This means that the same verbal knowledge may manifest itself differently depending on the moment-to-moment changes in internal states such as memory, attention, and fatigue and changes in key contextual parameters. Within this framework, only certain features of the external context may act as a control parameter.

Preliminary studies with typical adults and subgroups of children with specific language impairments suggest that timing demands may be one of many key external parameters. Specifically, studies of typical adults have demonstrated that increased timing demands result in breakdowns in syntactic processing that are the same as those observed in individuals with language disorders (Miyaki, Carpenter, & Just, 1994). The combined verbal and nonverbal demands of ongoing discourse also represent a second type of external constraint that has an impact on the verbal performance of the child with language disorder. For example, Evans (1996), in an investigation of the morphosyntactic impairment profiles of children with language impairments, observed significantly more morphosyntactic omissions in utterances with the greatest timing and turn-taking constraints as opposed to turn-internal utterances, which are affected less by these same external constraints.

In addition, the same external conditions may have a different impact at different times as a result of the changing state of the child, and the impact of this input on the system may have a nonlinear and unpredictable outcome that is only manifested much later in time. A possible example of this delayed manifestation is the interaction between memory impairments and the child's evolving language knowledge. A young child 2–3 years of age with a memory impairment who is unable to retain the order of words as in SVO constructions may never come to realize that the first noun in an SVO sentence is most often the agent. As a result, the child may never come to view word order as a salient cue in processing language in English (Bates & MacWhinney, 1987). This interaction between the state of the child's internal memory constraints and the external input early in the child's development results in a different knowledge state in which other cues are used to assign agency. If the child is assessed when he or she is much older, the child will not demonstrate a delayed pattern of language processing similar to younger typical children but will exhibit what appears to be a qualitatively different pattern of behavior because of the interaction between memory impairments and external input earlier in the child's development of a different set of processing cues. The emergence of an adaptive strategy would come to exist in the absence of the original impairment—the interaction between memory impairments and external verbal input. Once the strategy was learned, the child's memory impairments might improve, yet he or she would continue to use the alternative processing strategy and never acquire word order cues. For example, 7- to 8-year-old children with both expressive and receptive impairments appear to rely exclusively on animacy cues to assign the role of agent in contrast to both age-matched and younger typical children who rely on word order (Evans & MacWhinney, 1995). When assessed at age 7, these children demonstrated the ability to retain four to five items sequentially but were still using what appeared to be an adaptive processing strategy, which might have been acquired much earlier as the result of a state of the child's system at the time but which no longer exists.

CONCLUSION

The primary goal of using a spontaneous language sample in language assessment is to develop an understanding of the nature of a child's communicative impairments for the purpose of intervention. A dynamic systems account has two intriguing implications for intervention. The first is the relationship between the strength of an attractor basin and the energy required to move the system out of that particular attractor basin; the second is the nature of the impact of external input and the system's manifestation of this input at some later point in time.

A critical characteristic of dynamic systems is that as the system shifts from one attractor state to another, it will manifest a characteristic pattern of behavior. Specifically, the behavior of the system will become highly *unstable* just prior to its shift to the second attractor state. If the system is stable (i.e., in a strong attractor state), then changes in external constraints may perturb the system slightly, but the system will quickly return to its previous state. However, there is a critical value at which the system's behavior becomes so unstable that it will "jump" suddenly from one attractor state to another. This shift is rapid, resulting in what appears to be sudden, discontinuous behavior on the part of the system. What is important here is that it is the *strength* of the attractor basin that will affect the system's sensitivity to the external constraints. Thus, the more stable the system's behavior is, the *harder* it will be to change it, requiring more energy to shift it from one attractor basin to another.

With respect to intervention, a stable pattern will be more difficult to change because of either the presence of a very strong attractor basin, which might be represented, for example, by rare instances of the production of a particular form; or the absence of any attractor space as represented by the consistent omission of a particular form. Thus, a dynamic systems account suggests that a child who is exhibiting a highly unstable pattern of performance (e.g., 68% production of a particular structure) may be on the verge of shifting to a second attractor state. It also would predict that *less* energy would be required to shift this child to that second state in which the form is used consistently than to shift the child who exhibits a stable pattern of never having used the particular structure. The child's inconsistent use of a particular feature is problematic for competence-based accounts of language impairments because it is unclear how the child can produce a specific feature only some times and not others. From a dynamic systems account, the inconsistent production of a specific form suggests the emergence of a second, weaker, attractor state that is not strong enough for the child to settle into and stay in despite changes in external parameters such as production timing demands, ongoing discourse demands, or the demands inherent in different speaking contexts. The pattern of morphosyntactic impairment, which consistently has been reported in children with SLI but which has been represented by single summary measures of the percentage of occurrence in obligatory contexts, may actually reflect weak attractor basins that are particularly vulnerable to the demands of actual communication.

A dynamic systems account is not an extension of a competence-based structuralist's account, nor is it a return to behaviorism. Within the behaviorist paradigm, the form of the child's verbal behavior was viewed only as the result of external reinforcers; the language disorder was assumed to be the result of problems in this stimulus–response paradigm. Within the generative competence-based account, the form of the child's verbal behavior was exclusively the domain of internal linguistic knowledge, which was believed to generate the observed surface form of the child's utterance. In either of these accounts, the sampling context employed to collect a spontaneous language sample is only background, and the child's verbal behavior is separated from the sampling context and studied in isolation. In contrast to both of these theories, the observed form of the child's verbal behavior within a dynamic systems account is the result of the moment-to-moment interaction between the internal state of the child and external constraints on the child's system. The underlying mechanism of disorder, therefore, is the interaction between the internal state of the child at a given time and external conditions. Thus, the child's spontaneous language, when viewed from a dynamic systems account, can never be isolated and examined outside the context of ongoing discourse.

It appears, therefore, that the methodology that has been developed for studying dynamic complex systems in other domains may provide both a conceptual framework and the tools necessary to capture the dynamic behavior of children with language impairments. Using the traditional approach of comparing aggregated summary measures to characterize the child's performance can provide a measure of the stable patterns in the child's verbal performance, but it cannot capture changes over time, either moment to moment in ongoing language processing or developmentally. It is the change in the child's behavior over time that, from a dynamic systems account, provides clues to the outcome of interactions between external input and the evolving state of the child's system. With the use of phase portraits of state variables, which can reveal attractors in the child's verbal system, a dynamic systems framework can provide the techniques to capture this interaction as the child's verbal behavior changes moment to moment or developmentally over time (Evans, Stonick, & Schweizer, 1995).

As many researchers (Brinton, 1990; Craig, 1990, 1995; Miller, 1991; Skarakis-Doyle, 1990) have proposed, a new methodology is needed to analyze children with language impairments in a way that can capture the dynamic pattern of impairments evident in the child's use of language, be it phonological, morphological, syntactic, semantic, or pragmatic. The possibility that dynamical systems theory may provide a framework to accomplish this goal warrants attention in future research.

REFERENCES

Abraham, R.H., & Shaw, C.D. (1982). *Dynamics—The geometry of behavior. Part 1: Periodic behavior.* Santa Cruz, CA: Aerial Press.

Adams, M., & Pace, S. (1969). *A descriptive linguistic investigation of language problems in preschool children*. Paper presented at the American Speech-Language-Hearing Association.

Antinucci, F., & Parisi, D. (1973). Early language acquisition: A model and some data. In C. Ferguson & D. Slobin (Eds.), *Studies of child language development* (pp. 607–619). New York: Holt, Rinehart & Winston.

Arnold, V. (1983). *Geometrical methods in the theory of ordinary differential equations*. New York: Springer-Verlag.

Austin, J.L. (1962). *How to do things with words*. Cambridge, MA: Harvard University Press.

Bach, E., & Harms, R. (1968). *Universals in linguistic theory*. New York: Holt, Rinehart & Winston.

Bandura, A. (1977). *A social learning theory*. Englewood Cliffs, NJ: Prentice Hall.

Bates, E. (1976). Pragmatics and sociolinguistics in child language. In D.M. Morehead & A.E. Morehead (Eds.), *Normal and deficient child language* (pp. 411–463). Baltimore: University Park Press.

Bates, E. (1978). *Language and context: The acquisition of pragmatics*. New York: Academic Press.

Bates, E., Bretherton, I., & Snyder, L. (1988). *From first words to grammar: Individual differences and dissociable mechanisms*. Cambridge, MA: Cambridge University Press.

Bates, E., Camaioni, L., & Volterra, V. (1975). The acquisition of performatives prior to speech. *Merrill-Palmer Quarterly, 21*, 205–226.

Bates, E., & Carnevale, G. (1993). New directions in research on language development. *Developmental Review, 13*, 436–470.

Bates, E., Dale, P., & Thal, D. (1995). Individual differences and their implications for theories of language development. In P. Fletcher & B. MacWhinney (Eds.), *The handbook of child language* (pp. 96–151). Oxford: Blackwell Publishers.

Bates, E., Friederici, A., & Wulfeck, B. (1987). Comprehension in aphasia: A cross-linguistic study. *Brain and Language, 32*, 19–67.

Bates, E., & MacWhinney, B. (1979). A functional approach to the acquisition of grammar. In E. Ochs & B. Schieffelin (Eds.), *Developmental pragmatics* (pp. 167–211). New York: Academic Press.

Bates, E., & MacWhinney, B. (1982). Functionalist approaches to grammar. In E. Wanner & L. Gleitman (Eds.), *Language acquisition: The state of the art* (pp. 177–218). New York: Cambridge University Press.

Bates, E., & MacWhinney, B. (1987). Competition, variation, and language learning. In B. MacWhinney (Ed.), *Mechanisms of language acquisition* (pp. 157–194). Hillsdale, NJ: Lawrence Erlbaum Associates.

Bates, E., & MacWhinney, B. (1989). Functionalism and the competition model. In B. MacWhinney & E. Bates (Eds.), *The crosslinguistic study of sentence processing* (pp. 3–73). New York: Cambridge University Press.

Bates, E., Wulfeck, B., & MacWhinney, B. (1991). Cross-linguistic research in aphasia: An overview. *Brain and Language, 41*, 311–336.

Berko, J. (1958). The child's learning of English morphology. *Word, 14*, 150–177.

Berwick, R., & Weinberg, A. (1984). *The grammatical basis of linguistic performance*. Cambridge: MIT Press.

Bishop, D.V.M. (1985). Automated LARSP: Computer assisted grammatical analysis. *British Journal of Disorders of Communication, 19*, 78–87.

Blagden, C.M., & McConnell, N.L. (1985). *Interpersonal Language Skills Assessment*. Moline, IL: Lingui Systems.

Bloom, L. (1970). *Language development: Form and function in emerging grammars.* Cambridge: MIT Press.

Bloom, L., & Lahey, M. (1978). *Language development and language disorders.* New York: John Wiley & Sons.

Bloom, L., Lightbown, P., & Hood, L. (1975). Structure and variation in child language. *Monographs of the Society for Research in Child Development, 402*(106).

Bloom, L., Rocissano, L., & Hood, L. (1976). Adult sentence–child discourse: Developmental interaction between information processing and linguistic knowledge. *Cognitive Psychology, 8,* 521–552.

Boehm, A. (1971). *Boehm Test of Basic Concepts.* New York: The Psychological Corporation.

Bolinger, D. (1975). *Aspects of language.* New York: Harcourt Brace Jovanovich.

Bowerman, M.F. (1973). Structural relationships in children's utterances: Syntactic or semantic? In T. Moore (Ed.), *Cognitive development and the acquisition of language* (pp. 191–209). New York: Academic Press.

Bowerman, M.F. (1974). Learning the structure of causative verbs: A study in the relationship of cognitive, semantic, and syntactic development. *Papers and Reports on Child Language Development.*

Bowerman, M.F. (1976). Semantic factors in the acquisition of rules for word use and sentence construction. In D.M. Morehead & A.E. Morehead (Eds.), *Normal and deficient child language* (pp. 99–180). Baltimore: University Park Press.

Braine, M.D.S. (1963). The ontogeny of English phrase structure: The first phase. *Language, 39,* 3–13.

Braine, M.D.S. (1973). Three suggestions regarding grammatical analyses of children's language. In C.A. Ferguson & D.I. Slobin (Eds.), *Studies of child language development* (pp. 407–421). New York: Holt, Rinehart & Winston.

Bresnan, J. (Ed.). (1982). *The mental representation of grammatical relations.* Cambridge: MIT Press.

Bretherton, I., McNew, S., Snyder, L., & Bates, E. (1983). Individual differences at 20 months: Analytic and holistic strategies in language acquisition. *Journal of Child Language, 10,* 293–320.

Brinton, B. (1990). Peer commentary on "Clinical pragmatics: Expectations and realizations" by Tanya Gallagher. *Journal of Speech Language Pathology and Audiology, 14,* 8–9.

Brinton, B., Fujiki, M., Froem-Loeb, D., & Winkler, E. (1986). Development of conversational repair strategies in response to request for clarification. *Journal of Speech and Hearing Research, 29,* 75–81.

Brown, J., Redmond, A., Bass, K., Leibergott, J., & Swope, S. (1975). *Symbolic play in normal and language impaired children.* Washington, DC: American Speech and Hearing Association.

Brown, R. (1973). *A first language: The early stages.* Cambridge, MA: Harvard University Press.

Brown, R., & Bellugi, U. (1964). Three processes in the child's acquisition of syntax. In E.H. Lenneberg (Ed.), *New directions in the study of language* (pp. 133–151). Cambridge: MIT Press.

Brown, R., Cazden, C., & Bellugi, U. (1973). The child's grammar from I to III. In C.A. Ferguson & D.I. Slobin (Eds.), *Studies of child language development* (pp. 295–333). New York: Holt, Rinehart & Winston.

Brown, R., & Hanlon, C. (1970). Derivational complexity and order of acquisition in child speech. In J.R. Hayes (Ed.), *Cognition and the development of language* (pp. 155–207). New York: John Wiley & Sons.

Buder, E. (1991). A nonlinear dynamic model of social interaction. *Communications Research, 18,* 174–198.

Carrow, E. (1974). *Carrow Elicited Language Inventory.* Austin, TX: Learning Concepts.

Carter, A. (1974). *Communication in the sensorimotor period.* Unpublished doctoral dissertation, University of California, Berkeley.

Chafe, W. (1970). *Meaning and the structure of language.* Chicago: University of Chicago Press.

Chapman, R.S. (1981). Exploring children's communicative intents. In J. Miller (Ed.), *Assessing language production in children: Experimental procedures* (pp. 287–298). Baltimore: University Park Press.

Chomsky, N. (1957a). A review of verbal behavior, by B.F. Skinner. *Language, 35,* 26–58.

Chomsky, N. (1957b). *Syntactic structures.* Cambridge: MIT Press.

Chomsky, N. (1963). Formal properties of grammars. In R.D.R. Luce, R. Bush, & E. Galanter (Eds.), *Handbook of mathematical psychology* (pp. 528–550). New York: John Wiley & Sons.

Chomsky, N. (1964). Current issues in linguistic theory. In J.A. Fodor & J.J. Katz (Eds.), *The structure of language: Readings in the philosophy of language* (pp. 50–118). Englewood Cliffs, NJ: Prentice Hall.

Chomsky, N. (1965). *Aspects of the theory of syntax.* Cambridge: MIT Press.

Clark, E. (1973). What's in a word? On the child's acquisition of semantics in his first language. In T. Moore (Ed.), *Cognitive development and the acquisition of language* (pp. 65–110). New York: Academic Press.

Clark, E.V. (1974). Some aspects of the conceptual basis for first language acquisition. In R.L. Schiefelbusch & L.L. Lloyd (Eds.), *Language perspectives—Acquisition, retardation, and intervention* (pp. 105–128). Baltimore: University Park Press.

Craig, H. (1983). Pragmatic language models. In T. Gallagher & C. Prutting (Eds.), *Pragmatic assessment and intervention issues in language* (pp. 101–127). San Diego: College-Hill Press.

Craig, H. (1990). Peer commentary on "Clinical pragmatics: Expectations and realizations" by Tanya Gallagher. *Journal of Speech Language Pathology and Audiology, 14,* 8–9.

Craig, H. (1995). Pragmatic impairments. In P. Fletcher & B. MacWhinney (Eds.), *The handbook of child language* (pp. 623–640). Cambridge, MA: Blackwell Publishers.

Craig, H., & Evans, J. (1989). Turn exchange characteristics of SLI children's simultaneous and nonsimultaneous speech. *Journal of Speech and Hearing Disorders, 54,* 334–347.

Craig, H., & Evans, J. (1993). Pragmatics and SLI: Within-group variations in discourse behaviors. *Journal of Speech and Hearing Research, 36,* 777–789.

Craig, H., & Gallagher, T. (1983). Adult–child discourse: The conversational relevance of pauses. *Journal of Pragmatics, 7,* 347–360.

Craig, H., & Washington, J. (1993). Access behaviors of children with specific language impairment. *Journal of Speech and Hearing Research, 36,* 322–337.

Cromer, F. (1976). The cognitive hypothesis of language acquisition and its implications for child language deficiency. In D.M. Morehead & A.E. Morehead (Eds.), *Normal and deficient child language* (pp. 283–334). Baltimore: University Park Press.

Crystal, D. (1974). Review of R. Brown, "A first language: The early years." *Journal of Child Language, 1,* 289–307.

Crystal, D., Fletcher, P., & Garman, M. (1989). *Grammatical analysis of language disability.* London: Cole and Whurr.

Crystal, D., Fletcher, P., & Garman, M. (1990). *Grammatical analysis of language disabilities* (2nd ed.). San Diego: Singular.

Dailey, K., & Boxx, J. (1979). A comparison of three imitative tests of expressive language and a spontaneous language sample. *Language, Speech, and Hearing Services in Schools, 10,* 6–13.

Dale, P. (1976). *Language development: Structure and function* (2nd ed.). New York: Holt, Rinehart & Winston.

Darley, F., & Moll, K. (1960). Reliability of language measures of size of sample. *Journal of Speech and Hearing Research, 3,* 166–173.

de Ajuriaguerra, J., Jaeggi, A., Guinard, F., Kocher, F., Maquard, M., Roth, S., & Schmid, E. (1976). The development and prognosis of dysphasia in children. In D.M. Morehead & A.E. Morehead (Eds.), *Normal and deficient child language* (pp. 345–386). Baltimore: University Park Press.

Devany, R.L. (1989). *An introduction to chaotic dynamical systems.* Reading, MA: Addison-Wesley.

Dore, J. (1974). A pragmatic description of early language development. *Journal of Psycholinguistic Research, 3,* 343–351.

Dore, J. (1975). Holophrases, speech acts and language universals. *Journal of Child Language, 2,* 21–40.

Dunn, L. (1959). *Peabody Picture Vocabulary Test.* Minneapolis: American Guidance Service.

Dunn, L.M., & Dunn, L.M. (1981). *Peabody Picture Vocabulary Test–Revised.* Circle Pines, MN: American Guidance Service.

Edwards, D. (1973). Sensorimotor intelligence and semantic relations in early child grammar. *Cognition, 2,* 395–434.

Evans, J. (1996). SLI subgroups: Interaction between discourse constraints and morphological deficits. *Journal of Speech and Hearing Research, 39.*

Evans, J., & Craig, H. (1991, November). *SLI subgroups: Similarities and differences in turn-taking behaviors.* Paper presented at the Annual Convention of the American Speech-Language-Hearing Association, Atlanta.

Evans, J., & Craig, H. (1992). Language sampling collection and analysis: Interview compared to freeplay assessment contexts. *Journal of Speech and Hearing Research, 35,* 343–353.

Evans, J., & MacWhinney, B. (1995, June). *Maximum likelihood estimates of sentence processing skills of children with expressive and expressive receptive SLI.* Paper presented at the Symposium on Research in Child Language Disorders, Madison, WI.

Evans, J., Stonick, V., & Schweizer, S. (1995, December). *Linear and nonlinear dynamical models of specific language impairments.* Paper presented at the Annual Convention of the American Speech-Language-Hearing Association, Orlando, FL.

Feignbaum, M. (1980). Universal behavior in nonlinear systems. *Los Alamos Science, 1,* 4–27.

Fey, M., Leonard, L., & Wilcox, K. (1981). Speech-style modifications of language impaired children. *Journal of Speech and Hearing Disorders, 46,* 91–97.

Fillmore, C. (1968). The case for case. In E. Bach & R.T. Harms (Eds.), *Universals in linguistic theory* (pp. 1–90). New York: Holt, Rinehart & Winston.

Fletcher, P., & MacWhinney, B. (1995). *The handbook of child language.* Oxford: Blackwell Publishers.

Fodor, J., & Crain, S. (1987). Simplicity and generality of rules in language acquisition. In B. MacWhinney (Ed.), *Mechanisms of language acquisition* (pp. 35–62). Hillsdale, NJ: Lawrence Erlbaum Associates.

Fodor, J.A., Bever, T.G., & Garrett, M.F. (1974). *The psychology of language: An introduction to psycholinguistics and generative grammar.* New York: McGraw-Hill.

Freedman, P., & Carpenter, R. (1976). Semantic relations used by normal and language-impaired children at stage I. *Journal of Speech and Hearing Research, 19,* 784–795.

Fujiki, M., & Brinton, B. (1983). Sampling reliability in elicited imitation. *Journal of Speech and Hearing Disorders, 48,* 85–89.

Fujiki, M., & Brinton, B. (1987). Elicited imitation revisited: A comparison with spontaneous language production. *Language, Speech, and Hearing Services in Schools, 18,* 301–311.

Furrow, D., & Nelson, K. (1984). Environmental correlates of individual differences in language acquisition. *Journal of Child Language, 11,* 523–534.

Gallagher, T.M. (1981). Contingent query sequences within adult–child discourse. *Journal of Child Language, 8,* 51–62.

Gallagher, T. (1991). A retrospective look at clinical pragmatics. In T. Gallagher (Ed.), *Pragmatics of language: Clinical practice issues* (pp. 1–9). San Diego: Singular.

Gallagher, T., & Craig, H. (1982). An investigation of overlap in children's speech. *Journal of Psycholinguistic Research, 11,* 63–75.

Gallagher, T., & Craig, H. (1984). Pragmatic assessment: Analysis of highly frequent repeated utterances. *Journal of Speech and Hearing Disorders, 49,* 368–377.

Garvey, C. (1975). Requests and responses in children's speech. *Journal of Child Language, 2,* 41–63.

Garvey, C., & Hogan, R. (1973). Social speech and social interaction: Egocentrism revisited. *Child Development, 44,* 562–568.

Glass, L., & Mackey, M.C. (1988). *From clocks to chaos: The rhythms of life.* Princeton, NJ: Princeton University Press.

Gleason, H.A. (1961). *Introduction to descriptive linguistics.* New York: Holt, Rinehart & Winston.

Gleick, J. (1987). *Chaos: Making a new science.* New York: Penguin Press.

Goldfield, B., & Snow, C. (1985). Individual differences in language acquisition. In J. Gleason (Ed.), *Language development* (pp. 390–412). Columbus, OH: Charles E. Merrill.

Gordon, D., & Lakoff, G. (1971). Conversational postulates. *Papers from the seventh regional meeting.* Chicago: University of Chicago Press.

Greenfield, P., & Smith, J. (1976). *The structure of communication in early language development.* New York: Academic Press.

Greenfield, P., & Westerman, M. (1978). Some psychological relations between action and language structures. *Journal of Psycholinguistic Research, 7,* 453–473.

Grice, H. (1968). Utterer's meaning, sentence-meaning, and word-meaning. *Foundations of Language, 4,* 225–242.

Gruber, J.S. (1973). Correlations between the syntactic constructions of the child and of the adult. In C.A. Ferguson & D.I. Slobin (Eds.), *Studies of child language development* (pp. 4–9). New York: Holt, Rinehart & Winston.

Haken, H. (1978). *Synergistics: An introduction.* Heidelberg, Germany: Springer-Verlag.

Halliday, M. (1973). *Explorations in the functions of language.* London: Edward Arnold.

Halliday, M. (1975). Learning how to mean. In E.H. Lenneberg & E. Lenneberg (Eds.), *Foundations of language development: A multidisciplinary approach* (pp. 239–264). New York: Academic Press.

Hayles, K. (1991). *Chaos and order: Complex dynamics in literature and science.* Chicago: University of Chicago Press.

Hockett, C. (1960). The origin of speech. *Scientific American, 203,* 88–95.

Hughes, D., & Low, W. (1989, November). *Computer tutorial for learning DSS.* Paper presented at the Annual Convention of the American Speech-Language-Hearing Association, St Louis.

Ingram, D. (1971). Transitivity in child language. *Language, 47,* 888–910.

Ingram, D. (1972). The development of phrase structure rules. *Language Learning, 22,* 65–77.

Inhelder, B. (1976). Observations on the operational and figurative aspects of thought in dysphasic children. In D.M. Morehead & A.E. Morehead (Eds.), *Normal and deficient child language* (pp. 335–344). Baltimore: University Park Press.

Johnson, J., Miller, J., Curtiss, S., & Tallal, P. (1993). Conversations with children who are language impaired: Asking questions. *Journal of Speech and Hearing Research, 36,* 973–979.

Johnson, J., & Schery, T. (1976). The use of grammatical morphemes by children with communication disorders. In D.M. Morehead & A.E. Morehead (Eds.), *Normal and deficient child language* (pp. 239–258). Baltimore: University Park Press.

Johnson, N. (1965). Linguistic models of functional units of language behavior. In S. Rosenberg (Ed.), *New directions in psycholinguistics* (pp. 29–65). New York: Macmillan.

Johnson, W., Darley, F., & Spriestersbach, D.C. (1952). *Diagnostic methods in speech pathology.* New York: Harper & Row.

Johnson, W., Darley, F., & Spriestersbach, D.C. (1963). *Diagnostic methods in speech pathology* (2nd ed.). New York: Harper & Row.

Johnston, J., & Ramstadt, V. (1978). Cognitive development in pre-adolescent language impaired children. In M. Burns & J. Andrew (Eds.), *Selected papers in language and phonology* (pp. 49–55). Evanston, IL: Institute for Continuing Professional Education.

Johnston, J., & Slobin, D. (1979). The development of locative expressions in English, Italian, Serbo-Croatian and Turkish. *Journal of Child Language, 6,* 529–545.

Kaplan, R. (1963). *The conduct of inquiry.* Ann Arbor: University of Michigan Press.

Keenan, E.O. (1974). Conversational competence in children. *Journal of Child Language, 1,* 163–183.

Kelso, J., Ding, M., & Schöner, G. (1993). Dynamic pattern formation: A primer. In L. Smith & E. Thelen (Eds.), *A dynamic systems approach to development.* Cambridge: Bradford Books, MIT Press.

Kelso, J., Holt, K., Kugler, P., & Turvey, M. (1980). On the concept of coordinative structures as dissipative structures: II. Empirical lines of convergence. In J. Requin & G. Stelmach (Eds.), *Tutorials in motor neuroscience* (pp. 49–70). Amsterdam: Kluwer.

Kiefer, F. (1973). On presuppositions. In F. Kiefer & N. Ruwet (Eds.), *Generative grammar in Europe* (pp. 29–42). Dordrecht, The Netherlands: Reidel.

Kirchner, D., & Skarakis-Doyle, E. (1983). Developmental language disorders: A theoretical perspective. In T. Gallagher & C. Prutting (Eds.), *Pragmatic assessment and intervention issues in language* (pp. 215–246). San Diego: College-Hill Press.

Kirk, S., & McCarthy, J. (1961). *Illinois Test of Psycholinguistic Abilities.* Urbana: University of Illinois Press.

Klee, T. (1992). Measuring children's conversational language. In S.F. Warren & J. Reichle (Eds.), *Communication and language intervention series: Vol. 1. Causes and effects in communication and language intervention* (pp. 315–330). Baltimore: Paul H. Brookes Publishing Co.

Kramer, C., James, S., & Saxman, J. (1979). A comparison of language samples elicited at home and in the clinic. *Journal of Speech and Hearing Disorders, 44,* 7–18.

Kugler, P.N., Kelso, J., & Turvey, M. (1982). On the control and coordination of naturally developing systems. In G. Stelmach & J. Requin (Eds.), *Tutorials in motor behavior* (pp. 3–47). New York: North-Holland.

252 / EVANS

Kuhn, T.S. (1970). *The structure of scientific revolutions.* Chicago: University of Chicago Press.

Lakoff, G. (1971). On generative semantics. In D.D. Steinberg & L.A. Jakobovits (Eds.), *Semantics* (pp. 458–508). Cambridge, England: Cambridge University Press.

Lakoff, G., & Ross, J.R. (1967). *Is deep structure necessary?* Unpublished manuscript, Cambridge, MA.

Lakoff, R. (1972). Language in context. *Language, 48,* 907–927.

Lakoff, R. (1973). Questionable answers and answerable questions. In B.B. Kachru, R.B. Lees, Y. Malkiel, A. Pietrangeli, & S. Saporta (Eds.), *Issues in linguistic papers in honor of Henry and Renee Kahane* (pp. 45–80). Urbana: University of Illinois Press.

Lee, L. (1966). Developmental sentence types: A method for comparing normal and deviant syntactic development. *Journal of Speech and Hearing Disorders, 31,* 311–330.

Lee, L. (1971). *Northwestern Syntax Screening Test (NSST).* Evanston, IL: Northwestern University Press.

Lee, L. (1974). *Developmental Sentence Analysis.* Evanston, IL: Northwestern University Press.

Lee, L., & Cantor, S.M. (1971). Developmental Sentence Scoring: A clinical procedure for estimating syntactic development in children's spontaneous speech. *Journal of Speech and Hearing Disorders, 36,* 315–340.

Lee, L., & Koenigsknecht, R.A. (1974). *Developmental Sentence Analysis: A grammatical assessment procedure for speech and language disorders.* Evanston, IL: Northwestern University Press.

Leonard, L. (1972). What is deviant language? *Journal of Speech and Hearing Disorders, 37,* 427–446.

Leonard, L., Bolders, J., & Miller, J. (1976). An examination of the semantic relations reflected in the language usage of normal and language disordered children. *Journal of Speech and Hearing Research, 19,* 371–392.

Leonard, L., Camarata, S., Rowan, L., & Chapman, K. (1982). The communicative functions of lexical usage of language impaired children. *Applied Psycholinguistics, 3,* 109–127.

Leonard, L., Chapman, K., Rowan, L., & Weiss, A. (1983). Three hypotheses concerning young children's imitations of lexical items. *Developmental Psychology, 19,* 591–601.

Levison, S. (1983). *Pragmatics.* Cambridge, England: Cambridge University Press.

Liles, B. (1985). Production and comprehension of narrative discourse in normal and language disordered children. *Journal of Communication Disorders, 18,* 409–427.

Lock, A.J. (1972). *From out of nowhere.* Paper presented at the Second International Symposium on Child Language, Florence, Italy.

Long, S.H., & Fey, M.E. (1988). *Computerized profiling.* Ithaca, NY: Ithaca College.

Longhurst, T., & File, J. (1977). A comparison of developmental sentence scores from Head Start children collected in four conditions. *Language, Speech, and Hearing Services in Schools, 8,* 54–64.

Lorenz, E.N. (1963). Deterministic nonperiodic flow. *Journal of Atmospheric Science, 20,* 282–291.

Lund, N., & Duchan, J. (1983). *Assessing children's language in naturalistic contexts.* Englewood Cliffs, NJ: Prentice Hall.

Lund, N., & Duchan, J. (1988). *Assessing children's language in naturalistic contexts.* (2nd ed.). Englewood Cliffs, NJ: Prentice Hall.

MacDonald, M. (1978). *The Environmental Language Inventory*. Columbus, OH: Charles E. Merrill.

MacWhinney, B. (1991). *The CHILDES project: Tools for analyzing talk*. Hillsdale, NJ: Lawrence Erlbaum Associates.

MacWhinney, B. (1993). *The CHILDES database* (2nd ed.). Dublin, OH: Discovery Systems.

MacWhinney, B., & Bates, E. (Eds.). (1989). *The crosslinguistic study of sentence processing*. New York: Cambridge University Press.

MacWhinney, B., Bates, E., & Kliegel, R. (1984). Cue validity and sentence interpretation in English, German, and Italian. *Journal of Verbal Learning and Verbal Behavior, 23*, 127–150.

Mandelbrot, B.B. (1983). *The fractal geometry of nature*. San Francisco: W.H. Freeman.

McCarthy, D. (1954). Language development in children. In L. Carmichael (Ed.), *Manual of child psychology* (pp. 492–630). New York: John Wiley & Sons.

McCawley, J. (1968). The role of semantics in a grammar. In E. Bach & R.T. Harms (Eds.), *Universals in linguistic theory* (pp. 125–170). New York: Holt, Rinehart & Winston.

McNeill, D. (1966). The creation of language by children. In J. Lyons & R. Wales (Eds.), *Psycholinguistics papers* (pp. 99–126). Edinburgh, Scotland: University of Edinburgh Press.

McNeill, D. (1971). The capacity for the ontogenesis of grammar. In D.I. Slobin (Ed.), *The ontogenesis of grammar: A theoretical symposium* (pp. 17–40). New York: Academic Press.

McTear, M., & Conti-Ramsden, G. (1992). *Pragmatic disability in children*. London: Whurr Publishers.

Menyuk, P. (1964). Comparison of grammar of children with functionally deviant and normal speech. *Journal of Speech and Hearing Research, 7*, 109–121.

Menyuk, P., & Looney, P. (1972). Relationships among components of the grammar in language disorders. *Journal of Speech and Hearing Research, 15*, 395–406.

Miller, J. (1981). *Assessing language production in children: Experimental procedures*. Baltimore: University Park Press.

Miller, J. (1991). Research on language disorders in children: A progress report. In J. Miller (Ed.), *Research on child language disorders* (pp. 1–22). Austin, TX: PRO-ED.

Miller, J., & Chapman, R. (1983). *SALT: Systematic Analysis of Language Transcripts: User's manual*. Madison: University of Wisconsin Press.

Miller, J., Chapman, R., Branston, M., & Reichle, J. (1980). Language comprehension in sensorimotor stages V and VI. *Journal of Speech and Hearing Research, 23*, 284–311.

Miller, W.R., & Ervin, S.M. (1964). The development of grammar in child language. *Monographs of the Society for Research on Child Development, 29*, 9–34.

Miyaki, A., Carpenter, P., & Just, M. (1994). A capacity theory of syntactic comprehension disorders: Making normal adults perform like aphasic patients. *Cognitive Neuropsychology, 11*, 671–717.

Mordacai, D., Palin, M., & Palmer, C. (1985). *Lingquest I: Language sample analysis*. Napa, CA: Lingquest Software.

Morehead, D., & Ingram, D. (1973). The development of base syntax in normal and linguistically deviant children. *Journal of Speech and Hearing Research, 16*, 330–352.

Morehead, D.M., & Morehead, A.E. (1974). From signal to sign: A piagetian view of thought and language during the first two years. In R.L. Schiefelbusch & L.L. Lloyd (Eds.), *Language perspectives—Acquisition, retardation, and intervention* (pp. 153–190). Baltimore: University Park Press.

Morris, C. (1946). *Signs, language and behavior.* Englewood Cliffs, NJ: Prentice Hall.

Mowrer, O.H. (1952). Speech development in the young child: The autism theory of speech development and some clinical applications. *Journal of Speech and Hearing Disorders, 17,* 263–268.

Mowrer, O.H. (1954). The psychologist looks at language. *American Psychologist, 9,* 660–694.

Nelson, K. (1973). Structure and strategy in learning how to talk. *Monographs of the Society for Research in Child Development, 38,* 1–2.

Nelson, K. (1981). Individual differences in language development: Implications for development and language. *Developmental Psychology, 17,* 170–187.

Nicolis, G., & Prigogine, I. (1989). *Exploring complexity: An introduction.* San Francisco: W.H. Freeman.

Ochs, E. (1979). Transcription as theory. In E. Ochs & B. Schieffelin (Eds.), *Developmental pragmatics* (pp. 43–72). New York: Academic Press.

Olswang, L., & Carpenter, R. (1978). Elicitor effects of the language obtained from young language-impaired children. *Journal of Speech and Hearing Disorders, 43,* 76–88.

Osgood, C.E. (1957). *Method and theory in experimental psychology.* New York: Oxford University Press.

Osgood, C.E. (1963). On understanding and creating sentences. *American Psychologist, 18,* 735–751.

Parker, T.S., & Chua, L. (1989). *Practical numerical algorithms for chaotic systems.* New York: Springer-Verlag.

Peach, R. (1977, November). *Comprehension of relative and contrastive objectives by language disordered children.* Paper presented at the Annual Convention of the American Speech and Hearing Association, Chicago.

Peitgen, H.O., & Richter, P.H. (1986). *The beauty of fractals: Images of complex dynamical systems.* Berlin: Springer-Verlag.

Penn, C. (1988). The profiling of syntax and pragmatics in aphasia. *Clinical Linguistics and Phonetics, 2,* 179–207.

Pinker, S. (1984). *Language learnability and language development.* Cambridge, MA: Harvard University Press.

Pinker, S. (1989). *Learnability and cognition: The acquisition of argument structure.* Cambridge: MIT Press.

Pollio, H. (1968). Associative structure and verbal behavior. In T. Dixon & D. Horton (Eds.), *Verbal behavior and general behavioral theory* (pp. 37–65). Englewood Cliffs, NJ: Prentice Hall.

Postal, P. (1972). The best theory. In S. Peters (Ed.), *Goals in linguistic theory* (pp. 179–201). Englewood Cliffs, NJ: Prentice Hall.

Prigogine, I., & Stengers, I. (1984). *Order out of chaos: Man's new dialogue with nature.* New York: Bantam.

Prutting, C., Gallagher, T., & Mulac, A. (1975). Imitation: A closer look. *Journal of Speech and Hearing Disorders, 41,* 412–422.

Prutting, C., & Kirchner, D. (1983). Applied pragmatics. In T. Gallagher & C. Prutting (Eds.), *Pragmatic assessment and intervention issues in language* (pp. 29–64). San Diego: College-Hill Press.

Retherford, K., Schwartz, B., & Chapman, R. (1982). Semantic roles and residual grammatical categories in mother and child speech: Who tunes into whom? *Journal of Child Language, 8,* 583–608.

Reynell, J. (1969). *Reynell Expressive Developmental Language Scale.* Slough, England: National Foundation for Educational Research.

Rice, M.L. (1995). Grammatical categories of children with specific language impairments. In R.V. Watkins & M.L. Rice (Eds.), *Communication and language intervention series: Vol. 4. Specific language impairments in children* (pp. 69–89). Baltimore: Paul H. Brookes Publishing Co.

Robertson, S., Cohen, A., & Meyers-Kress, G. (1993). Behavioral chaos: Beyond the metaphor. In L. Smith & E. Thelen (Eds.), *A dynamic systems approach to development* (pp. 119–150). Cambridge, MA: Bradford Books, MIT Press.

Ross, J.R. (1970). On declarative sentence. In R.A. Jakobs & P.S. Rosenbaum (Eds.), *Readings in English transformational grammar* (pp. 139–152). Waltham, MA: Ginn.

Roth, F., & Spekman, N. (1984). Assessing the pragmatic abilities of children: Part I. Organizational framework and assessment parameters. *Journal of Speech and Hearing Disorders, 49,* 2–11.

Ruelle, D. (1989). *Elements of differentiable dynamics and bifurcation theory.* New York: Academic Press.

Sacks, H., Schegloff, E., & Jefferson, G. (1974). A simplest systematics for the organization of turn-taking for conversation. *Language, 50,* 696–735.

Scarborough, H. (1990). Index of Productive Syntax (IPSyn). *Applied Psycholinguistics, 11,* 1–22.

Schiefelbusch, R. (1963). Language studies of mentally retarded children. *Journal of Speech and Hearing Disorders, 10,* 4–15.

Schlesinger, I.M. (1971). Production of utterances and language acquisition. In D.I. Slobin (Ed.), *The ontogenesis of grammar* (pp. 63–102). New York: Academic Press.

Schlesinger, I.M. (1974). Relational concepts underlying language. In R.L. Schiefelbusch & L.L. Lloyd (Eds.), *Language perspectives—Acquisition, retardation, and intervention* (pp. 129–152). Baltimore: University Park Press.

Scott, C., & Taylor, A. (1978). A comparison of home and clinic gathered language samples. *Journal of Speech and Hearing Disorders, 43,* 482–495.

Searle, J. (1969). *Speech acts: An essay in the philosophy of language.* Cambridge, England: Cambridge University Press.

Shanon, C., & Weaver, W. (1949). *The mathematical theory of communication.* Urbana: University of Illinois Press.

Shulman, B. (1986). *Test of Pragmatic Skills–Revised.* Tucson, AZ: Communication Skill Builders.

Sinclair, H. (1971). Sensorimotor action patterns as a condition for the acquisition of syntax. In R. Huxley & E. Ingram (Eds.), *Language acquisition: Models and methods* (pp. 121–130). New York: Academic Press.

Skarakis, E., & Greenfield, P. (1982). The role of new and old information in the verbal expressions of language disabled children. *Journal of Speech and Hearing Research, 25,* 462–467.

Skarakis-Doyle, E. (1990). Peer commentary on "Clinical pragmatics: Expectations and realizations" by Tanya Gallagher. *Journal of Speech Language Pathology and Audiology, 14,* 8–9.

Skinner, B.F. (1954). *Science and human behavior.* New York: Macmillan.

Skinner, B.F. (1957). *Verbal behavior.* New York: Appleton-Century-Crofts.

Sloane, H.N., & MacAulay, B.D. (1968). *Operant procedures in remedial speech and language training.* Lanham, MD: Universities of America Press.

Slobin, D. (1970). Universals of grammatical development in children. In G.B. Flores d'Arcais & J.M. Levelt (Eds.), *Advances in psycholinguistics* (pp. 174–186). Amsterdam: Elsevier/North Holland.

Smith, M. (1933a). Grammatical errors in the speech of preschool children. *Child Development, 4,* 183–190.

Smith, M. (1933b). The influence of age, sex, and situation on the frequency, form and function of questions asked by preschool children. *Child Development, 4,* 201–213.

Snyder, L. (1975). *Pragmatics in language disordered children: Their prelinguistic and early verbal performatives and presuppositions.* Unpublished doctoral dissertation, University of Colorado.

Stalnaker, L., & Craighead, N. (1982). An examination of language samples obtained under three experimental conditions. *Language, Speech, and Hearing Services in Schools, 13*(2), 121–128.

Templin, M.C. (1957). *Certain language skills in children.* Minneapolis: University of Minnesota Press.

Templin, M.C., & Darley, D. (1960). *The Templin-Darley Test of Articulation.* Iowa City: University of Iowa Bureau of Educational Research.

Thelen, E., Kelso, J., & Fogel, A. (1987). Self-organizing systems and infant motor development. *Developmental Review, 7,* 39–65.

Thelen, E., & Smith, B. (1994). *A dynamic systems approach to the development of cognition and action.* Cambridge: MIT Press.

Tyack, D., & Gottsleben, R. (1974). *Language sampling, analysis, and training: Baseline analyses and goal.* Los Angeles: Consulting Psychologists Press.

Vallacher, R., & Nowark, A. (1994). *Dynamical systems in social psychology.* New York: Academic Press.

van Geert, O. (1991). A dynamic systems model of cognitive and language growth. *Psychological Review, 98,* 3–53.

van Kleeck, A., & Frankel, T. (1981). Discourse devices used by language disordered children: A preliminary investigation. *Journal of Speech and Hearing Disorders, 46,* 250–257.

von Neumann, J. (1950). The character of the equation. In A.H. Taub (Ed.), *Recent theories of turbulence: Collected works* (pp. 437–450). New York: Pergamon Press.

Watkins, R.V., & Rice, M.L. (Eds.). (1995). *Communication and language intervention series: Vol. 4. Specific language impairments in children.* Baltimore: Paul H. Brookes Publishing Co.

Whitehurst, G., Fischel, J., Arnold, D., & Lonigan, C. (1992). Evaluating outcomes with children with expressive language delay. In S.F. Warren & J. Reichle (Eds.), *Communication and language intervention series: Vol. 1. Causes and effects in communication and language intervention* (pp. 277–313). Baltimore: Paul H. Brookes Publishing Co.

11

Assessing Children's Language in Meaningful Contexts

Angela Notari-Syverson and Angela Losardo

THE PROCESS OF ASSESSING LANGUAGE involves making inferences about the nature of underlying competencies from a select sample of children's behaviors in specific situations judged to be representative of a broader construct (Cicchetti & Wagner, 1990; McCune, Kalmanson, Fleck, Glazewski, & Sillari, 1990). For assessments to be meaningful, they must draw on a broader understanding of learning and development across domains (Meisels, 1994). One of the most important purposes of assessment is to yield information about the contexts in which children learn best and how children respond to instruction (Lahey, 1988; Nelson, 1994). Practitioners must be knowledgeable about child development and theories of how children learn in order to choose appropriate assessment tools and procedures (Anstey & Bull, 1991).

This chapter focuses on assessing children's language in meaningful contexts such as home, school, and community environments. This chapter reviews theoretical language acquisition perspectives that have had considerable influence on assessment approaches used with children, examines the different types and purposes of assessment, defines key terms, explores issues and limitations of language assessment practices, and identifies promising approaches and models for assessing language and communication across multiple contexts and perspectives.

ASSESSMENT AND THEORIES OF LANGUAGE LEARNING

The approaches used in identifying and remediating language and communication problems in children have been influenced over the years by changing views of the nature of language acquisition. During the 1950s, assessment of the communicative abilities of children largely focused on the development of speech sounds, size of vocabulary, and sentence structure in preschool and school-age populations (Johnson, Darley, & Spriestersbach, 1952; Templin, 1957). Although extensive normative data were available, the results from these assessments provided little direction to interventionists designing instructional programs. A second approach prevalent during this time was deeply rooted in the medical model. Proponents of this model argued that knowing the etiology of a disorder would assist in ameliorating the problem (Emerick & Haynes, 1986). Using this approach, children were classified according to communicative disability, but, again, the assessments used to categorize children provided little useful information to service providers developing appropriate intervention goals and content.

During the late 1950s, the assessment focus, driven by the nativistic position, shifted from studying speech to examining structural aspects of language. Proponents of the nativistic position asserted that the infant is born with the innate ability to learn language and that the environment plays a limited role in development (Chomsky, 1957). Both auditory processing and psycholinguistic models of language assessment were emerging (Lund & Duchan, 1983). Although the focus of these models was on developing a direct relationship between test performance and intervention, which was a step forward, service providers using results from this type of assessment still found it difficult to design functional intervention programs. Test items, selected on the basis of their ability to discriminate between typically developing children of different ages (e.g., discrimination of individual phonemes), were not contextually relevant and consisted of isolated skills believed to be relatively unaffected by environmental experiences (Johnson, 1982; Nelson, 1993).

During the 1960s, clinicians and researchers with a behavioral orientation began conducting research that demonstrated the important role of environmental variables in language acquisition. Language was viewed strictly as a behavior that children learn from adults according to principles of classical and operant conditioning. Approaches to assessment emerged that involved quantitative measurement of specific skills in prescriptive and highly controlled teaching sequences (e.g., programmed instruction, precision teaching). These models emphasized imitating adult language and using contingent reinforcement. Behavior analysts generated important and useful applications to assessment practices, such as behavioral observation methods and criterion-referenced tests still in use in the mid-1990s.

In the 1970s, several investigators drew attention to the need to understand semantic content in order to describe children's utterances in terms of their syntactic structures (e.g., Bloom, 1970). Subsequent approaches to assessment reflected the growing emphasis on semantic content and presumed cognitive prerequisites of language, rather than on the syntactic structure (McCormick & Schiefelbusch, 1984; Schlesinger, 1974). Also emerging in the 1970s was an approach to language assessment that addressed pragmatics. The development of syntax and semantics in children was viewed as dependent, in part, on the social interactions of children with their environment. Young children's utterances were classified according to their functions in various social contexts.

Attention was directed toward assessing language functions and contexts, but little systematic information was provided to practitioners developing intervention programs.

An approach to language learning and assessment has emerged as a synthesis of syntactic, semantic, and pragmatic theory and research on the social reciprocity of the child–caregiver interaction. This perspective draws heavily on Vygotsky's (1978) social-constructivist approach, which considers language acquisition an active and social process. The social-constructivist approach focuses on the social and communicative aspects of language in meaningful and real-life situations. Children actively construct their understanding of language and how it is used through interactions with adults and peers. Children's meanings, forms, and uses of language vary depending on their social and cultural backgrounds. Assessment procedures based on this perspective tend to be descriptive and informal and emphasize children's learning potential in relation to their social interactions with adults.

Assessment approaches over the years have tended to reflect the predominant theory of language acquisition and communicative competence. A major challenge exists for developing and adopting contextually relevant assessment instruments and procedures that reflect theories of language learning. To understand the issues and limitations of adopting such models, knowledge of the types and purposes of assessment is necessary.

TYPES AND PURPOSES OF ASSESSMENT

Assessment is the process of obtaining information to make evaluative decisions (Meisels, 1994). Assessments can be divided into two broad categories: formal and nonformal. *Formal assessments* are standardized tests that yield specifically defined information on a preset content and have specified guidelines for administration. Information usually is collected on a one-time basis and is compared with normative data. *Nonformal assessments* are structured and systematic observations of behaviors within meaningful, context-bound activities (e.g., children's narratives, conversations about books, oral reports, dramatic enactments, participation in class discussions) in multiple settings. Information collection is ongoing. Using Silliman and Wilkinson's (1991) classification, structured observational tools are grouped into three main categories: categorical, narrative, and descriptive.

Categorical tools have predetermined categories into which all events and behaviors are coded during the observation. This type of observation can be quantified and summarized by a numerical representation. Typical examples of categorical tools are rating scales and checklists. They are relatively easy and inexpensive to use, but they are not suitable when detailed information is needed on qualitative aspects of behaviors. *Narrative tools* include journals, running records, anecdotal notes of observations of critical incidents, and ethnographic notes recorded during participant observations. These tools are systematic and detailed written descriptions of behaviors. They are easy to record and share with others; however, the accuracy and the selection of information may be subject to interpretive biases. *Descriptive tools* are verbatim accounts of actual language use and provide a detailed record of behaviors and a description of various contexts. Their use requires trained staff and usually employs technological tools such as audio recording and videotaping. Analysis of a descriptive record is time consuming.

Before choosing formal or nonformal assessment procedures, practitioners must understand for which purposes they are measuring a child's performance. Measurement can involve at least four processes with the following uniquely different purposes: screening, diagnostic assessment, program assessment, and evaluation.

Screening is a brief procedure that determines whether a child's performance is sufficiently different from the performance of other children of the same chronological age to warrant more comprehensive testing. Following an initial suspicion of a delay, a *diagnostic assessment* provides in-depth information on the specific nature of the problem. These tools are used to qualify children for special education services and to make referral and placement decisions. Screening and diagnostic instruments generally are norm referenced. Traditional norm-referenced instruments, constructed primarily for screening and diagnosing, do not yield direct information for making program decisions or for choosing curricular content, nor have they proved sensitive to intervention efforts (Darby, 1979; Garwood, 1982). Items on standardized tests are selected because of their capacity to discriminate between groups of children of different ages, not necessarily because of their educational relevance.

Program assessment specifically addresses the need to obtain educationally relevant information and to provide guidance in developing educational programs. Program assessment serves at least three functions (Bricker & Littman, 1982). First, it provides information for identifying appropriate intervention content. Second, caregivers may use results from program assessments to compare their goals for children with those of the service providers. Third, it may be used to document children's progress over time. Used as an *evaluation* tool, results of children's performance on a program assessment are compared before and after intervention. Program assessments generally are criterion referenced. Rather than comparing a child's performance to a norm or standardized sample, criterion-referenced tests measure mastery of specific objectives defined by predetermined standards of criteria. Because these instruments are not standardized, adaptations are allowed and encouraged in order to elicit a representative sample of children's behavior in optimal conditions.

One limitation of criterion-referenced tests is that many were developed by selecting isolated items from various norm-referenced instruments. This procedure invalidates age-equivalency scores for individual items and limits their educational relevance (Johnson, 1982). Items drawn from standardized tests do not necessarily represent functional behaviors that can be used to develop educational goals. Also, many criterion-referenced assessments are based on a fragmented-skill, test–teach–retest approach, which does not reflect models of the way children learn language.

Curriculum-based assessments (CBAs) are a direct application of criterion-referenced assessment strategies to educational content (Notari, Slentz, & Bricker, 1991). CBA is a form of criterion-referenced measurement whereby curricular objectives serve as the criteria for identifying educational targets (Bagnato & Neisworth, 1991). Because of the direct congruence among testing, teaching, and progress evaluation, CBA is the most direct means for identifying a child's entry point within an educational program and for refining and readjusting instruction. Assessment and curricular content are coordinated to address the same skills and abilities, and repeated testing occurs over time to measure the child's progress on these skills.

Bagnato and Neisworth (1991) distinguished two types of CBA: curriculum-referenced scales, which include skills common to most educational programs but which are not particular to any specific curriculum (e.g., the Brigance Diagnostic Inventory of Early Development–Revised [Brigance, 1991]); and curriculum-embedded scales in which assessment items are identical to skills included in a specific curriculum (e.g., the Assessment, Evaluation, and Programming System for Infants and Children: AEPS Measurement for Birth to Three Years [Bricker, 1993]). Curriculum-embedded assessments provide specific guidelines for assessment, developing intervention goals and objectives, and conducting educational activities to facilitate the acquisition of functional skills.

Administering assessments in a single session using standardized procedures often results in underestimating the capabilities of children with disabilities (Bagnato & Neisworth, 1991). The advantage of using CBAs is that they emphasize the learning process. CBAs are uniquely suited for ongoing collection of information over the course of the school year rather than for the portrayal of a specific instance of the child's behavior. Most important, they allow service providers to monitor children's learning in order to plan curricula and adjust teaching strategies to the individual characteristics of the child. However, empirical data on psychometric properties and educational relevance of CBAs are very limited.

FIVE KEY ISSUES IN ASSESSING LANGUAGE IN MEANINGFUL CONTEXTS

The issues related to assessing children's language in meaningful contexts are 1) the influence of context and culture on language, 2) the relationship between language and literacy, 3) how children respond to instruction, 4) the importance of a transdisciplinary approach to assessment, and 5) the need for a multidimensional approach to assessment.

Influence of Context and Culture

Research and theoretical models (e.g., Barker, 1968; Bronfenbrenner, 1979) have drawn attention to the strong influences of the physical and social environments on all aspects of child development. Assessing language must expand from analyzing the three basic dimensions of language—content, form, and use—to analyzing contextual and cultural influences that either facilitate or hinder language understanding and use.

CBAs sometimes are used to measure children's language use in restricted settings (e.g., resource rooms) with little, if any, information collected on learning processes and potential in the general classroom environment. An underlying assumption of this practice is that children with disabilities should be removed from the contexts that are giving them difficulty and taught a special curriculum using approaches that differ from those of the general classroom (Nelson, 1994). This approach has not met with much success as children fail to generalize skills learned in therapy sessions to other more natural contexts (Warren & Kaiser, 1988).

Nelson (1994) used the term *curriculum-based language assessment* to refer to the process of determining whether children have the language skills and strategies for processing information within the context of the school curriculum. Traditional curriculum-based approaches are concerned only with the children's mastery of the official curriculum, without considering that children must learn many other kinds of "hidden" curricula in order to succeed in school (Nelson, 1994). These hidden curricula include various unspoken expectations for children in terms of knowledge and familiarity with mainstream culture, rules for communication and behavior in school settings, and rules for peer acceptance and interaction (Nelson, 1989).

Language use in the context of the school curriculum is the most significant factor that puts certain groups at a disadvantage (Miller, 1984). Differences exist between language spoken at home and language required in school (Adler, 1981; Barrera, 1993; Cazden, 1988; Heath, 1982; Labov, 1972; Snow, 1983). For example, Caucasian, middle-class culture that predominates in school settings emphasizes a formal style of language and early orientation toward the written word, neglecting areas that African Americans are oriented toward such as oral language expressed through drama, poetry, and song (Hale, 1992; Kochman, 1972). Verbal and nonverbal discrepancies often occur when teachers and children are from different cultural backgrounds. African American children, for example, tend to use a topic-associating narrative style in contrast to the topic-centered discourse style used by teachers (Michaels, 1986). Also, teachers expect direct eye contact and answers to direct questions; some Asian and Native American children, however, do not consider these interactions appropriate ways of communicating with adults (Gilmore, 1984; Locust, 1988).

Assessing the language of children from diverse cultural and linguistic backgrounds must include consideration of the influences of contextual and cultural factors on language (Adler, 1981; Gutierrez-Clellen & Quinn, 1993; Labov, 1972; Miller, 1984). For example, the use of culturally appropriate pictures improved the language scores of African American children (Cazden, 1970). Children from lower-income families achieved the same level of performance as did children from middle-class families when they received additional adult support during assessment in the form of probes and questions (Heider, Cazden, & Brown, 1968, cited in Cazden, 1970). Au and Mason (1981) found that native Hawaiian children understood written texts better when read in the "talk-story" conversational format typical of their culture, as compared with turn-taking reading groups. Barrera (1993) found that children with disabilities responded differently when their non-English home language was introduced into the intervention setting.

Assessing pragmatic aspects such as the organization of language in terms of style, genre, speech acts, and narratives that deal with the use of language across contexts is increasingly important for understanding language and communication skills of children from diverse cultural frameworks. For these children, language assessment must differentiate language development from the mastery of language as the primary medium for instruction and for learning (Bartoli & Botel, 1988; Westby, 1985). Children may score below norms not because they have speech and language impairments, but because of a sociocultural mismatch between their language experiences in the home and the academic language used in school (Nelson, 1993). External biases of tests resulting from differences in general aspects of the environment, child rearing, schooling, and sociocultural status may hinder the differentiation of language variations due to cultural and stylistic differences from language development problems. Traditional tests, for example, focus on written language and ignore many oral language skills by which African American children may demonstrate greater competence (Hale, 1992). Also, responses to the stress caused by acculturation factors can be easily confused with learning disabilities (Adler, 1981; Gavillàn-Torres, 1984). Because children display language and communicative competence differently across school and other social settings, information from family members is critical in making decisions about the need for language intervention services (Nelson, 1993).

The nondiscriminatory evaluation required by PL 94-142, the Education for All Handicapped Children Act of 1975 (since updated as PL 101-476, the Individuals with Disabilities Education Act [IDEA] of 1990), acknowledges cultural and linguistic differences, stating that assessments should be administered in the language the person understands best (Gavillàn-Torres, 1984). Tests translated into other languages, however, must be used with caution because of the unproved assumption that bilingual children's language development and use are similar to those of monolingual children (Miller, 1984). Children with limited proficiency in the language used for instruction must pay attention to both instructional content and the language used to convey the content. This becomes even more challenging for children with disabilities who are bilingual and who also are dealing with learning difficulties in general (Barrera, 1993).

Language and Literacy

Theory and research show that literacy development begins in the very early years (e.g., Morrow, 1989; Snow, 1983). Language and literacy develop simultaneously and in an interrelated manner. Both involve symbolic representational abilities and meaning-making activities (Meadows, 1993; Sawyer, 1991). Within the context of the school curriculum, oral and written language can be viewed broadly as linguistic strategies for gaining knowledge and processing information and are the most important means of acquiring and communicating knowledge (Norris, 1989; Silliman & Wilkinson, 1991).

School curricula lack integration of oral language and literacy. The focus is on oral language in the preschool and early elementary years. Children must learn to process language that is more complex and decontextualized than language that is used at home and must learn the rules of communicative interactions that are typical of the classroom (Berlin, Blank, & Rose, 1980; Heath, 1982). The traditional "reading readiness" approach leads to the misconception that young children, especially those with disabilities, are not ready to interact with print. Data from early literacy interventions with preschoolers and kindergartners have shown that children with disabilities can learn early literacy skills (Katims, 1991; O'Connor & Notari-Syverson, in press). Storybook reading has been associated with improved language outcomes for young children who are developing typically (Whitehurst et al., 1988) and for children with disabilities (Dale, Crain-Thoreson, Notari-Syverson, & Cole, in press; Swinson & Ellis, 1988). Expanding early childhood assessment to include early literacy experiences could provide useful information on children's early experience with books, a strong predictor of school success (Wells, 1985).

In elementary classrooms, the curriculum focuses primarily on reading and writing skills, and children learn new information from increasingly decontextualized written language texts (Nelson, 1994). Studies have shown, however, that literacy incorporates a broad set of skills that include speaking and listening as well as reading and writing (Silliman & Wilkinson, 1991). There is a growing recognition of the influence of oral language and communication on the acquisition of literacy. Children who experience problems in oral language development are very likely to develop literacy-learning difficulties (Aram & Nation, 1980; Catts & Kamhi, 1987) and to need classroom-based models of language intervention that integrate both oral and written language activities into the school curriculum (Silliman & Wilkinson, 1991).

Responsiveness to Instruction

Although traditional CBAs provide teachers with information on when a child is not meeting performance criteria, they rarely provide information on how to change instruction and adjust teaching strategies to the individual needs of the child (Mehrens & Clarizio, 1993). Most tests cover lower-level basic skills rather than higher-level thinking skills such as integrating information and decision making (Bartoli & Botel, 1988). Little, if any, information is provided on the child's ability to learn. Still worse, in many classrooms the curriculum is actually driven by the assessment, as teachers focus on preparing their students for successful performance on standardized tests (Darling-Hammond, 1989). Assessment should focus on identifying what a child needs to do to succeed in a given context, including the context of social interaction, and what a child can learn when proper support is provided by an adult or a more experienced peer (Nelson, 1994; Palincsar, Brown, & Campione, 1994). One promising approach, dynamic assessment, is described later in this chapter.

Transdisciplinary Approach

The choice of assessment procedures should be determined, in part, by the respective roles of the teacher, specialists, and families in gathering information and making decisions about curricula. Traditionally, communication specialists have adopted one of two approaches to assessment: multidisciplinary or interdisciplinary. Using a multidisciplinary approach, communication specialists conduct diagnostic assessment activities in isolation from other professionals. The communication specialist who adopts the interdisciplinary approach conducts assessment activities separate from other team members but periodically meets with them to share information. Communication specialists typically have used assessment tools and procedures that are standardized and that yield information of questionable use to classroom teachers.

One serious consequence of these two approaches is the lack of coordination and formal input from teachers, other service providers, and families (Silliman & Wilkinson, 1991). Collaboration with families consists mostly of one-way communication from the teacher or communication specialist to the parent, usually only to report test results or negative behavior (Thomas, 1993). The lack of connection among teacher, specialist, school, and family results in judgments about the child being made from incomplete information, which can lead to placement errors (Bartoli & Botel, 1988). A transdisciplinary approach to service delivery addresses the inadequacies of the other two models. Using a transdisciplinary model, families and service providers work collaboratively and reach all decisions through consensus. Adopting this model facilitates the use of more integrated, curriculum-based assessment activities and procedures.

Multidimensional Approach

The most important consideration in choosing an assessment is whether it provides a valid portrayal of how children use language in real situations (Brown, Collins, & Duguid, 1989). Assessment planning should follow two main guidelines. First, an accurate and comprehensive picture of children's language and communication abilities across settings must be obtained (Bricker, 1992). Language and communication assessment and intervention must take into account the curricular contexts in which children are experiencing problems and draw upon opportunities in those contexts when devising interventions (Nelson, 1994). Assessing and intervening across contexts calls for a comprehensive plan of assessment that uses multiple methods and sources across multiple contexts and involves collaboration among disciplines and with the family (Neisworth & Bagnato, 1988; Silliman & Wilkinson, 1991; Thomas, 1993).

Second, procedures must be individualized to match unique characteristics of children and families (Bagnato & Neisworth, 1991; Lahey, 1988). Classroom teachers face increasing variability in children's language and literacy skills because of cultural diversity and inclusion of children with disabilities (Wilkinson & Silliman, 1993). Plans of assessment must be individualized to allow for the different ways in which these children may respond to assessment procedures (Lahey, 1988). Assessment procedures should draw from positivistic, quantitative frameworks (e.g., tests) used by specialists to gain information about the child's developmental status and from phenomenological perspectives that use approaches derived from ethnographic and linguistic anthropology to gain qualitative information about the perspectives of others, such as parents, peers, and the child (Nelson, 1994). Comprehensive and individualized plans of assessment should be developed by selecting a combination of procedures ranging from formal, standardized tests to informal, naturalistic observations (Lahey, 1988; Silliman, Wilkinson, & Hoffman, 1993).

INNOVATIVE APPROACHES AND MODELS

This section provides specific examples of state-of-the-art models that can be used to assess language and literacy skills of young children in preschool settings and of older, school-age children. These innovative models of assessment include 1) embedded approaches, 2) alternative approaches, 3) dynamic approaches, and 4) comprehensive models.

Embedded Approaches

Research has shown that contexts such as low-structured, child-centered, and familiar routine activities are best for obtaining an accurate picture of children's language. Generally, young children use more complex language during low-structured situations than during elicited-production tests (Lahey, Launer, & Shiff-Myers, 1983; Longhurst & Grubb, 1974; Prutting, Gallagher, & Mulac,

1975) and when they talk about a self-initiated topic (Strandberg & Griffith, 1968, cited in Cazden, 1970). Similarly, young children with disabilities talk more when questions are embedded within a conversational context, and they are more likely to address questions about child-initiated topics than they are questions about a new topic (Yoder, Davies, & Bishop, 1992). Also, children's language is more complex during routine interactions than during nonroutine interactions (Yoder & Davies, 1990).

Observational assessment activities can be embedded in child-initiated activities (e.g., conversation, brainstorming, exploratory talk, problem solving, storytelling) during meaningful daily routines (Anstey & Bull, 1991). Observing children's spontaneous behaviors, however, is not always practical or time efficient, and relevant behaviors will not necessarily appear. Adults can manipulate the environment to create opportunities to assess specific skills. Following are some applications of embedded approaches to assessment.

Nonstandardized Elicitations Lahey (1988) referred to nonstandardized elicitations in which the adult takes an active role in naturalistic situations by suggesting certain tasks and probes in order to elicit particular responses. To assess sentence construction, for example, the adult may manipulate puppets and ask the child to describe specific actions performed by the puppet. Similarly, the adult may prepare specific materials for an art project to elicit labeling of colors, shapes, and sizes.

Concentrated Encounters Cazden (1977) proposed assessment through concentrated encounters. These situations are representative of real-life events and familiar interaction experiences, but they are condensed and focused by teacher direction to yield more information in less time. Instead of conducting separate tests, for example, the teacher may condense the assessment of early language and literacy skills into a single observation of a child's behaviors during storybook reading. If the book is carefully selected, then the teacher will be able to elicit a variety of skills from book-handling behaviors and picture labeling to knowledge of story structure and nursery rhymes, as well as word and letter recognition and letter sounds.

Play-Based Models The context of play is particularly suited for observing language and communication skills of young children; the familiar and pleasurable nature of play is conducive to the expression of children's optimal abilities and provides many opportunities for children to practice a variety of skills. CBAs such as the transdisciplinary play-based assessment (Linder, 1993) provide interventionists with a useful framework for observing a range of skills including modalities or methods of communication, components of language (e.g., pragmatics, phonology, syntax, semantics), receptive language skills, and oral-motor skills.

Milieu Approaches Milieu approaches refer to a group of naturalistic strategies for teaching language in its functional context to young preschool children (Kaiser, Yoder, & Keetz, 1992). Milieu teaching draws from applied behavioral technology and uses child-responsive interaction styles and environmental arrangement to provide a social and physical context for teaching. These language intervention techniques are supported by a strong database on their efficacy in improving children's acquisition of language in instructional settings (Kaiser et al., 1992); however, limited support is available on their utility for generalizing skills across settings (Losardo & Bricker, 1994).

One naturalistic approach—activity-based intervention—provides specific guidelines for assessment activities (Bricker & Cripe, 1992). Activity-based intervention is part of a larger framework that links assessment, intervention, and evaluation activities. Training on children's goals and objectives is embedded in child-directed, routine, and planned activities that occur at home and in center-based programs. A series of seven assessment activity plans has been developed and used successfully in center-based programs. These plans can be used to provide comprehensive and detailed information about children's behavioral repertoires. Each plan contains assessment items from several developmental domains that are likely to be observed during specific activities. For example, the following behaviors of children may be observed during a snack activity: getting into and out of a child-size chair (gross motor); putting the lid back on a jar (fine motor); assigning one object to two or more people (cognitive); transferring food with a spoon (adaptive); using two-word utterances (social-communication); and taking turns (social). Each activity plan has an associated recording form or CBA-type checklist. Children should have multiple opportunities to perform skills with different people using different materials in multiple settings.

Watson, Layton, Pierce, and Abraham (1994) described a similar approach to the assessment of early literacy skills in which skills are embedded within specific classroom activities. For example, concepts of books and print can be assessed during storybook reading at opening circle, story structure can be assessed during dramatic play, and phonological awareness can be assessed during writing and library time.

Critical Experiences   For older school-age children, similar approaches to assessment have been developed. Bartoli and Botel (1988) proposed a framework for observing children's oral and written language during routine events in the classroom. The teacher structures observations of children's learning around selected critical experiences such as transactions with text, independent reading and writing, and oral and written composing. Within these experiences, observations are made of children's oral and written language skills (e.g., narrative structure, syntactic complexity) that can serve as a basis for developing individualized education programs (IEPs). Subsequent intervention also takes place around the same critical learning events.

Alternative Approaches

Performance assessments and authentic assessments have been developed in response to the dissatisfaction with standardized, norm-referenced tests and multiple-choice tests for assessing student outcomes (Marzano, Pickering, & McTighe, 1993). *Performance assessment* is a broad term that refers to tasks whereby students demonstrate and apply their knowledge (e.g., tell a story, build a model, draw a map, make a presentation about a researched topic). *Authentic assessment* is similar to performance assessment and refers to the completion of a task in a real-life context (e.g., write a letter to a friend or the newspaper, read a list of products to buy at the grocery store) (Cohen & Spenciner, 1994). The focus of this approach is to document how and why instructional procedures work or do not work to achieve "authentic" changes in language learning and development. Informal, systematic observational tools (e.g., categorical, narrative, descriptive) are the most useful strategies to evaluate progress in various aspects of children's language as used in meaningful situations. Adults can easily create opportunities for assessing language skills during daily events and activities by asking children to provide explanations for an action, for how an object was made, or for a conclusion reached; asking children to make plans for activities and predict events; and encouraging children to obtain and exchange information about a topic or procedure. The critical issue is whether the observed changes reflect a transfer of responsibility from teacher to student (Silliman et al., 1993), as the ultimate goal is for children to perform these tasks with minimal, if any, adult support.

Portfolio assessment is a tool used to systematically collect and evaluate the data yielded from performance and authentic assessments, as well as from curriculum-based and norm-referenced tests; it documents the student's efforts, progress, or achievement, particularly in the area of communication (e.g., writing, reading, speaking, listening) (Arter & Spandel, 1991). Portfolios primarily compile actual work samples that reflect real tasks (e.g., essays, reports, list of books read, dictations) and provide a more authentic representation of children's application of knowledge than would test scores or observations of directly elicited behaviors in contrived testing situations. Young children's portfolios may contain samples of artwork, self-portraits, drawings, photographs of block constructions, videotapes and audio recordings of conversations, anecdotal notes of teacher observations, and interviews with parents (Cohen & Spenciner, 1994). School-age children's portfolios also may include writing samples, as well as work samples in reading and mathematics. Methods specifically for documenting language behaviors include verbatim transcriptions of children's dictations, audiotapes or videotapes of children's dialogues, checklists and anecdotal notes on language behaviors across a variety of situations (e.g., lunch, dramatic play), and parent reports on language used in the home and other social settings.

Portfolios should reflect the broad goals of the general classroom curriculum, and the criteria used to evaluate projects or products should be similar to those used every day in the classroom. In special education, the goals of the portfolio can be those outlined in the IEP. One important feature of portfolio assessment is the student's participation in collecting and evaluating work samples.

Additional support from teachers may be needed to help children collect, review, and evaluate their work (Schutt & McCabe, 1994). Adults should encourage children to systematically place samples of their work (e.g., drawings, writings) into their portfolio folder at school and at home. Teachers and children should review the collection of work together. Teachers can provide guidance by asking children to select their favorite work, to impart what they learned from an activity, to indicate which work was the most difficult, and to assess what they would do differently the next time (Puckett & Black, 1994).

Limitations of portfolios are that the work in the portfolio may not be representative of what the student knows and can do, and conclusions drawn by teachers about the work may be subjective. Also, developing clear and objective criteria for judging performance has been troublesome; expectations and standards may not always be available for different types of data that are generated under various conditions (e.g., use of language at school during free play and during direct testing, use of language at home [Rivera, 1994]). Using portfolios for large-scale assessment requires standardization of criteria across grade levels and schools, and implementation necessitates teacher training. In general, teachers who have used portfolios have reported positive changes in their practices and student outcomes. Limited empirical data, however, are available on the technical qualities (e.g., interrater reliability), student outcomes, and feasibility (e.g., time constraints) (Herman & Winters, 1994).

Dynamic Approaches

Assessment through teaching is the collection of information by participating directly in student–teacher interactions, observing student–student interactions, and watching students use language when working with ideas and materials (Brookes & Brookes, 1993). This type of assessment provides information on children's responsivity to instruction, a powerful predictor of future outcomes. Dynamic assessments (e.g., Brown & Ferrara, 1985; Feuerstein, 1979; Lidz, 1991; Olswang, Bain, & Johnson, 1992; Palincsar et al., 1994) focus on the child's responsivity to instruction (versus static profiles) and on learning and metacognitive processes. Programs based on Feuerstein's mediated learning model (Feuerstein, 1979), which focuses on teaching children problem-solving strategies and providing differing levels of adult support for child learning, have been successful for improving outcomes in language and literacy of preschool children with disabilities (Cole, Dale, & Mills, 1991; Haywood, Brookes, & Burns, 1986; Notari, Cole, & Mills, 1992) and of older children with disabilities (e.g., Englert, Raphael, & Mariage, 1994; Palincsar & Klenk, 1992).

Available dynamic assessment instruments (e.g., Learning Potential Assessment Device [Feuerstein, 1979]; Preschool Learning Assessment Device [Lidz & Thomas, 1987]) are complex and are not designed for use by teachers in classroom settings (Bricker, 1992; Palincsar et al., 1994). There is a need for functional, user-friendly dynamic assessment procedures. One promising approach is that described by Gutierrez-Clellen and Quinn (1993) for assessing narratives of children from diverse cultural backgrounds. The focus of process and learning potential over mastery makes this approach extremely appropriate for testing in cross-cultural settings (Hegarty & Lucas, 1978; Miller, 1984).

Comprehensive Models

Two comprehensive models have been developed that translate state-of-the-art theory into practical and comprehensive assessment frameworks. These models are a combination of assessment approaches and procedures.

Primary Language Record   The Primary Language Record (PLR) (Barrs, Ellis, Hester, & Thomas, 1988) originally was developed in England. The model is being piloted in New York Public Schools (Falk, MacMurdy, & Darling-Hammond, 1994) and in California (California Learning Record) (Thomas, 1993). This assessment framework is designed to evaluate and support the comprehensive development of children, particularly the developmental areas related to language and literacy. The PLR provides multiple perspectives on children and their learning and appears especially suited for use with children from diverse cultural backgrounds and children with learning disabilities (Falk et al., 1994). Information about children's culture, languages, experiences, and interests is obtained through focused interviews with the children and their families. The PLR provides specific guidelines and a structure for teachers to systematically record observations of children's behaviors and collect samples of children's work. Rating scales also are included to assess children's literacy development.

The major purpose of the PLR is to assist teachers with identifying learning experiences and teaching strategies that will help children develop skills. Developing IEPs takes an innovative approach; rather than enumerating skills and criteria for mastery, educational objectives focus on recommendations for types of instructional supports. Sample objectives from Falk et al. (1994) include 1) providing familiar texts and simple-pattern language books around themes of interest, 2) making copies of these books in both Spanish and English for home, and 3) providing opportunities for involvement in school plays and presentations to foster oral language.

Pennsylvania Comprehensive Reading and Communication Plan A second comprehensive approach, the Pennsylvania Comprehensive Reading and Communication Plan (Bartoli & Botel, 1988), is based on an ecological approach to language and literacy. Disabilities are viewed as contextually bound and dependent on the interactions among home, school, and community. Ecological evaluations include classroom observations during critical experiences, collaborative staff evaluations, family interviews, portfolios, and student participation in the evaluation.

Although these innovative models have important implications for assessment and intervention, developing and adopting practical assessment procedures have been slow for a number of reasons (Bricker, 1992). Collecting information in real-life settings requires additional time and training not always available to practitioners. Innovative instruments have not been sufficiently field tested, and too little is known about their technical qualities. Some instruments (e.g., dynamic assessments) have been developed for research purposes and are not suited for use in daily intervention settings. Others, particularly those based on qualitative approaches, may conflict with traditional quantitative conceptualizations of measurement (Darling-Hammond, 1989).

CULTURE, HOME, AND COMMUNITY

The social-constructivist perspective emphasizes the role of the social and cultural environment on children's acquisition and use of language. To respond to the needs of children from diverse cultural backgrounds, practitioners must look beyond individual characteristics and integrate sociocultural realities into early intervention and assessment practices (Barrera, 1993; Bernheimer, Gallimore, & Weisner, 1990). Few assessment models provide specific guidelines for the systematic collection and integration of information from outside of the classroom.

Culture and world view of homes and communities remain a part of children's lives when they come to school. Schools need to know, understand, and validate a child's social experience (Bartoli & Botel, 1988; Kochman, 1972). The most appropriate methods for collecting information about a child's culture use ethnographic approaches such as parent interviews to understand parents' views about their children and their own experiences with school (Crago & Cole, 1991; Duchan, 1991). Parent involvement requires two-way communication in which parents are included in a truly collaborative manner in observations and discussions at school (Thomas, 1993).

For children who are bilingual, assessment also must provide information about their knowledge of languages other than English so that the assessment of language development can be differentiated from the use of language as a medium for instruction (Westby, 1985). Barrera (1993) recommended examining several aspects of language: presence of receptive and expressive skills in non-English language, use of diverse rules and styles of language usage, second-language learning, and concept and skill learning through a nonnative language. Assessment practices should include an "ethnography" of the child's own language, taking advantage of tools such as videotapes and audio recordings (Gavillàn-Torres, 1984) and using culture-language mediators (interpreters) when appropriate.

Two conditions are essential for successfully implementing the previously discussed innovative and promising approaches to assessment of children's language. One is interdisciplinary collaboration, including a change in the traditional role of communication specialists and teachers (Losardo, 1996; Marvin, 1987; Miller, 1989; Silliman & Wilkinson, 1991). The other is appropriate professional development offered both at the preservice and in-service levels. At the preservice level, information should be provided on language acquisition, learning styles, child development, and culture and learning (Anstey & Bull, 1991). Personnel preparation training programs should be interdisciplinary in focus and should train students to work on teams (Bricker, Losardo, & Straka, 1995). At the in-service level, professionals in the field need ongoing instruction and support to learn alternative approaches to assessment (e.g., structured observational methods) and need opportunities to exchange information and experiences with other colleagues both within and across disciplines (Falk et al., 1994; Silliman & Wilkinson, 1991).

CONCLUSION

Changing views of the nature of language acquisition and the increasing diversity in cultural makeup of school populations have contributed to the development of new approaches to language assessment. The social-constructivist perspective stresses the importance of assessing children's language within the context of meaningful events that reflect real-life situations, shifting the emphasis from paper-and-pencil tests and standardized measures to naturalistic, activity-based approaches and authentic assessments.

Ultimately, the purpose of assessment is to provide children with appropriate language-learning experiences and instructional support. Dynamic assessment is a promising approach designed to provide information on children's responsivity to instruction and to help teachers identify teaching strategies that support language learning.

Language learning is intrinsically related to the cultural context, and children display language skills differently across school, home, and community settings. Most important, language assessment should be conducted within a comprehensive, contextually relevant framework that guides the collection of information using a variety of methods across multiple settings and diverse sources.

REFERENCES

Adler, S. (1981). *Poverty children and their language: Implications for teaching and treating.* New York: Grune & Stratton.

Anstey, M., & Bull, G. (1991). From teaching to learning: Translating monitoring into practice. In E. Daly (Ed.), *Monitoring children's language development: Holistic assessment in the classroom* (pp. 3–15). Portsmouth, NH: Heinemann.

Aram, D.M., & Nation, J.E. (1980). Preschool language disorders and subsequent language and academic difficulties. *Journal of Communication Disorders, 13,* 159–170.

Arter, J.A., & Spandel, V. (1991). *Using portfolios of student work in instruction and assessment.* Portland, OR: Northwest Regional Educational Laboratory.

Au, K.H., & Mason, J.M. (1981). Social organizational factors in learning to read: The balance of rights hypothesis. *Reading Research Quarterly, 17,* 115–152.

Bagnato, S.J., & Neisworth, J.T. (1991). *Assessment for early intervention: Best practices for professionals.* New York: Guilford Press.

Barker, R. (1968). *Ecological psychology.* Palo Alto, CA: Stanford University Press.

Barrera, I. (1993). Effective and appropriate instruction for all children: The challenge of cultural/linguistic diversity and young children with special needs. *Topics in Early Childhood Special Education, 13*(4), 461–487.

Barrs, M., Ellis, S., Hester, H., & Thomas, A. (1988). *The Primary Language Record.* London: ILEA/Centre for Language in Primary Education.

Bartoli, J., & Botel, M. (1988). *Reading/learning disability: An ecological approach.* New York: Teachers College Press.

Berlin, L.J., Blank, M., & Rose, S.A. (1980). The language of instruction: The hidden complexities. *Topics in Language Disorders and Learning Disabilities, 1*, 47–58.

Bernheimer, L., Gallimore, R., & Weisner, T. (1990). Ecocultural theory as a context for the individual family service plan. *Journal of Early Intervention, 14*(3), 219–233.

Bloom, L. (1970). *Language development: Form and function in emerging grammars.* Cambridge: MIT Press.

Bricker, D. (1992). The changing nature of communication and language intervention. In S.F. Warren & J. Reichle (Eds.), *Communication and language intervention series: Vol. 1. Causes and effects in communication and language intervention* (pp. 361–375). Baltimore: Paul H. Brookes Publishing Co.

Bricker, D. (Ed.). (1993). *Assessment, evaluation, and programming system for infants and children: AEPS measurement for birth to three years.* Baltimore: Paul H. Brookes Publishing Co.

Bricker, D., & Cripe, J.W. (1992). *An activity-based approach to early intervention.* Baltimore: Paul H. Brookes Publishing Co.

Bricker, D., & Littman, D. (1982). Intervention and evaluation: The inseparable mix. *Topics in Early Childhood Special Education, 1*(4), 23–33.

Bricker, D., Losardo, A., & Straka, E. (1995). *Description and evaluation of an early intervention/early childhood special education personnel preparation program.* Manuscript submitted for publication.

Brigance, A.H. (1991). *Brigance Diagnostic Inventory of Early Development–Revised.* North Billerica, MA: Curriculum Associates.

Bronfenbrenner, U. (1979). *The ecology of human development: Experiments by nature and design.* Cambridge, MA: Harvard University Press.

Brookes, J.G., & Brookes, M. (1993). *In search of understanding: The case for constructivist classrooms.* Alexandria, VA: Association for Supervision and Curriculum Development.

Brown, A.L., & Ferrara, R.A. (1985). Diagnosing zones of proximal development. In J.V. Wertsch (Ed.), *Culture, communication, and cognition* (pp. 273–305). Cambridge, MA: Cambridge University Press.

Brown, P., Collins, A., & Duguid, P. (1989). Situated cognition and the culture of learning. *Educational Researcher, 17*(1), 32–42.

Catts, H., & Kamhi, A. (1987). Relationship between language and reading disorders: Implications for the speech-language pathologist. *Topics in Language Disorders, 8*, 377–392.

Cazden, C.B. (1970). The neglected situation in child language research and education. In F. Williams (Ed.), *Language and poverty: Perspectives on a theme* (pp. 81–101). Chicago: Markham.

Cazden, C.B. (1977). Concentrated versus contrived encounters: Suggestions for language assessment in early childhood. In A. Davies (Ed.), *Language and learning in early childhood* (pp. 40–59). London: Heinemann.

Cazden, C.B. (1988). *Classroom discourse: The language of teaching and learning.* Portsmouth, NH: Heinemann.

Chomsky, N. (1957). *Syntactic structures*. The Hague, Holland: Mouton.

Cicchetti, D., & Wagner, S. (1990). Alternative assessment strategies for the evaluation of infants and toddlers: An organizational perspective. In S.J. Meisels & J.P. Shonkoff (Eds.), *Handbook of early childhood intervention* (pp. 246–277). New York: Cambridge University Press.

Cohen, L.G., & Spenciner, L.J. (1994). *Assessment of young children*. New York: Longman.

Cole, K., Dale, P., & Mills, P. (1991). Individual differences in language delayed children's responses to direct and interactive preschool instruction. *Topics in Early Childhood Special Education, 11*(1), 99–124.

Crago, M.B., & Cole, E.B. (1991). Using ethnography to bring children's communicative and cultural worlds into focus. In T. Gallagher (Ed.), *Pragmatics of language: Clinical practice issues* (pp. 99–131). San Diego: Singular Publishing Group.

Dale, P., Crain-Thoreson, C., Notari-Syverson, A., & Cole, K. (in press). Parent–child storybook reading as an intervention technique for young children with language delays. *Topics in Early Childhood Special Education*.

Darby, B.L. (1979). Infant cognition: Considerations for assessment tools. In B.L. Darby & M.J. Mays (Eds.), *Infant assessment: Issues and applications* (pp. 103–111). Seattle: WESTAR.

Darling-Hammond, L. (1989). Curiouser and curiouser: Alice in testingland. *Rethinking Schools, 3*(2), 1–17.

Duchan, J.F. (1991). Everyday events: Their role in language assessment and intervention. In T.M. Gallagher (Ed.), *Pragmatics of language: Clinical practice issues* (pp. 43–98). San Diego: Singular Publishing Group.

Education for All Handicapped Children Act of 1975, PL 94-142, 20 U.S.C. § 1401 *et seq.*

Emerick, L., & Haynes, W. (1986). *Diagnosis and evaluation in speech pathology*. Englewood Cliffs, NJ: Prentice Hall.

Englert, C.S., Raphael, T.E., & Mariage, T.V. (1994). Developing a school-based discourse for literacy learning: A principled search for understanding. *Learning Disability Quarterly, 17*(1), 2–32.

Falk, B., MacMurdy, S., & Darling-Hammond, L. (1994, April). *Taking a different look: How the Primary Language Record supports teaching for diverse learners*. Paper presented at the Annual Meeting of the American Educational Research Association, New Orleans.

Feuerstein, R. (1979). *Dynamic assessment of retarded performers*. Baltimore: University Park Press.

Garwood, S.G. (1982). (Mis)use of developmental scales in program evaluation. *Topics in Early Childhood Special Education, 1*(4), 61–69.

Gavillàn-Torres, E. (1984). Issues of assessment of limited-English-proficient students and of truly disabled in the United States. In N. Miller (Ed.), *Bilingualism and language disability: Assessment and remediation* (pp. 131–153). London: Croom Helm.

Gilmore, P. (1984). Research currents: Assessing sub-rosa skills in children's language. *Language Arts, 61*, 384–391.

Gutierrez-Clellen, V.F., & Quinn, R. (1993). Assessing narratives of children from diverse cultural/linguistic groups. *Language, Speech, and Hearing Services in Schools, 24*, 2–9.

Hale, J. (1992). Dignifying black children's lives. *Dimensions, 20*(3), 8–9, 40.

Haywood, C., Brookes, P., & Burns, S. (1986). Stimulating cognitive development at developmental level: A tested, non-remedial preschool curriculum for preschoolers and older retarded children. *Special Services in the Schools, 3*(1–2), 127–147.

Heath, S.B. (1982). What no bedtime story means: Narrative skills at home and at school. *Language in Society, 11*, 49–78.

Hegarty, S., & Lucas, D. (1978). *Able to learn? The pursuit of culture fair assessment.* Windsor, England: National Foundation for Educational Research.

Herman, J.L., & Winters, L. (1994). Portfolio research: A slim collection. *Educational Leadership, 52*(2), 48–55.

Individuals with Disabilities Education Act (IDEA) of 1990, PL 101-476, 20 U.S.C. § 1400 *et seq.*

Johnson, N.M. (1982). Assessment paradigms and atypical infants: An interventionist's perspective. In D. Bricker (Ed.), *Intervention with at-risk and handicapped infants: From research to application* (pp. 63–76). Baltimore: University Park Press.

Johnson, W., Darley, F., & Spriestersbach, D.C. (1952). *Diagnostic manual in speech correction.* New York: Harper and Row.

Kaiser, A.P., Yoder, P.J., & Keetz, A. (1992). Evaluating milieu teaching. In S.F. Warren & J. Reichle (Eds.), *Communication and language intervention series: Vol. 1. Causes and effects in communication and language intervention* (pp. 9–47). Baltimore: Paul H. Brookes Publishing Co.

Katims, D. (1991). Emergent literacy in early childhood special education: Curriculum and instruction. *Topics in Early Childhood Special Education, 11*(1), 69–84.

Kochman, T. (1972). Black American speech events and a language program for the classroom. In C.B. Cazden, V.P. John, & D. Hymes (Eds.), *Functions of language in the classroom* (pp. 135–151). New York: Teachers College Press.

Labov, W. (1972). *Language in the inner city: Studies in the Black English vernacular.* Philadelphia: University of Pennsylvania Press.

Lahey, M. (1988). *Language disorders and language development.* New York: Macmillan.

Lahey, M., Launer, P., & Shiff-Myers, N. (1983). Prediction of production: Elicited imitation and spontaneous speech productions of language-disordered children. *Applied Psycholinguistics, 4,* 319–343.

Lidz, C. (1991). *Practitioner's guide to dynamic assessment.* New York: Guilford Press.

Lidz, C., & Thomas, C. (1987). The Preschool Learning Assessment Device: Extension of a static approach. In C. Lidz (Ed.), *Dynamic assessment: An interaction approach to evaluating learning potential* (pp. 288–326). New York: Guilford Press.

Linder, T.W. (1993). *Transdisciplinary play-based assessment: A functional approach to working with young children* (Rev. ed.). Baltimore: Paul H. Brookes Publishing Co.

Locust, C. (1988). Wounding the spirit: Discrimination and traditional American Indian belief systems. *Harvard Educational Review, 58*(3), 315–330.

Longhurst, T., & Grubb, S. (1974). A comparison of language samples collected in four situations. *Language, Speech, and Hearing Services in Schools, 5,* 71–78.

Losardo, A. (1996). Preparing communication specialists. In D. Bricker & A. Widerstrom (Eds.), *Preparing personnel to work with infants and young children and their families: A team approach* (pp. 91–113). Baltimore: Paul H. Brookes Publishing Co.

Losardo, A., & Bricker, D. (1994). A comparison study: Activity-based intervention and direct instruction. *American Journal on Mental Retardation, 98*(6), 744–765.

Lund, N.J., & Duchan, J.F. (1983). *Assessing children's language in naturalistic contexts.* Englewood Cliffs, NJ: Prentice Hall.

Marvin, C. (1987). Consultation services: Changing the roles for SLPs. *Journal of Childhood Communication Disorders, 11,* 1–15.

Marzano, R.J., Pickering, D., & McTighe, J. (1993). *Assessing student outcomes: Performance assessment using the dimensions of learning model.* Alexandria, VA: Association for Supervision and Curriculum Development.

McCormick, L., & Schiefelbusch, R. (1984). *Early language intervention.* Columbus, OH: Charles E. Merrill.

McCune, L., Kalmanson, B., Fleck, M.B., Glazewski, B., & Sillari, J. (1990). An interdisciplinary model of infant assessment. In S.J. Meisels & J.P. Shonkoff (Eds.),

Handbook of early childhood intervention (pp. 219–245). New York: Cambridge University Press.

Meadows, S. (1993). *The child as thinker: The development and acquisition of cognition in children.* New York: Routledge.

Mehrens, W.A., & Clarizio, H.F. (1993). Curriculum-based measurement: Conceptual and psychometric considerations. *Psychology in the Schools, 30,* 241–254.

Meisels, S. (1994). Designing meaningful measurements for early childhood. In B.L. Mallory & R.S. New (Eds.), *Diversity and developmentally appropriate practices: Challenges for early childhood education* (pp. 202–222). New York: Teachers College Press.

Michaels, S. (1986). Narrative presentations: An oral preparation for literacy. In J. Cook-Gumperz (Ed.), *The social construction of literacy* (pp. 94–116). New York: Cambridge University Press.

Miller, L. (1989). Classroom-based language intervention. *Language, Speech, and Hearing Services in Schools, 20,* 153–169.

Miller, N. (1984). Some observations concerning formal tests in cross-cultural settings. In N. Miller (Ed.), *Bilingualism and language disability: Assessment and remediation* (pp. 107–114). London: Croom Helm.

Morrow, L.M. (1989). *Literacy development in the early years: Helping children read and write.* Englewood Cliffs, NJ: Prentice Hall.

Neisworth, J.T., & Bagnato, S.J. (1988). Assessment in early childhood special education: A typology of dependent measures. In S.L. Odom & M.B. Karnes (Eds.), *Early intervention for infants and children with handicaps: An empirical base* (pp. 23–49). Baltimore: Paul H. Brookes Publishing Co.

Nelson, N.W. (1989). Curriculum-based language assessment and intervention. *Language, Speech, and Hearing Services in Schools, 20,* 170–184.

Nelson, N.W. (1993). Language intervention in school settings. In D.K. Bernstein & E. Tiegerman (Eds.), *Language and communication disorders in children* (3rd ed., pp. 273–324). New York: Macmillan.

Nelson, N.W. (1994). Curriculum-based language assessment and intervention across grades. In E. Wallach & K. Butler (Eds.), *Language learning disabilities in school-age children and adolescents* (pp. 104–131). New York: Macmillan.

Norris, J.A. (1989). Providing language remediation in the classroom: An integrated language-to-reading intervention method. *Language, Speech, and Hearing Services in Schools, 20,* 205–218.

Notari, A., Cole, K., & Mills, P. (1992). Facilitating cognitive and language skills of young children with disabilities: The mediated learning program. *International Journal of Cognitive Education and Mediated Learning, 2*(2), 169–179.

Notari, A., Slentz, K., & Bricker, D. (1991). Assessment–curriculum systems for early childhood/special education. In D. Mitchell & R.I. Brown (Eds.), *Early intervention studies for children with special needs* (pp. 160–205). London: Chapman and Hill.

O'Connor, R., & Notari-Syverson, A. (in press). Ladders to literacy: The effects of teacher-led phonological activities for kindergarten children with and without disabilities. *Exceptional Children.*

Olswang, L.B., Bain, B.A., & Johnson, G.A. (1992). Using dynamic assessment with children with language disorders. In S.F. Warren & J. Reichle (Eds.), *Communication and language intervention series: Vol. 1. Causes and effects in communication and language intervention* (pp. 187–215). Baltimore: Paul H. Brookes Publishing Co.

Palincsar, A., Brown, A., & Campione, J.C. (1994). Models and practices of dynamic assessment. In E. Wallach & K. Butler (Eds.), *Language learning disabilities in school-age children and adolescents* (pp. 132–144). New York: Macmillan.

Palincsar, A., & Klenk, L. (1992). Fostering literacy learning in supportive environments. *Journal of Learning Disabilities, 25*(4), 211–225.

Prutting, C., Gallagher, T., & Mulac, A. (1975). The expressive portion of the NSST compared to a spontaneous language sample. *Journal of Speech and Hearing Disorders, 40*, 40–49.

Puckett, M.B., & Black, J.K. (1994). *Authentic assessment of the young child.* New York: Macmillan.

Rivera, D. (1994). Portfolio assessment. *LD Forum, 19*(4), 14–16.

Sawyer, D. (1991). Whole language in context: Insights into the current debate. *Topics in Language Disorders, 11*(3), 1–13.

Schlesinger, I. (1974). Relational concepts underlying language. In R.L. Schiefelbusch & L. Lloyd (Eds.), *Language perspectives: Acquisitions, retardation, and intervention* (pp. 129–151). Baltimore: University Park Press.

Schutt, P.W., & McCabe, V.M. (1994). Portfolio assessment for students with disabilities. *Learning Disabilities, 5*(2), 81–85.

Silliman, E.R., & Wilkinson, L.C. (1991). *Communicating for learning: Classroom observation and collaboration.* Rockville, MD: Aspen Publishers, Inc.

Silliman, E.R., Wilkinson, L.C., & Hoffman, L.P. (1993). Documenting authentic progress in language and literacy learning: Collaborative assessment in classrooms. *Topics in Language Disorders, 11*(3), 58–71.

Snow, C. (1983). Literacy and language: Relationships during the preschool years. *Harvard Educational Review, 53*, 165–189.

Swinson, J., & Ellis, C. (1988). Telling stories to encourage language. *British Journal of Special Education, 15*, 169–171.

Templin, M. (1957). *Certain language skills in children.* Minneapolis: University of Minnesota Press.

Thomas, S. (1993). Rethinking assessment: Teachers and students helping each other through the "sharp curves of life." *Learning Disability Quarterly, 16*(4), 257–279.

Vygotsky, L. (1978). *Mind in society: The development of higher psychological process.* (M. Cole, S. Schribern, V. John-Steiner, & E. Souberman, trans.). Cambridge, MA: Harvard University Press.

Warren, S.F., & Kaiser, A.P. (1988). Research in early language intervention. In S.L. Odom & M.B. Karnes (Eds.), *Early intervention for infants and children with handicaps: An empirical base* (pp. 89–108). Baltimore: Paul H. Brookes Publishing Co.

Watson, L.R., Layton, T.L., Pierce, P., & Abraham, L. (1994). Enhancing emerging literacy in a language preschool. *Language, Speech, and Hearing Services in Schools, 25*, 136–145.

Wells, G. (1985). Preschool literacy-related activities and success in school. In D.R. Olson, N. Torrance, & A. Hildyard (Eds.), *Literacy, language, and learning* (pp. 229–255). Cambridge, MA: Cambridge University Press.

Westby, C.E. (1985). Learning to talk—Talking to learn: Oral-literate language differences. In C. Simon (Ed.), *Communication skills and classroom success* (pp. 81–218). San Diego: College-Hill Press.

Whitehurst, G., Falco, F.L., Lonigan, C.J., Fischel, J.E., DeBaryshe, B.D., Valdez-Menchaca, M.C., & Caulfield, M. (1988). Accelerating language development through picturebook reading. *Developmental Psychology, 24*, 552–559.

Wilkinson, L.C., & Silliman, E. (1993). Assessing students' progress in language and literacy: A classroom approach. In L. Morrow, L. Wilkinson, & J. Smith (Eds.), *Integrated language arts: Controversy to consensus* (pp. 241–269). Needham, MA: Allyn & Bacon.

Yoder, P., & Davies, B. (1990). Do parental questions and topic continuations elicit replies from developmentally delayed children? A sequential analysis. *Journal of Speech and Hearing Research, 23*, 513–573.

Yoder, P., Davies, B., & Bishop, K. (1992). Getting children with developmental disabilities to talk to adults. In S.F. Warren & J. Reichle (Eds.), *Communication and language intervention series: Vol. 1. Causes and effects in communication and language intervention* (pp. 255–275). Baltimore: Paul H. Brookes Publishing Co.

12

Dynamic Assessment
The Model and Its Language Applications

Elizabeth D. Peña

STANDARDIZED LANGUAGE TESTS ARE USED primarily for classifying children based on performance and for predicting future performance (Lidz, 1981; Wolf, Bixby, Glenn, & Gardner, 1991). Professionals who perform language assessments have become increasingly dissatisfied with these assessment practices because of their limited predictive validity (Lahey, 1990; McCauley & Swisher, 1984a, 1984b) and their limited prescriptive uses (Neisworth & Bagnato, 1986). Specifically, psychoeducational tests do not predict response to instruction (Lidz, 1981, 1987), nor do they predict ability (Lahey, 1990). Haywood, Brown, and Wingenfeld (1990) argued that standardized tests do not have good predictive validity in individual cases even if they do for group data. In addition, variables such as test-taking experience, setting, and examiner may influence test performance. Thus, children who do not perform well on a standardized language test may not necessarily have a language disorder (Lahey, 1990). For example, a child may perform poorly on a standardized test because of unfamiliarity with the specific test content or with the examiner. In addition, standardized language tests are not designed to help plan intervention. Items on standardized tests are selected to maximize differences among children (Lidz, 1981). Because of this, a standardized test may be used to make comparisons with the norm, but it does not give enough detail about a specific child's error pattern (Lidz, 1981; McCauley & Swisher, 1984b).

Dynamic assessment is an interactive approach to the assessment process based on direct intervention, and it yields information that typically is limited in traditional (static) testing: predictive and prescriptive information (Lidz, 1987, 1991). Generally, dynamic assessment utilizes a test–teach–retest model. The pretest functions as a baseline and is considered the starting point of the assessment. This baseline directs the intervention phase of the assessment. Intervention may consist of graduated prompts (Campione & Brown, 1987) or mediated learning experiences (MLEs) (e.g., Feuerstein, 1979; Lidz, 1987, 1991). Reassessment is the final stage of the process. Rather than measuring a single performance before and after intervention, dynamic assessment measures the change that is constantly created by the assessment process itself.

Dynamic assessment procedures typically are contrasted with static assessment practices (Haywood et al., 1990). Static tests are those that systematically sample products of learning at one point in time and report the results in terms of a standardization group or external criteria. Both standardized (norm-referenced) tests and criterion-referenced tests are considered static. In static assessment, the role of the examiner is that of neutral observer and recorder; the child is viewed as a passive respondent (Meyers, 1987). An assumption of static assessment is that variation in performance represents variation in ability (Anastasi, 1983; McCauley & Swisher, 1984b). A standardized language test score, then, is assumed to provide an adequate and valid estimate of language ability (Adler, 1990; Damico, 1990; Duran, 1988, 1989; McCauley & Swisher, 1984b). Criterion-referenced tests do not classify children by comparing them with their peers; rather, they compare a child's performance against a standard of mastery in a specific domain (Bailey & Harbin, 1980; Lidz, 1981). An advantage of criterion-referenced tests is that they can be linked directly with intervention (Lidz, 1981; Neisworth & Bagnato, 1986); however, these tests yield little information concerning the reason for examinees' errors or directions for remediation.

In contrast to static assessment, dynamic assessment is an interactive process that fosters change. If language learning is primarily a socially mediated process, then dynamic language assessment is the observation of language learning during mediation. This process of inducing a change and then measuring that change is the core of dynamic assessment.

Characteristics that define dynamic assessment are its interactive nature, its focus on learning processes, and the type of information that is gained (Campione, 1989; Haywood et al., 1990; Lidz, 1995). Dynamic assessment yields information about children's abilities that traditional psychometric assessment practices do not and provides information regarding the amount and nature of examiner investment necessary to produce a desired change in the learner. The examiner responds to the child in specific ways during the assessment in order to modify the child's response to the task. One important assumption of dynamic assessment is that all children are capable of learning; if the dynamic assessment does not produce a change, then the examiner must continue to provide MLE to effect a change. Thus, the examiner's role shifts from a passive to an interactive and process-oriented one in a teaching relationship (Feuerstein, Rand, Jensen, Kaniel, & Tzuriel, 1987; Haywood et al., 1990; Lidz, 1987, 1991; Meyers, 1987). Traditional diagnostic methods have always recommended diagnostic teaching or testing for stimulability as part of the data-gathering phase during assessment (Darley, 1979; Tomblin, Morris, & Spriestersbach, 1994); however, dynamic assessment differs from diagnostic teaching in that it focuses on inferred learning processes as well as on content. Dynamic assessment emphasizes the learning process rather than the products of past learning (Haywood et al., 1990; Lidz, 1987, 1991). Because of this deemphasis on the products of previous experience, researchers have advocated dynamic assessment to reduce bias in psychological testing (Carlson & Wiedl, 1979; Feuerstein et al., 1987; Figueroa, 1989; Haywood et al., 1990; Lidz, 1982, 1987; Sewell, 1987). Most important, dynamic assessment links assessment with intervention by providing information about how the learners respond to the intervention that is provided during dynamic assessment.

The teaching phase of dynamic assessment is individually designed, with the examiner responding contingently to the child's responses. Instead of assuming that the child's poor performance equates poor ability, the examiner gives the child learning experiences and strategies and the opportunity to demonstrate learning ability. Because the child is given the opportunity to learn strategies that apply to the test situation, dynamic assessment minimizes test bias. In addition, dynamic assessment directly assesses the learning process providing strong construct validity because the examiner directly observes the learning process (Haywood et al., 1990). Prescriptive recommendations are derived from the strategies that the child learns and uses during mediation. For example, observing that a child was able to complete a puzzle once he or she learned to use the strategy of comparing leads directly to making classroom recommendations for focusing on using comparison strategies to facilitate further learning.

THE MODEL

The theoretical basis for dynamic assessment can be traced to Vygotsky's concept of the *zone of proximal development* (ZPD). Vygotsky (1978) demonstrated that children's achievement levels, under a teacher's guidance, improved when the teacher varied the tasks slightly and in deliberate ways. When a child could successfully perform a previously difficult task, with minimal modification from the teacher, the task was considered to be in the zone of proximal development. Vygotsky's ZPD concept has been applied to dynamic assessment. Vygotsky (1978) viewed intellectual development as a socially created combination of heredity, environment, and human interaction involving adults or older children. Within these human interactions, Vygotsky described two simultaneous levels of development: the actual—what the the child can do without adult help—and the potential—what the child can do with adult help. Vygotsky proposed that ZPD was the difference between the two levels and concluded that this zone should be assessed in order to measure true ability.

Building on this orientation toward interaction, Rey (cited in Haywood et al., 1990) proposed that process-oriented tests could be used to assess the processes of learning. He argued that assessment should extend beyond simply whether the child could find the correct answer with assistance. He suggested that an intentional interaction between the examiner and examinee would help determine the nature of the process contributing to low test performance.

The concept of dynamic assessment incorporating interactive teaching strategies received its greatest impetus from the work of Feuerstein (1979) and his colleagues (Feuerstein, Rand, & Hoffman, 1979; Haywood & Tzuriel, 1992; Lidz, 1987, 1991). Feuerstein (1979) argued that lack of experience often is mistaken for lack of ability (Feuerstein et al., 1987). Through the assessment of modifiability (i.e., change through mediation), examiners can gain insight into *how* a child learns a task and *what* is needed for that child to learn and generalize the task. One of the primary outcomes of dynamic assessment is the modifiability of the child. Through mediation, examiners gain information about how modifiability in the child can be induced (Feuerstein et al., 1987). Determining modifiability involves three factors: child responsiveness (i.e., how the child responds to and uses new information), examiner effort (i.e., the quantity and quality of effort necessary to induce change), and transfer (i.e., generalization of new skills) (Lidz, 1987, 1991).

APPLYING THE CONSTRUCT TO LANGUAGE ASSESSMENT

In a social constructivist model, language learning is viewed as interactive and contextualized within a social domain (Bates, 1976; Blount, 1982; Heath, 1983, 1986; Schieffelin & Ochs, 1986; van Kleeck, 1985). For example, researchers have examined how mothers support learning for their children through guided participation (Rogoff, 1990), scaffolding (Bruner, 1978), and/or mediation (Vygotsky, 1978, 1986). Through guided participation, children learn what is expected of them within their community. Meaning is created jointly; through this joint construction of meaning, children learn about the uses of language (Rogoff, 1990). Heath (1983) provided rich descriptions of different communities in which adults, through interactions, help children create meaning and convey expectations. In one example, Heath described an interaction between Sally, 2 years old, and her Aunt Sue. "While peeling tomatoes, Aunt Sue asked Sally, 'What is that?' Sally persisted in responding 'red,' although Aunt Sue emphasized the label 'tomato'" (p. 141). Through this type of interaction, children learn that the names of things are important. Bruner (1978) noted that the more competent adult uses scaffolding to break down learning for the child so that the child is able to accomplish more difficult tasks. In narrative events, for example, adults may use prompts (e.g., What happens next? How did he feel?), thus giving structure to the child's story. This type of interaction has been characterized as joint creation of meaning requiring participation of both the adult and the child. Language learning, then, is socially mediated within the cultural context (Vygotsky, 1978).

Lee (1966) suggested that children with language disorders fail to make linguistic generalizations that guide language development. Thus, a child with a language disorder, by definition, has poor language-learning ability. Traditionally, a language disorder is defined as performance significantly below the mean for age peers (Bloom & Lahey, 1978; Launer & Lahey, 1981; McCauley & Swisher, 1984b; Schery, 1981). This normative view of language development assumes equivalent language, learning, and teaching experiences for all children. However, children have different home-language experiences because of the variety of socialization practices found within and across cultures (Blount, 1982; Heath, 1983, 1986; Schieffelin & Ochs, 1986). In addition, language demands vary according to the situation, the speaker, and the roles of interactants. Children who score low on standardized tests may be reflecting a wide variation in language experiences and not simply differences in ability. Thus, it is difficult to distinguish children academically at risk without language disorder from those with language disorder on the basis of standardized language assessment procedures alone. Dynamic assessment makes this differentiation by taking into account a child's experiences, repertoire of language skills, and the potential to learn new skills. As an interactive assessment, dynamic assessment is used to teach children the skills and strategies that they need to perform optimally on standardized tests.

CONTINUUM OF DYNAMIC APPROACHES

Dynamic assessment should 1) profile the learner's abilities or performance strengths and identify weak processing areas; 2) observe the learner's modifiability; 3) induce active, self-regulated learning; and 4) recommend interventions that appear to benefit performance (Lidz, 1991). The specific techniques and content used to assess children's language abilities vary according to the amount of standardization of the procedure and the area targeted for assessment. Some approaches to dynamic assessment utilize standardized tests and instructions; others use a set of tools that are applied differently for each child. Most available literature focuses on mediation of cognitive and reading skills. There are only a few studies that focus on language assessment.

Specific applications of dynamic assessment can be viewed on a continuum of structure—high, or standardized, to low, or open ended. Different approaches, by their nature, yield different kinds of information. At the more structured end of the continuum, reliability of intervention is a goal; procedures ensure that reliability is maintained. At the other end, reliability is not an issue because procedures spontaneously evolve in response to the child. The high-structure approaches focus on prediction, response to standardized instruction, and accurate identification of children with low ability. The low-structure approaches focus on diagnostic prescription, individualized instruction, and modifiability. Both approaches focus on teaching within the assessment, but they do so differently. The high-structure approach typically utilizes predetermined cues or prompts that are organized in increasing amounts of contextual or examiner support. The cues are concluded when the child is able to independently solve the task. MLE, by contrast, typically is used in the more low-structure approaches. MLE describes the quality of the interaction between the examiner and the child within the teaching phase of the assessment. In the role of the mediator, the examiner guides the child through the task by helping the child select and organize information. Each approach contributes differently to the growing literature on dynamic assessment.

High-Structure, "Standardized" Approaches

Campione (1989) and colleagues (Campione & Brown, 1977, 1978, 1984, 1987; Campione, Brown, & Bryant, 1985; Campione, Brown, & Ferrara, 1982) have contributed significantly to the literature on dynamic assessment. They have attempted to operationalize Vygotsky's zone of proximal development as a series of graduated prompts. The model focuses on assessing assisted learning and transfer, or generalization (Campione, 1989; Campione & Brown, 1987). The main goal is to improve the predictive ability of the intervention process for the purpose of profiling the learner's readiness to learn within a specific domain. Brown and Campione (1981, 1984, 1986) and colleagues try to specify the processes involved in change or learning during instruction and evaluate how these processes operate. Skills underlying learning are directly evaluated in a given situation in a pretest–intervention–posttest design. Standardized procedures are used for the pretests and posttests. During the intervention phase, the learner initially is given weak, general hints, progressing to more detailed instruction as needed. Learning is defined by how much instruction (i.e., number of prompts) is needed before the learner responds correctly. Transfer is defined by how much instruction is necessary before the learned information is applied to new settings.

Brown and Campione (1981, 1984, 1986) and colleagues have demonstrated the relationships among learning, transfer, and ability (Brown & French, 1979; Brown & Palincsar, 1982, 1986; Campione & Brown, 1987; Campione et al., 1982; Campione, Brown, Ferrara, Jones, & Steinberg, 1985; Palincsar & Brown, 1984). Using a variation of the Raven's Progressive Matrices task (Raven, Court, & Raven, 1977), Campione, Brown, Ferrara, et al. (1985) demonstrated transfer differences between children with mental retardation and their typically developing peers. Children participated in instruction sessions using computers. During the learning phase, they learned to solve problems using rules (e.g., rotation, imposition, subtraction) of increasing difficulty. During the maintenance phase, children were presented with novel but similar tasks in random order of difficulty. The third phase (transfer) consisted of similar tasks and transfer problems, which required the use of combined rules. The groups were similar in the learning phase but were differentiated in the maintenance and transfer phases. In addition, the differences between the two groups of children became more apparent as the similarity to the learning phase decreased. The results suggest that transferring learning to a new task may be a powerful indicator of ability.

In another study, Ferrara, Brown, and Campione (1986) used letter series completions to demonstrate differences in transfer between third- and fifth-grade children of average IQ and high IQ. Children with high IQ needed fewer hints to learn the initial problems. As the transfer distance increased, greater differences manifested in the number of hints needed by the children with high IQ and by the children with average IQ.

Brown and Campione's (1981, 1984, 1986) approach contributes to the predictive validity of dynamic, or interactive, assessment approaches. Because of the predictive information obtained, this approach represents an improvement over static tests. A drawback to this approach is in translating the derived information to prescription and intervention (Campione, 1989). The number of cues required to facilitate a correct response is not sufficient to derive an intervention plan for a specific child. Lidz (1991) suggested that providing cues from the general to the specific level is not grounded in a theory of learning or instruction. She argued that the steps between each prompt are not necessarily equal and may not form a hierarchy of complexity because the cues are based on degree of specificity rather than on complexity. Finally, Lidz (1991) noted that focusing on the task rather than on the learner limits the approach's prescriptive power. Knowing that a child needed a high number of prompts to correctly respond to a task does not assist in planning intervention. However, knowing the nature of the prompts that helped the child solve the task could be incorporated into an intervention plan.

High-structure approaches also use various types of feedback as an approach to dynamic assessment (Carlson, 1983; Carlson & Wiedl, 1979, 1980). Using a test–teach–retest paradigm, Carlson and Wiedl (1979) explored the effects of various feedback conditions on the performance of school-age children from three cultural backgrounds: European American, Mexican American, and African American. The studies demonstrate the differential performance of the three groups on traditionally administered static tests, in contrast to test performance under feedback conditions (verbalization during and after solution, verbalization after solution, simple feedback, elaborated feedback, and elaborated feedback plus verbalization during and after solution). A sample of 147 fourth- and fifth-grade students from 15 elementary schools participated in the study. Tests of cognitive functioning included a series of nonverbal problem-solving tests. These measures were administered under standard, verbalization, and elaborated feedback conditions. Results indicate that children's scores differed depending on the feedback condition. In the standard test condition, scores differed among the three groups across age. However, the 5- to 6-year-olds demonstrated virtually no differences in the three groups under the self-talk plus elaborated feedback condition. In addition, the self-talk plus elaborated feedback condition (compared with the other conditions) yielded the highest test scores for all three groups. Because interactive approaches improved scores for all three groups over those from static tests, the authors concluded that the higher scores represented the children's true ability.

A third dynamic assessment approach proposed by Budoff (1987) uses coaching procedures during the teaching phase to classify children on the basis of ability. Although Budoff's method approaches a more low-structure approach, it is included here because of the emphasis on classification and the use of progressively simplified presentations of the teaching task. Pre–post tests consist of standardized cognitive measures. The role of the examiner during coaching is to direct student attention, explain attributes, and guide the student from concrete responses to abstract thinking. Children are expected to demonstrate improved performance on the posttest so that "optimal" performance is reflected in posttest scores. The tasks include the Kohs Learning Potential Task (KLPT) (Budoff & Corman, 1974), the Raven Learning Potential Test (Corman & Budoff, 1973), the Series Learning Potential Test (Budoff, 1987), and the Picture Word Game (Gimon, Budoff, & Corman, 1974). The KLPT teaches strategies for constructing block designs. The coaching materials consist of 3 four-block designs and 2 nine-block designs with stimulus cards. Initially, the child must solve a problem from a stimulus card using undifferentiated blocks. If the child is unable to solve the problem, then one row of the design is presented at a time. If the child still is unable to construct the target row, then the blocks are progressively outlined. In addition to task simplification, teaching procedures include frequent praise, comparison of the construction against the stimulus card, and emphasis on the elements of the block design.

Studies using Budoff's procedures have included children in general education and special education and children from a variety of cultures. Budoff (1967, 1969) adapted the Kohs Block Designs (Kohs, 1923) in a test–teach–retest design with adolescents who were classified as having educable mental retardation (EMR). Using these procedures, Budoff and Corman (1974) sampled 627 children with EMR in segregated classes ($n = 471$), residents of state institutions for people with mental retardation ($n = 134$), and participants in a community workshop ($n = 22$). Results indicated that training minimized socioeconomic class differences. This conclusion supported the procedure as a less-biased measure of intelligence. Budoff (1967) used this procedure with samples of institutionalized and community special-class adolescents with EMR. Results indicated high correlation between immediate and delayed (1 month) posttraining scores. These results were used to support claims of stability and reliability of the KLPT as an assessment of reasoning ability. Budoff and Corman (1973) used a similar procedure utilizing the Raven Progressive Matrices as the pretest and posttest. They sampled 403 children with EMR, ranging in age from 7 to 15 years, attending segregated special classes. Although the pretest and posttest scores were not influenced by ethnicity and social class, a disproportionate number of African American and female subjects continued to fall into the low-ability group. In this work, Budoff (1987) and colleagues observed three response patterns in the children. High scorers were those children who demonstrated mastery of the test task at the pretest. Gainers were those children who did not score well initially but were able to improve their performance after training. Nongainers were those children who were unable to improve their test scores after training. Criticisms of this procedure have focused on the inherent problems of the categories. Specifically, the researchers had difficulty resolving test gain relative to initial performance level (Lidz, 1991). A child starting at a higher score and demonstrating little gain would be considered a nongainer, whereas a child starting at a lower score and demonstrating high gain would be considered a gainer but may or may not reach the same score as the first child. Subsequently, Budoff and colleagues have used three scores in their analyses of learning potential: pretraining score, posttraining score, and posttraining score adjusted for pretest level (residualized gain score).

Budoff (1987) focused on providing a method for accurately classifying children for special education, particularly children who are likely to be misclassified because of differences in experiences. He had dropped the "gainer" and "nongainer" categories. Consistent with his earlier approach, Budoff stressed the child's ability to profit from learning. After a pretest, children were provided with training experiences related to the test tasks. Although these studies have provided support for predictive validity of dynamic measures, leading to more accurate classification, they have limited prescriptive value.

Low-Structure, Prescriptive Approaches

Low-structure approaches focus on cognitive functions and have the objective of prescribing intervention rather than classifying. Feuerstein (1979) and his colleagues have proposed a model of dynamic assessment that incorporates MLE in a test–teach–retest paradigm. In the mediation process, the adult modifies incoming information so that the child (learner) can use the information meaningfully (Tzuriel & Klein, 1987). Rather than using prompts, coaching, or differential feedback, mediation is the purposeful teaching of skills and strategies for problem solving (Lidz, 1991). This parallels the natural process of socialization (i.e., learning one's culture through meaningful interactions with adults and older children).

Lidz (1987, 1991) discussed several aspects of an MLE based on Feuerstein (1979; Klein & Feuerstein, 1985). The MLE focuses on the role of the adult mediator or examiner and includes mediation of intentionality, meaning, transcendence, and competence. These are believed to be the most crucial components of MLE (C.S. Lidz, personal communication, October 1995). *Mediation of intentionality* means that the examiner consciously tries to engage the child in the interaction for the purpose of teaching. Specifically, the examiner communicates to the child the purpose for the interaction (Lidz, 1991). For example, the mediator might say, "Today we are going to work together to compare and think about why comparisons are important." Mediation of intentionality focuses on cognitive functions such as comparison (Haywood, Brooks, & Burns, 1983; Lidz, 1991). *Mediation of meaning* focuses the child's attention on what is important in a given context and helps the child understand its value and relevance within the culture. In a matching activity, the mediator may point out the model and explain why it is important that the item matches. For example, the mediator might say, "Comparison helps us to organize what we see and helps you to sort correctly." *Mediation of transcendence* bridges concepts and events beyond the immediate task and inducts abstract ideas. The examiner relates specifics of the interaction to other experiences that the child has had or may have in the future. Mediation of transcendence promotes conceptual, inferential, or hypothetical thinking (Lidz, 1991). An example of transcendence in teaching the cognitive function of comparison is to discuss when it might be important to use a model and systematic scanning. For example, the mediator might say, "When you put your toys away, how do you know where they belong? If you don't know where to put something, what are some ways that you can figure it out?" *Mediation of competence* encourages a strategic, deliberate approach to problem solving. In using competence within a comparison activity, the mediator may point out relevant cues that help the child search for and select items that match (e.g., "You need to look at each picture and compare it to the model"). MLE, using these components, helps the child become a self-regulated, active learner and symbolic thinker (Lidz, 1991).

Mediation, in the context of dynamic assessment, means that the examiner's response to the child is intended to provide the child with information and strategies to enable the child to meet task demands more successfully and to give meaning and organization to the child's world. Modifiability is determined by how readily the child learns and uses the mediated information (Feuerstein, 1979; Haywood et al., 1990; Lidz, 1987). Feuerstein's Learning Potential Assessment Device (LPAD) (Feuerstein, 1979) was developed to evaluate an individual's ability to benefit from instruction. The LPAD battery consists of a variety of verbal and nonverbal tasks that are used to evaluate analogical reasoning, numerical reasoning, categorization, and memory (Lidz, 1991). Given optimal MLE, all individuals presumably can learn; it is up to the mediator to find out how. The implementation and tasks selection for the LPAD is highly individualized. Lidz (1991) stated that the LPAD involves three central components. The first component is the learner's behavior regarding what Feuerstein calls *deficient cognitive functions*. Deficiencies at the input phase consist of the processes concerned with data gathering. At the elaboration phase, deficiencies pertain to the ability to use the data that have been gathered. At the output phase, deficiencies manifest in the communication of responses (Jensen, Robinson-Zañartu, & Jensen, 1992; Lidz, 1991). The second component is the behavior of the assessor. MLE is used to give the learner task-specific experience and focus. The third component is that the LPAD tasks are distinguished by use of a "cognitive map" composed of seven dimensions: 1) familiarity of content; 2) modality; 3) cognitive deficiencies; 4) input, elaboration, and output; 5) task complexity; 6) abstractness; and 7) efficiency.

Feuerstein, Miller, Rand, and Jensen (1981) demonstrated the differential performance of "disadvantaged" students on a static test versus dynamic assessment (using the LPAD). Their results showed that these students performed better during dynamic testing than on static testing. This demonstrates that the static assessment alone fails to fully capture a child's ability. Feuerstein et al. (1979) discussed applying dynamic assessment to students whose scores fell in the range for a diagnosis of mental retardation and who also were culturally or linguistically different. They suggested that the LPAD can be used to rule out low performance as a result of cultural and linguistic differences. In their discussion, they used anecdotal evidence to illustrate the process of assessment.

The LPAD model has, however, been criticized in two areas. First, because it is highly individualized, its reliability and stability are in question (Lidz, 1991); Campione (1989) suggested that the LPAD is highly subjective and lacking in consistency. The second criticism is its link to educational objectives (M.R. Jensen, personal communication, August 1994). There are mixed results on the transfer from Instrumental Enrichment (Feuerstein, 1980) (the intervention follow-up based on the LPAD) to school subjects. Jitendra and Kameenui (1993) stated that the inductive reasoning tasks used on the LPAD are "far removed from classroom tasks" (p. 14).

In response to these criticisms, Lidz (1987, 1991) proposed two complementary applications to dynamic assessment. The first approach utilizes a standardized cognitive assessment as the pre–post measure; the second approach consists of a curriculum-based adaptation of dynamic assessment. In the first approach, Lidz and Thomas (1987) provided a dynamic extension of the Kaufman Assessment Battery for Children (K–ABC) (Kaufman, 1983) called the Preschool Learning Assessment Device (PLAD). Two subtests from the K–ABC serve as pre- and postmeasures: the Triangles subtest and the Matrices subtest. On the Triangles subtest, children must assemble two-sided plastic triangles (blue and yellow) to match a design on a stimulus card. On the Matrices subtest, children complete a 2-by-2 visual analogy by selecting the correct picture or design. Intervention utilizing figure drawing, block building, and parquetry as the mediation tasks targets the cognitive functions needed to successfully accomplish the two subtests. Research using this approach has demonstrated the differential performance of preschool children, with and without mediation (Lidz & Thomas, 1987). The mediated group achieved higher scores on the posttest than did the nonmediated group. Furthermore, correlation of the Triangles posttest scores with measures of social competency differed significantly for mediated and nonmediated groups. No differences in correlation of the Matrices posttest scores and social competency for the two groups were found. Applying the principles used in developing and administering the PLAD, Lidz (1991) provided guidelines for adapting dynamic assessment to curriculum-derived tasks. The curriculum content that the child may be having trouble with is used to develop testing and teaching tasks. Three versions of the target task are developed and used to test and mediate. The target tasks are analyzed according to content, processes, operations, complexity, abstraction, efficiency, and modalities. The first version of the task is used as a pretest. MLE is used to intervene on the second version of the task. Observation of learning is based on a Luria (1966) "planning–arousal–simultaneous–successive" model (Lidz, 1991, p. 126). Finally, the posttest is the third version of the task.

Studies using this test–teach–retest model have compared mediated and nonmediated groups. In a test–teach–retest paradigm, Missiuna and Samuels (1989) found that children receiving mediated learning performed better compared with a control group on posttest measures of language and cognition. Reinharth (1989) also demonstrated the effects of mediation on young children with developmental delay. In addition to better performance by the mediated group compared with the control group, follow-up testing 2 weeks later showed additional gains for the mediated group.

DYNAMIC APPROACHES TO LANGUAGE ASSESSMENT

Limited research exists on dynamic assessment applications to language. However, the studies that apply dynamic and interactive dynamic-like procedures parallel the procedures previously described.

Diagnostic Therapy

Although not strictly dynamic assessment, diagnostic, or trial, therapy is sometimes completed as part of a diagnostic battery to "test the limits" and to predict response to intervention. Diagnostic therapy differs from dynamic assessment in its focus on the child's behaviors given context and support, as opposed to the child's metacognitive ability. Specifically, trial therapy focuses on a particular content and observes a child's response to contextual cues. For example, analysis of tasks requiring more and less evaluator support can be used to develop trial therapy. The examiner may manipulate a language task, providing more or less context, cues, or prompts. The child is observed under these conditions, and the information is used to develop an intervention plan. Diagnostic therapy can serve as a link between static assessment and recommendations for intervention based on the trial therapy (Haynes, Pindzola, & Emerick, 1992; Weiss, Tomblin, & Robin, 1994).

In one study, two different intervention methods were used in a trial therapy session to predict how three toddlers would perform in two treatment conditions: modeling versus modeling plus evoked productions (Weismer, Murray-Branch, & Miller, 1993). Specifically, assessments before treatment were designed to evaluate the children's ability to learn targeted lexical items in each of the two conditions. For each assessment, two object labels (different from the treatment words) were targeted. Following teaching, probes were administered twice for each of the target words presented during the assessment. None of the children recognized or produced the words taught in the modeling-only condition. One of the three children recognized and produced two of the four target words taught through modeling plus evoked production. Overall, these results were not predictive of or correlated to the use of specific teaching methods. Nevertheless, Weismer et al. suggested that these procedures may be useful in selecting treatment objectives during ongoing therapy.

Successive Cueing

Olswang and Bain (1991; Bain & Olswang, 1995; Olswang, Bain, & Johnson, 1992) applied an approach similar to that of Brown and Campione (1981, 1984, 1986; Campione & Brown, 1978, 1984, 1987). They outlined an approach that uses a hierarchy of cues to determine a child's readiness to benefit from intervention. In one study (Olswang, Bain, Rosendahl, Oblak, & Smith, 1986), dynamic assessment was used with two children who presented similar profiles on static tests. Dynamic assessment consisted of teaching the children single words using three types of cues: modeling (e.g., "This is a baby"), modeling with an elicitation question (e.g., "This is a baby. What is it?"), and modeling with an object obstacle (e.g., withholding the object until the child attempted to produce the word) (Olswang & Bain, 1991, p. 260). The two children responded differently to the three intervention cues. One child was much more responsive than the other during dynamic assessment. During intervention, the two children again responded differently. Dynamic assessment showed a relationship to children's differential response to treatment.

Olswang and Bain (1991) discussed three possible outcomes of this type of dynamic assessment procedure. First, there may be no differences in performance between static and dynamic assessments. This would suggest that the child either is unable to benefit from intervention at this time or may already be functioning at an optimal level. Second, the child needs few cues to improve performance. This child may be entering a growth spurt and may not need intervention at this time. Third, the child may need many cues to improve performance. This child most likely needs intervention and is ready to benefit from intervention.

Learning Measures

Roseberry and Connell (1991) suggested a language-teaching procedure to distinguish language disorder from language difference. Although the teaching procedure is different from the MLE suggested by the dynamic assessment literature, it is similar in its test–teach–retest methodology. A modeling approach was used to teach an invented morpheme to typically developing bilingual children and children with specific language impairment (SLI). Teaching consisted of two individual sessions (15–20 minutes each) of pretest–teach–generalization probing. Each session began by establishing whether the children knew the labels for 20 pictures. When the children could name the 20 pictures, the teaching session began. The children were taught the invented morpheme /ə/, meaning "part of," using another set of pictures. The teacher named the picture of the whole object and then the picture of part of the object using the noun plus the invented morpheme /ə/. Next, the generalization probe assessed whether the children were able to transfer the learned morpheme to the first set of pictures. Results indicated that the typically developing children easily transferred the invented morpheme, whereas the children with SLI had more difficulty transferring. These results indicate that bilingual children with SLI and typically developing bilingual children can be differentiated based on their responses to language teaching.

Although the literature suggests that dynamic assessment potentially differentiates between children who have different learning experiences and those who have language-learning disabilities, few studies address this potential.

Mediated Language-Learning Experience

Another approach to dynamic assessment of language is using MLE as the teaching procedure. Using MLE in the assessment process is not intended to teach test items (i.e., teaching to the test) but rather to mediate strategies that will enable children to become self-regulated and active learners by teaching them the cognitive-linguistic skills needed to perform optimally on language tests, thus tapping ability. There are several researchers who are applying MLE to language assessment in a test–teach–retest approach similar to that used by Lidz (1987, 1991).

Brown (1994) applied MLE to the language assessment of Spanish-speaking adolescents with learning disabilities focusing on improving performance with synonyms. The Antonym-Synonym Subtest of the Woodcock Language Proficiency Battery–Spanish Form (WLPB–S) (Woodcock, 1981) was used as a pre–post test. Mediation tasks focused on vocabulary words; students were asked to define, categorize (by action, object, or description), compare, and provide a synonym. Mediation learning utilized MLE components of mediation of competence, transcendence, meaning, and intentionality and regulation of behavior (based on Lidz, 1991). For example, students were told the mediation goal and why the chosen goal was important (intentionality and meaning): "We will talk about how we describe objects, actions, and feelings.... It's important to know these words for school to read and write better" (Brown, 1994, p. 36). Cognitive functions targeted include comparative behavior, precision and accuracy, using two or more sources of information, and hypothesis testing. Comparative behavior was mediated using a word list. Students compared and categorized words. The investigator asked the students what makes certain kinds of words action, object, or description words. Then, they discussed how comparing words and placing them in these categories could assist in determining synonyms. Following mediation, there were significant differences between pretest and posttest scores on the WLPB–S. Significant correlations between modifiability ratings and posttest scores supported the usefulness of MLE in identifying children who were less modifiable.

Totten (1994) used dynamic language assessment via the Language Screening Assessment Tool–Primary (LSAT–P) (Austin Independent School District) with a second-grade student. On the pretest, the student performed poorly on the verbal absurdities, similarities and differences, and question formulations subtests of the LSAT–P. Three 30-minute MLE sessions were used to teach strategies in these three weak areas. Activities included analyzing and discussing the task, modeling expected responses, and generating original examples. Posttesting revealed improvement on all three subtests. In addition, the student was able to increase frustration thresholds when interacting with the examiner and did not avoid tasks that were difficult for him.

A number of studies have applied dynamic assessment to differentiate between language differences and language disorders in culturally and linguistically diverse children. A test–mediate–retest approach is used for assessing language-learning ability and for developing intervention.

Gutierrez-Clellen and Quinn (1993) proposed using MLE in dynamic assessment of school-age children's narratives. Their approach includes mediation as well as use of prompts during elicitation of a narrative. Gutierrez-Clellen, Peña, and Quinn (1995) applied Lidz's (1991) components of MLE to the assessment of narrative skills in preschool classrooms. After a baseline observation of narrative learning opportunities and demands in the classroom, it is suggested that the evaluator use mediation of intentionality, transcendence, and meaning to teach targeted features of narratives. A posttest can be used to analyze the children's ability to transfer the learned narrative structures to different contexts.

Peña, Quinn, and Iglesias (1992) applied MLE in a dynamic assessment to differentiate between typically developing children and children with possible language disorder. Children were Puerto Rican and African American. They were enrolled in Head Start and demonstrated below-average performance on a standardized test of expressive vocabulary. MLE consisted of teaching children that it was important to pay attention to "special names." Activities consisted of play with puzzles, books, and objects, in which the value of noun labels was emphasized. For example, meaning was mediated by explaining that "special names help us to tell things apart." Transcendence was mediated by talking about what would happen if their teacher did not know the children's names. Finally, competence was mediated by helping each child develop a plan for working out the games and remembering to name the items that each child saw. Typically developing children and children with possible language disorder did not receive significantly different scores on the pretest. After mediated learning experiences, typically developing children scored higher on the posttest compared with the children with possible language disorder. Repeated measures ANOVA indicated different pre–post test patterns for the two groups. Because the children were given experiences and strategies to help them increase their performance, assessment moved beyond what the children already knew to what they were able to do with help. These findings lend support to dynamic assessment as a potentially nonbiased method.

Lidz and Peña (in press) discuss the differential responses to MLE of two children who tested similarly on the Expressive One-Word Picture Vocabulary Test (EOWPVT) (Gardner, 1981). The first child was highly responsive to MLE during two 20-minute sessions. This child quickly learned that the goal of the sessions was to label using "special names" and learned to use labeling when pictures were presented. The second child had more difficulty recalling the goal of the session and had difficulty paying attention and self-monitoring. This child needed significant examiner support in order to label pictures presented during MLE. On the posttest, the child who learned to label scored higher than on the pretest; the child who was less modifiable showed little change from pretest to posttest.

In a follow-up study, Peña (1993) added a control (no treatment) group and two test tasks (pre- and post-MLE). Results indicated significant differences between control and experimental (MLE) groups' pre–post test patterns. Specifically, the experimental group scored significantly higher than did the control group on the Expressive One-Word Picture Vocabulary Test–Revised (EOWPVT–R) (Gardner, 1990), the Preschool Language Scale (modified) (Zimmerman, Steiner, & Pond, 1979), and the Comprehension Subtest of the Stanford-Binet Intelligence Scale (Thorndike, Hagen, & Sattler, 1986). Comparison of children with high and low language ability on each of the tasks indicated that the pre–post test patterns differentiated the groups. In a multiple regression analysis, modifiability measures (e.g., attention to task, awareness of goal, transfer, ability to seek help) differentiated high and low groups. Analysis of response types of the EOWPVT–R from pretest to posttest revealed that children with high and low language ability benefited from MLE. After MLE, children with high language ability used fewer unrelated or nonresponses, fewer descriptions and gestures, and fewer incorrect labels; the use of correct labels increased. Children with low language ability used fewer unrelated or nonresponses and fewer descriptions and gestures. They used about the same proportion of incorrect responses from pretest to posttest, but they used a higher proportion of labels (although some were incorrect). The study suggested that MLE has benefits beyond the specific intervention. Although MLE was designed only to teach labeling skills (the EOWPVT–R), scores on two other language tests also improved from pretest to posttest. This is consistent with the "snowball effect" of mediation, enabling children to become active learners (Haywood & Wingenfeld, 1992; Lidz, 1987). In addition, that both groups benefited from MLE when response types were analyzed underscores the need for careful observation of the changes that children with low language ability make in response to treatment.

LIMITATIONS OF DYNAMIC ASSESSMENT APPROACHES

There is a growing database of literature on the applications of dynamic assessment to language; however, many issues still must be considered. One issue is the time investment needed for dynamic assessment procedures. A second issue is its psychometric reliability and validity (Baine & Olswang, 1995; Embretson, 1992; Haywood et al., 1990; Lidz, 1995).

Language test procedures must reflect referral questions. Dynamic language assessment provides a way to observe the learning process. This observation yields authentic, valid information about the child in the process of learning. The philosophy that drives dynamic assessment focuses on optimal learning. Thus, classifying by ability or program placement is not the main focus or use for dynamic assessment (Feuerstein et al., 1987). In fact, it has been suggested that a contribution of dynamic assessment is to keep children out of special education (Haywood et al., 1990; Jensen et al., 1992). The goal of dynamic assessment is to identify areas in which intervention is needed and to describe how to support the intervention.

Observing the child in the process of learning and prescribing intervention based on that observation represents a paradigm shift that affects underlying assumptions about assessment, namely reliability and validity. Typically, reliability is sought by minimizing error. However, the nature of dynamic assessment does not lend itself well to such analysis; in fact, change or "error" is actively sought (Haywood et al., 1990; Lidz, 1995). Because dynamic assessment seeks to change functioning, an effective dynamic assessment would be indicated by low correlation between pretest and posttest. Therefore, test–retest reliability is an inappropriate criterion for evaluating dynamic assessment. Some attempts have been made to establish interobserver reliability. For example, Vaught (1989) conducted a study in which 10 dynamic assessment experts independently observed and scored videotaped sessions of administration of LPAD instruments. Vaught found consistent agreement on identifying specific cognitive deficiencies; however, she found low to moderate agreement on severity ratings and level of required mediation.

Haywood et al. (1990) suggested that "construct validity may be inherent in the dynamic approach" (p. 418). Because dynamic assessment observes the learning process itself and works to remediate limitations, the assessment is directly related to ability. Embretson (1987) suggested that incremental validity involving pretest-to-posttest comparisons may be useful for dynamic assessment. In this approach, validity is tested by comparing pretest and posttest results with learning. If the posttest correlates more highly with ability than does the pretest, then incremental validity is supported. Children should score higher after MLE. Incremental validity would demonstrate that dynamic assessment generates new and important information about a child's functioning. Embretson (1992) suggested that it is difficult to obtain appropriate validity criteria for dynamic assessment. She has addressed this issue in a psychometric model, a multidimensional Rasch model for learning and change (MRMLC) (Embretson, 1991). This model addresses psychometric difficulties with change measurement (e.g., simple gain scores). In this model, individual differences in modifiability compared with initial ability are estimated. Modifiability is derived from item response patterns rather than from a linear derivation of a total score. This yields individual measures of ability not based on group correlations.

The relatively few attempts to establish reliability and validity in dynamic assessment have focused on psychometric models (e.g., Babad & Budoff, 1974; Carlson & Wiedl, 1979; Lidz & Thomas, 1987; Rand & Kaniel, 1987). Because dynamic assessment does not purport to hold static properties nor seek them, static measures of reliability and validity are not ideal measures. At best, most of these studies have established weak to moderate support for dynamic assessment (Embretson, 1992). However, because dynamic assessment focuses on individual change and involves the mediator as the instrument of that change, models of naturalistic inquiry can establish guidelines for reliability and validity. Naturalistic inquiry can help retain depth and richness of dynamic assessment that may be lost otherwise.

Figure 1 represents the pattern of dynamic assessment as a naturalistic inquiry. Dynamic assessment, in effect, becomes a naturalistic inquiry in that the mediator is the instrument inducing, responding to, and observing change. Guba and Lincoln (1981) discussed seven characteristics that qualify "human as instrument of choice" (Lincoln & Guba, 1985, p. 193): responsiveness, adaptability, holistic emphasis, knowledge-base expansion, processual immediacy, opportunities for clarification and summarization, and opportunity to explore atypical or idiosyncratic responses. By interposing him- or herself between content and child in a dynamic assessment, the mediator becomes the assessment instrument. This allows for sensitivity and intimate involvement that can never be obtained in a static approach to assessment. Lincoln and Guba (1985) suggested that there is a "trade-off between perfection and adaptability" (p. 193) in qualitative analysis and observation. Although dynamic assessment may lose some of its psychometric (static) perfection, it has the potential to gain significantly over traditional static tests in terms of the adaptability and flexibility it can provide. Dynamic assessment seeks to produce change. The change is observed across instruments and situations to establish consistency and validity of the phenomenon.

Reliability in static assessment typically is established through replicability. Because it is highly individualized, and the examiner works to change the child's functioning, dynamic assessment cannot be replicated. Naturalistic inquiry, however, provides an alternative test of reliability. Guba and Lincoln (1981) dis-

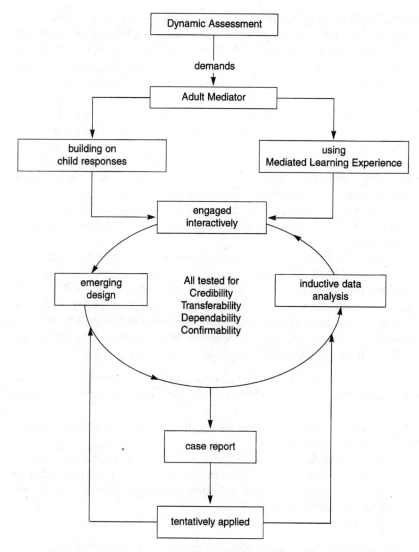

Figure 1. Dynamic assessment as a naturalistic inquiry. (Adapted from Lincoln & Guba, 1985.)

cussed the "trustworthiness" of information derived from naturalistic inquiry. Trustworthiness is tested within the context of the inquiry through the constructs of credibility, transferability, dependability, and confirmability. They suggested that for a naturalistic inquiry, a test of consistency, or "auditability," is equivalent to psychometric reliability. They argued that consistency in a naturalistic inquiry can be established by having a second evaluator or team examine the work. Guba and Lincoln (1981) explained that in a naturalistic inquiry, a second researcher cannot replicate the assessment "without knowing the decisions made by the original investigators at every step of the process" (p. 122). But evaluators can review the decisions made and verify that the decisions made were methodologically sound. Credibility is established through triangulation and/or repeated observations. Thus, for reliability, a second evaluator is asked whether he or she would have reached the same conclusion given the perspective and the data. This is contrasted with the psychometric procedure of establishing intertester reliability, in which the observers are asked to *independently* come to the same conclusion. In evaluating reliability of dynamic assessment, a second evaluator may inspect the examiner's notes and compare them with the final report. The evaluator may question why certain tasks were targeted for mediation and how the data were organized. The process of dynamic assessment is then compared with the assumptions of the model to establish agreement. Accordingly, the trustworthiness of dynamic assessment might be established, in part, through naturalistic methodology.

Maxwell (1992) argued that validity involves the relationship between the account and what that account is about—that is, the *interpretation* of the data. The data and methods are not, in and of themselves, valid or invalid. The critical issue in validity of an account is how the data are explained. He argued that the validity of an account does not depend on "absolute truth" (p. 283) because it is possible to have different accounts from different perspectives. He discussed five different types of validity, increasing in level of abstraction:

1. Descriptive validity involves factual accuracy or reporting.
2. Interpretive validity involves reporting the account from the participant's perspective.
3. Theoretical validity refers to the explanatory nature or theoretical understanding of an account. This is similar to construct validity.
4. Generalizability involves the usefulness of the theory of the account for another similar situation; generalizability can be either internal (within the community, person, or situation studied) or external (other *similar* communities, people, situations).
5. Evaluative validity is a critical evaluation of what was observed.

These types of validity can be applied to dynamic assessment through development of a "theory" of what is observed during the mediated learning experience. The interpretation of the observation emerges from the socially constructed interaction and is developed into a tentative case report.

CONCLUSION

Although few studies have applied dynamic assessment to assessment of language, results thus far are promising. Dynamic and dynamic-like procedures can be used to evaluate language learning. Some critical issues continue to be what is derived from the dynamic assessment and psychometric properties of the approach.

The structure (high to low) of the dynamic assessment method employed yields different sorts of information. At the more structured end of dynamic assessment, validity and information are gained about the child's ability to transfer to similar school tasks. However, the dynamic nature of interactive assessment is lost by making it too structured, resulting in "snapshots" of performance, given certain kinds of cues. By focusing on reliability and validity, dynamic assessment becomes static because of the statistical constraints. The information gained through such observations is not enough to serve as the basis for planning and predicting (i.e., surface description). However, unstructured approaches gain in authenticity but may lose out in replicability (i.e., reliability). Naturalistic approaches may yield some alternatives for examining the dynamic assessment procedure.

Language assessors are constantly challenged to provide assessments that capture language ability. Children come to school with different experiences, values, and goals; thus, there is a need to provide assessments that do not penalize students for lack of experience. In addition to identification, assessment must provide direction for intervention. Dynamic assessment allows a form of assessment that is authentic and useful and that promises to link assessment with instruction and intervention.

REFERENCES

Adler, S. (1990). Multicultural clients: Implications for the SLP. *Language, Speech, and Hearing Services in Schools, 21*(3), 135–139.

Anastasi, A. (1983, November). *The nature of intelligence: A view from the 1980's.* Invited address, Minority Assessment Conference, Arizona Conference on Applied Psychological Issues, Tucson.

Austin Independent School District. (n.d.). *Language Screening Assessment Tool– Primary.* Austin, TX: Author.

Babad, E.Y., & Budoff, M. (1974). Sensitivity and validity of learning-potential measurement in three levels of ability. *Journal of Educational Psychology, 66,* 434–447.

Bailey, D., & Harbin, G. (1980). Nondiscriminatory evaluation. *Exceptional Children, 46,* 590–596.

Bain, B., & Olswang, L. (1995). Examining readiness for learning two-word utterances by children with specific expressive language impairment: Dynamic assessment validation. *American Journal of Speech-Language Pathology, 4*(1), 81–92.

Bates, E. (1976). *Language and context: The acquisition of pragmatics.* New York. Academic Press.

Bloom L., & Lahey, M. (1978). *Language development and language disorders.* New York: John Wiley & Sons.

Blount, B. (1982). Culture and the language of socialization: Parental speech. In D.A. Wagner & H.W. Stevenson (Eds.), *Cultural perspectives on child development* (pp. 55–76). San Francisco: W.H. Freeman.

Brown, A., & Campione, J. (1981). Inducing flexible thinking: A problem of access. In M. Friedman, J.P. Das, & N. O'Connor (Eds.), *Intelligence and learning* (pp. 515–529). New York: Plenum.

Brown, A., & Campione, J. (1984). Three faces of transfer: Implications for early competence, individual differences, and instruction. In M. Lamb, A. Brown, & B. Rogoff (Eds.), *Advances in developmental psychology* (Vol. 3, pp. 143–192). Hillsdale, NJ: Lawrence Erlbaum Associates.

Brown, A., & Campione, J. (1986). Cognitive science and learning disabilities. *American Psychologist, 41*(10), 1059–1068.

Brown, A., & French, L. (1979). The zone of potential development: Implications for intelligence testing in the year 2000. *Intelligence, 3*, 253–271.

Brown, A., & Palincsar, A. (1982). Inducing strategic learning from texts by means of informed, self-control training. *Topics in Learning and Learning Disabilities, 2*(1), 1–15.

Brown, A.L., & Palincsar, A.S. (1986). Reciprocal teaching of comprehension strategies: A natural history of one program for enhancing learning. In J. Borkowski & J.D. Day (Eds.), *Intelligence and cognition in special children: Comparative studies of giftedness, mental retardation, and learning disabilities.* New York: Ablex.

Brown, S. (1994). *A comparison of dynamic and standardized procedures in the language assessment of Spanish speaking learning disabled adolescents.* Unpublished master's thesis, San Diego State University, San Diego, CA.

Bruner, J.S. (1978). Learning how to do things with words. In J.S. Bruner & R.A. Garton (Eds.), *Human growth and development* (pp. 62–84). Oxford, England: Oxford University Press.

Budoff, M. (1967). Learning potential among institutionalized young adult retardates. *American Journal of Mental Deficiency, 72*, 404–411.

Budoff, M. (1969). Learning potential: A supplementary procedure for assessing the ability to reason. *Seminars in Psychiatry, 1*, 278–290.

Budoff, M. (1987). The validity of learning potential assessment. In C.S. Lidz (Ed.), *Dynamic assessment: An interactional approach to evaluating learning potential* (pp. 52–81). New York: Guilford Press.

Budoff, M., & Corman, L. (1973). *The effectiveness of a group training procedure on the Raven Learning Potential measure with children of diverse racial and socioeconomic backgrounds* (RIEPrint #58). Cambridge, MA: Research Institute for Educational Problems.

Budoff, M., & Corman, L. (1974). Demographic and psychometric factors related to improved performance on the Kohs Learning Potential procedure. *American Journal of Mental Deficiency, 78*, 578–585.

Campione, J. (1989). Assisted assessment: A taxonomy of approaches and an outline of strengths and weaknesses. *Journal of Learning Disabilities, 22*(3), 151–165.

Campione, J., & Brown, A. (1977). Memory and metamemory development in educable retarded children. In R.V. Kail, Jr., & J.W. Hagen (Eds.), *Perspectives on the development of memory and cognition* (pp. 367–406). Hillsdale, NJ: Lawrence Erlbaum Associates.

Campione, J., & Brown, A. (1978). Toward a theory of intelligence: Contributions from research with retarded children. *Intelligence, 2*, 279–304.

Campione, J., & Brown, A. (1984). Learning ability and transfer propensity as sources of individual differences in intelligence. In P.H. Brooks, R.D. Sperber, & C. McCauley (Eds.), *Learning and cognition in the mentally retarded* (pp. 265–294). Baltimore: University Park Press.

Campione, J., & Brown, A. (1987). Linking dynamic assessment with school achievement. In C.S. Lidz (Ed.), *Dynamic assessment: An interactional approach to evaluating learning potential* (pp. 82–115). New York: Guilford Press.

Campione, J., Brown, A., & Bryant, N. (1985). Individual differences in learning and memory. In R.J. Sternberg (Ed.), *Human abilities: An information processing approach* (pp. 103–126). San Francisco: W.H. Freeman.

Campione, J., Brown, A., & Ferrara, R. (1982). Mental retardation and intelligence. In R.J. Sternberg (Ed.), *Handbook of human intelligence* (pp. 392–490). Cambridge, MA: Harvard University Press.

Campione, J., Brown, A., Ferrara, R., Jones, R., & Steinberg, E. (1985). Differences between retarded and non-retarded children in transfer following equivalent learning performances: Breakdowns in flexible use of information. *Intelligence, 9,* 297–315.

Carlson, J. (1983). *Applications of dynamic assessment to cognitive and perceptual functioning of three ethnic groups. Final report.* Riverside: University of California at Riverside. (ERIC Document Reproduction Service No. ED 233 040)

Carlson, J., & Wiedl, K. (1979). Toward a differential testing approach: Testing the limits employing the Raven matrices. *Intelligence, 3,* 323–344.

Carlson, J., & Wiedl, K. (1980). Applications of a dynamic testing approach in intelligence assessment: Empirical results and theoretical formulations. *Seitschrift fur Differentiele und Diagnostische Psychologie, 1,* 303–318.

Corman, L., & Budoff, M. (1973). *A comparison of group and individual training procedures on the Raven Learning Potential measure with black and white special class students.* (REIPrint #57). Cambridge, MA: Research Institute for Educational Problems.

Darley, F. (1979). *Evaluation of appraisal techniques in speech and language pathology.* Reading, MA: Addison-Wesley.

Damico, J. (1990). Descriptive assessment of communicative ability in limited English proficient students. In E.V. Hamayan & J.S. Damico (Eds.), *Limiting bias in the assessment of bilingual students* (pp. 157–217). Austin, TX: PRO-ED.

Duran, R. (1988). Testing of linguistic minorities. In R. Linn (Ed.), *Educational measurement* (3rd ed., pp. 573–587). New York: Macmillan.

Duran, R. (1989). Assessment and instruction of at-risk Hispanic students. *Teaching Exceptional Children, 56*(2), 145–152.

Embretson, S.E. (1987). Toward development of a psychometric approach. In C.S. Lidz (Ed.), *Dynamic assessment: An interactional approach to evaluating learning potential* (pp. 141–170). New York: Guilford Press.

Embretson, S.E. (1991). Implications of a multidimensional latent trait model for measuring change. In L.M. Collins & J.L. Horn (Eds.), *Best methods for the analysis of change: Recent advances, unanswered questions, future directions* (pp. 184–197). Washington, DC: American Psychological Association Books.

Embretson, S.E. (1992). Measuring and validating cognitive modifiability as an ability: A study in the spatial domain. *Journal of Educational Measurement, 29*(1), 25–50.

Ferrara, R., Brown, A., & Campione, J. (1986). Children's learning and transfer of inductive reasoning rules: Studies in proximal development. *Child Development, 57,* 1089–1099.

Feuerstein, R. (1979). *The dynamic assessment of retarded performers. The Learning Potential Assessment Device, theory, instruments, and techniques.* Baltimore: University Park Press.

Feuerstein, R. (1980). *Instrumental enrichment.* Baltimore: University Park Press.

Feuerstein, R., Miller, R., Rand, Y., & Jensen, M. (1981). Can evolving techniques better measure cognitive change? *Journal of Special Education, 15,* 201–219.

Feuerstein, R., Rand, Y., & Hoffman, M. (1979). *The dynamic assessment of retarded performers: The Learning Potential Assessment Device.* Baltimore: University Park Press.

Feuerstein, R., Rand, Y., Jensen, M.R., Kaniel, S., & Tzuriel, D. (1987). Prerequisites for assessment of learning potential: The LPAD model. In C.S. Lidz (Ed.), *Dynamic assessment: An interactional approach to evaluating learning potential* (pp. 35–51). New York: Guilford Press.

Figueroa, R. (1989). Psychological testing of linguistic-minority students: Knowledge gaps and regulations. *Exceptional Children, 56,* 145–152.

Gardner, M.F. (1981). *Expressive One-Word Picture Vocabulary Test.* Novato, CA: Academic Therapy Publications.

Gardner, M.F. (1990). *Expressive One-Word Picture Vocabulary Test–Revised.* Novato, CA: Academic Therapy Publications.

Gimon, A., Budoff, M., & Corman, L. (1974). Learning potential measurement with Spanish-speaking youth as an alternative to IQ tests: A first report. *Interamerican Journal of Psychology, 8,* 233-246.

Guba, E., & Lincoln, Y. (1981). *Effective evaluation.* San Francisco: Jossey-Bass.

Gutierrez-Clellen, V., Peña, E., & Quinn, R. (1995). Accommodating cultural differences in narrative style: A bilingual perspective. *Topics in Language Disorders, 15*(4), 54–67.

Gutierrez-Clellen, V., & Quinn, R. (1993). Assessing narratives in diverse cultural-linguistic populations: Clinical implications. *Language, Speech, and Hearing Services in Schools, 24*(1), 2–9.

Haynes, W., Pindzola, R., & Emerick, L. (1992). *Diagnosis and evaluation in speech pathology.* Englewood Cliffs, NJ: Prentice Hall.

Haywood, H.C., Brooks, P., & Burns, S. (1983). *Cognitive curriculum for young children: Experimental version.* Nashville, TN: Vanderbilt University.

Haywood, H.C., Brown, A.L., & Wingenfeld, S. (1990). Dynamic approaches to psychoeducational assessment. *School Psychology Review, 19,* 411–422.

Haywood, H.C., & Tzuriel, D. (1992). *Interactive assessment.* New York: Springer-Verlag.

Haywood, H.C., & Wingenfeld, S. (1992). Interactive assessment as a research tool. *Journal of Special Education, 26*(3), 253–268.

Heath, S.B. (1983). *Ways with words: Language, life, and work in communities and classrooms.* Cambridge, England: Cambridge University Press.

Heath, S.B. (1986). Sociocultural contexts of language development. In California State Department of Education (Ed.), *Beyond language: Social and cultural factors in schooling language minority children* (pp. 143–186). Los Angeles: Evaluation, Dissemination and Assessment Center, California State University.

Jensen, M.R., Robinson-Zañartu, C., & Jensen, M.L. (1992). *Dynamic assessment and mediated learning: Assessment and intervention for developing cognitive and knowledge structures—An alternative in the era of reform.* Atlanta: Cognitive Education Systems.

Jitendra, A., & Kameenui, E. (1993). Dynamic assessment as a compensatory assessment approach: A description and analysis. *Remedial and Special Education, 15*(5), 8–18.

Kaufman, A.S. (1983). *Kaufman Assessment Battery for Children (K–ABC).* Circle Pines, MN: American Guidance Service.

Klein, P.S., & Feuerstein, R. (1985). Environmental variables and cognitive development: Identification of the potent factors in adult–child interaction. In S. Harel & N.J.

Anastasiow (Eds.), *The at-risk infant: Psycho/socio/medical aspects* (pp. 369–377). Baltimore: Paul H. Brookes Publishing Co.

Kohs, R. (1923). *Intelligence measurement*. New York: Macmillan.

Lahey, M. (1990). Who shall be called language disordered? Some reflections and one perspective. *Journal of Speech and Hearing Disorders, 55,* 612–620.

Launer, P., & Lahey, M. (1981). Passages: From the fifties to the eighties in language assessment. *Topics in Language Disorders, 1,* 11–30.

Lee, L. (1966). Developmental sentence types: A method for comparing normal and deviant syntactic development. *Journal of Speech and Hearing Disorders, 31,* 311–330.

Lidz, C.S. (1981). *Improving assessment of schoolchildren*. San Francisco: Jossey-Bass.

Lidz, C.S. (1982, April). *Psychological assessment of the preschool disadvantaged child*. Paper presented at the annual international convention of the Council for Exceptional Children, Houston, TX. (ERIC Document Reproduction Service No. 219 912)

Lidz, C.S. (1987). *Dynamic assessment: An interactional approach to evaluating learning potential*. New York: Guilford Press.

Lidz, C.S. (1991). *Practitioner's guide to dynamic assessment*. New York: Guilford Press.

Lidz, C.S. (1995). Dynamic assessment and the legacy of L.S. Vygotsky. *School Psychology International, 16*(2), 143–154.

Lidz, C.S., & Peña, E. (in press). Dynamic assessment: The model, its relevance as a non-biased approach, and its application to Latino-American preschool children. *Language, Speech, and Hearing Services in Schools*.

Lidz, C.S., & Thomas, C. (1987). The Preschool Learning Assessment Device: Extension of a static approach. In C.S. Lidz (Ed.), *Dynamic assessment: An interactional approach to evaluating learning potential* (pp. 288–326). New York: Guilford Press.

Lincoln, Y., & Guba, E. (1985). *Naturalistic inquiry*. Beverly Hills: Sage Publications.

Luria, A.R. (1966). *Human brain and psychological processes* (B. Haigh, trans.). New York: Harper & Row.

Maxwell, J. (1992). Understanding and validity in qualitative research. *Harvard Educational Review, 62*(3), 279–300.

McCauley, R., & Swisher, L. (1984a). Psychometric review of language and articulation tests for preschool children. *Journal of Speech and Hearing Disorders, 49,* 34–42.

McCauley, R., & Swisher, L. (1984b). Use and misuse of norm-referenced tests in clinical assessment: A hypothetical case. *Journal of Speech and Hearing Disorders, 49,* 338–348.

Meyers, J. (1987). The training of dynamic assessors. In C.S. Lidz (Ed.), *Dynamic assessment: An interactional approach to evaluating learning potential* (pp. 288–326). New York: Guilford Press.

Missiuna, C., & Samuels, M. (1989). Dynamic assessment of preschool children with special needs: Comparison of mediation and instruction. *Remedial and Special Education, 10*(2), 53–62.

Neisworth, J., & Bagnato, S. (1986). Curriculum-based developmental assessment: Congruence of testing and teaching. *School Psychology Review, 15*(2), 180–199.

Olswang, L., & Bain, B. (1991). When to recommend intervention. *Language, Speech, and Hearing Services in Schools, 22,* 255–263.

Olswang, L.B., Bain, B.A., & Johnson, G.A. (1992). Using dynamic assessment with children with language disorders. In S.F. Warren & J. Reichle (Eds.), *Communication and language intervention series: Vol. 1. Causes and effects in communication and language intervention* (pp. 187–215). Baltimore: Paul H. Brookes Publishing Co.

Olswang, L., Bain, B., Rosendahl, P., Oblak, S., & Smith, A. (1986). Language learning: Moving performance from context dependent to independent state. *Child Language Teaching and Therapy, 2,* 180–210.

Palincsar, A., & Brown, A. (1984). Reciprocal teaching and comprehension-fostering and monitoring activities. *Cognition and Instruction, 1,* 117–175.

Peña, E. (1993). *Dynamic assessment: A non-biased approach for assessing the language of young children.* Unpublished doctoral dissertation, Temple University, Philadelphia.

Peña, E., Quinn, R., & Iglesias, A. (1992). The application of dynamic methods to language assessment: A non-biased procedure. *Journal of Special Education, 26*(3), 269–280.

Rand, Y., & Kaniel, S. (1987). Group administration of the LPAD. In C.S. Lidz (Ed.), *Dynamic assessment: An interactional approach to evaluating learning potential* (pp. 196–214). New York: Guilford Press.

Raven, J.C., Court, J.H., & Raven, J. (1977). *Raven's Progressive Matrices and Vocabulary Scales.* London: H.K. Lewis & Co. Ltd.

Reinharth, B.M. (1989). *Cognitive modifiability in developmentally delayed children.* Unpublished doctoral dissertation, Yeshiva University, New York.

Rogoff, B. (1990). *Apprenticeship in thinking: Cognitive development in social context.* New York: Oxford University Press.

Roseberry, C., & Connell, P.J. (1991). The use of an invented language rule in the differentiation of normal and language-impaired Spanish-speaking children. *Journal of Speech and Hearing Research, 34,* 596–603.

Schery, T. (1981). Selecting assessment strategies for language disordered children. *Topics in Language Disorders, 1*(3), 59–73.

Schieffelin, B.B., & Ochs, E. (1986). *Language socialization across cultures.* Cambridge, England: Cambridge University Press.

Sewell, T.E. (1987). Dynamic assessment as a nondiscriminatory procedure. In C.S. Lidz (Ed.), *Dynamic assessment: An interactional approach to evaluating learning potential* (pp. 426–443). New York: Guilford Press.

Thorndike, R.L., Hagen, E.P., & Sattler, J.M. (1986). *Stanford-Binet Intelligence Scale* (4th ed.). Chicago: Riverside.

Tomblin, J.B., Morris, H., & Spriestersbach, D. (1994). *Diagnosis in speech-language pathology.* San Diego: Singular.

Totten, G. (1994). *The dynamic language assessment of culturally and linguistically diverse school-age children: A proposed protocol.* Unpublished master's thesis, University of Texas at Austin.

Tzuriel, D., & Klein, P. (1987). Assessing the young child: Children's analogical thinking modifiability. In C.S. Lidz (Ed.), *Dynamic assessment: An interactional approach to evaluating learning potential* (pp. 268–287). New York: Guilford Press.

van Kleeck, A. (1985). Issues in adult–child interaction: Six philosophical orientations. *Topics in Language Disorders, 3,* 1–13.

Vaught, S. (1989). *Interjudge agreement in dynamic assessment: Two instruments from the Learning Potential Assessment Device.* Unpublished master's thesis, Vanderbilt University, Nashville, TN.

Vygotsky, L.S. (1978). *Mind in society: The development of higher psychological processes* (M. Cole, V. John-Steiner, S. Scribner, & E. Souberman, Eds.). Cambridge, MA: Harvard University Press.

Vygotsky, L.S. (1986). *Thought and language* (A. Kozulin, trans.). Cambridge: MIT Press.

Weismer, S., Murray-Branch, J., & Miller, J. (1993). Comparison of two methods for promoting productive vocabulary in late talkers. *Journal of Speech and Hearing Research, 36*(5), 1037–1050.

Weiss, A., Tomblin, J.B., & Robin, D. (1994). Language disorders. In J.B. Tomblin, H. Morris, & D. Spriestersbach (Eds.), *Diagnosis in speech-language pathology* (pp. 99–134). San Diego: Singular.

Wolf, D., Bixby, J., Glenn, J., III, & Gardner, H. (1991). To use their minds well: Investigating new forms of student assessment. *Review of Research in Education, 17*, 31–74.

Woodcock, R.W. (1981). *Woodcock Language Proficiency Battery–Spanish Form.* Chicago: Riverside.

Zimmerman, I., Steiner, V., & Pond, R. (1979). *Preschool Language Scale.* Columbus, OH: Charles E. Merrill.

13

Progress in Assessing, Describing, and Defining Child Language Disorder

Jon F. Miller

THE FIRST STEP IN DEVELOPING the science of any field is careful observation and description (Tukey, 1977). Observations provide data on the range of performance for the behavior being studied. Through the process of observing and recording the behavior of individual children over time or groups of children in similar contexts and across contexts, consistency and variation of performance can be described. Developing the science of investigating language disorder has not followed this process; rather, the field has skipped the observational stage, moving directly to hypothesis-testing research. Hypotheses for research have been derived directly from developmental theory proposed as explanations for the development of typical children or from linguistic theories characterizing adult competence, not from language acquisition. Much of this work appears to be testing each new linguistic theory on populations with disorders in hopes of finding a fit rather than building a theory of disordered performance from the bottom up, observation to theory. In contrast, the modern era of research on typical language development was introduced by Brown's (1973) careful observation of three children acquiring their primary language. There are several aspects of Brown's work that are relevant to a discussion of assessment tools used in developing the science of disordered performance.

After Brown's remarkable descriptions of three children learning language during the 1960s and 1970s, researchers came to understand that the language-learning process was much more complicated than adding words to vocabulary or picking up sentences from adults through imitation. Children seemed to be constructing their language system as they progressed through the stages of development. This language-learning process required a rich language environment and the child's own cognitive skills. Brown's detailed descriptions of children learning their language brought into focus the complexities of human cognition and the role that language learning could play in gaining insight into developing cognitive skills. Brown's work produced new measures to describe language progress. One of the most innovative was the use of mean length of utterance (MLU) as a way of exploring grammatical development over time and across children. Brown reasoned that children cannot add syntactic complexity early in development without adding words or morphemes to their sentences. He then demonstrated that children with the same MLUs were using similar grammatical rules to formulate their utterances and that syntactic development could be charted as a series of stages defined by MLU. MLU through four to five morphemes has become an index of language development of individual children and the basis of comparison of development between children. Most studies of language development through the early 1980s used MLU rather than age to document developmental stage and the equivalence of subject groups because, as Brown had argued, MLU was independent of age. The language development of the three children seemed to progress at a rate independent of the children's age. Although researchers later learned that this was not entirely correct (Miller & Chapman, 1981), Brown's work provided a tool—MLU—for researchers to define equivalent language status of children participating in group studies. MLU also proved to be an ideal mechanism for comparing the outcomes of different studies through the mid-1980s (Miller, 1981). This single measure has been used more than any other to document developmental progress and also has been used as a sensitive indicator of disordered performance (Aram, Morris, & Hall, 1993). Brown's work demonstrated the power of description as a process for exploring the potential of individual measures to capture the specific language behaviors. The future of assessment aimed at documenting disordered performance will require a similar descriptive process as that used by Brown to identify new measures and to explore their descriptive utility and validity in characterizing disordered language performance through the developmental period.

STATE OF THE ART

This book has reviewed the status of the assessment of language and communication behavior and has provided a summary of the progress of research in understanding child language disorder. The chapters in this book brought together research covering every aspect of assessing language performance. Each chapter provided a detailed review of the literature and insightful summaries of the state of the art in measurement for early and later language development, across linguistic levels, discussing specific issues and methodologies, the impact of cultural and linguistic differences, and alternative models to the commonly used assessment process. This chapter highlights several points made throughout the book and discusses a long-term program of research aimed at overcoming some fundamental problems that have limited researchers' understanding of disordered language performance.

The most fundamental problem for the field, according to Thal and Katich (see Chapter 1), is that there is no agreement on the definition of specific language impairment (SLI) or even whether the construct of SLI is productive. SLI cannot easily be separated from mild intellectual impairments; researchers do not know whether SLI is a unitary phenomenon with a single cause or is a number of different syndromes each with a unique cause. Another issue that Thal and Katich raise is that single measures of language performance are consistently inadequate for determining whether a child of any age has typical or delayed development. Yet another issue is that the features of disordered performance change over time as the result of advancing development and adaptive strategies.

Taken together, these issues point to the need for more descriptive work to help define the parameters of language disorder and its scope; sequence; and associated perceptual, cognitive, and motor abilities. This will require new measures, old measures used in combination, and measures that can be used hierarchically to describe and ultimately define disordered language performance. It should be clear after reading this volume that developing individual measures requires documenting their validity through descriptive studies of children with language disorders. As has often been pointed out, most of the standardized tests use items that discriminate performance between and among children on language tasks at different ages. Standardized tests, by definition, cannot describe children's language performance because they do not use items that all children perform. They define a language disorder as poor performance on the items on the test. An examination of the items on these tests will leave any researcher dismayed and discouraged.

The solution to improving the definition of disorder is to develop measures that address the performance problems observed in children with disorder, find the performance range of typical children as a comparison base, and examine the power of these measures taken together to describe disordered performance. The steps are the same ones that Brown (1973) used, developing the measures to start the process, then documenting their validity and reliability through descriptive study. Before examining a long-term project that addresses these issues, a review of the theoretical discussion so fluently presented by Evans (see Chapter 10) is helpful because this chapter describes the theoretical and analytical processes that ultimately may be used to quantify disordered performance through the use of linear and nonlinear dynamical models.

THEORETICAL PROGRESS

Assessment methods are both the outcome of theory and the tools required for theoretical development. Evans (see Chapter 10) traces the evolution of the theory-assessment method from the mid-1950s as it relates to the study of language development and disorder. She proposes that dynamic systems theory best captures the accounts of children with language impairment across phonological, morphological, syntactic, semantic, or pragmatic levels of performance.

Evans views disordered performance as dynamic, changing relative to context and speaker demands as well as over time. This proposal is important for two reasons. First, it recognizes that language disorder is not a single entity described by a single metric but rather several distinct yet related impairments affecting one or more levels of the language system. Each of these disorders will change over time as the child makes accommodations for specific impairments to overcome the language limitation and improve everyday communication. Evans argues that dynamic modeling provides the tools to explore this view of disorder and provides the statistical methods to test changing relationships among variables for different communication tasks and to model the linear and nonlinear changes in performance over time. According to Evans, the substance of dynamic modeling theory is evaluating simultaneous data derived from a language sample. The basic assumption of this theory is that a language is the sum of several linguistic levels interacting to form messages. Although each language level can be shown to operate on a set of rules, the language levels are not independent in the sense that an impairment at one level will have consequences for other levels. It is in the predicting and testing of these impairments that dynamic modeling shows promise. To implement this model, sufficient data must be collected from children with language disorders. Given the lack of agreement on the defining characteristics of disordered performance, this appears to be out of reach for the language disorders research community, not to mention the funding agencies. A description of a project initiated some years ago to address several issues in assessing language disorder may be useful here as an example of how language-sample analysis can provide the descriptive platform for evaluating new measures of performance, exploring the relationship among measures within and across language levels, and describing different patterns of disordered language performance.

LANGUAGE-SAMPLE ANALYSIS PROJECT

The goal of the language-sample analysis (LSA) project was to implement LSA in school and clinical settings. The project assumed that LSA was the most informative measurement process available to both clinicians and researchers (Miller, 1981). LSA holds the most promise for yielding valid indicators of developmental progress and disordered performance because the sampling and transcription process provides direct access to primary language data. At the time that this project began, the Blue Book had just been published (Miller, 1981) detailing an extensive array of analysis procedures that could be performed on language samples to document performance. At the same time, very few clinicians used LSA routinely in their clinical work, either as an identification tool or to document intervention progress, not because they did not believe it was useful or had not had appropriate training but because it took too much time to transcribe and analyze the sample. No consistent transcription or analysis standards existed, which limited communication of the results even within the same school district, and there were no data to compare performance of school-age children to document specific impairments. The first step in implementing this methodology required solutions for the time limitations, consistency, and a basis for comparison. At the same time, it appeared that the measures being used were not addressing the language performance impairments that clinicians identified for intervention in order to improve educational performance. As researchers worked to reduce the barriers to using LSA, they began to see that the measures that described typical language development were not sufficient to describe the range of disordered language performance observed in school-age children. The development of an efficient LSA tool would provide access to the descriptive data necessary to better understand the disordered language behavior that clinicians were dealing with each day. The major step in developing the analyses was the development of SALT—computer programs for the systematic analysis of language transcripts. Early versions of SALT implemented measures that typically had been done by hand (Miller, 1981), saving considerable analysis time, and then began to exploit the power of the computer to yield solutions to problems that could not be obtained any other way. The evolution of this effort to make LSA accessible to clinicians has yielded new measures of disordered performance, descriptive profiles of hundreds of children with language disorder, and a hierarchical assessment strategy using general measures calculated by the computer to identify areas requiring more detailed analyses. The following section reviews the collaborative process that was devised and implemented to make LSA accessible to speech-language pathologists (SLPs) throughout the state of Wisconsin.

Solutions to the Problems Confronting Implementation of LSA

Time The time limitation surfaced in two areas: 1) transcribing the sample and 2) analyzing the sample. The time it takes to transcribe a language sample can range from 1 to 3 hours, effectively limiting the use of this technique to a very few children for even the most motivated clinician. Professional time is too valuable to spend in transcription. Since 1990, the concept of transcription laboratories has been successfully implemented, first in Madison and, subsequently, statewide. These labs use nonprofessionals to transcribe samples recorded on audiotapes into computer text files using a standard format developed for SALT analysis. The basic SALT format requires no coding or analysis requiring professional judgment. With about 20 hours of training, an experienced word processor with good English-language skills can reliably transcribe clinical samples. The lab in the Madison schools transcribed more than 500 samples a year for 6 years. The additional time-saving device is computer analysis routines using SALT. SALT produces a variety of quantitative analyses at the word and utterance levels that can be calculated accurately without coding. Most recent has been the development of a clinical report module that automatically compares the target child with a reference database of more than 250 children between

3 and 13 years of age in either a conversation or a narrative sampling context. The computer analyses save considerable time and free the clinician to interpret the results in combination with other assessment results.

Reducing analysis time was one of the first goals in developing SALT. Computers can perform a variety of analyses very quickly compared with paper-and-pencil methods. The first versions of SALT were implemented on a main-frame computer and could calculate MLU, Type-Token Ratio (TTR), and the number of different words almost instantly. This was revolutionary at the time. Later, as other measures were added, it became apparent that the individual measures could not capture the performance variation of the children with disorder, but their performance across measures produced profiles describing clusters of performance impairments. Using computer language analysis is a double-edged sword; the computer can calculate measures very quickly for large numbers of variables, but it is very literal, counting only what it is instructed to count. Much of language requires context for interpretation, both linguistic and nonlinguistic. Computers do not make decisions in context; they require specific coding for much of syntax, semantic, and pragmatic analysis. Humans, however, excel at interpreting context. The approach, therefore, has been to focus on calculations of variables that the computer can count accurately without additional coding to exploit the power of the computer for what it does best. Clinical profiles use these measures exclusively to provide an efficient initial description of performance. To follow up the initial description, extensive computer software routines have been developed supporting the detailed coding of transcripts for linguistic or nonlinguistic features at any language level. The detailed coding of transcripts cannot be done automatically; it requires human decisions about linguistic features in context.

Consistency   The computer-analysis approach has forced the use of a consistent transcription protocol. Adding the requirement that the transcript be readable by teachers and parents has improved accessibility of the process and has improved communication among professionals. It has even allowed the use of transcripts in therapy to discuss specific areas of difficulty. A second area in which consistency has been improved is in selecting specific sampling contexts. Two have been chosen: conversation and narration—*conversation* because there has been considerable research using this context in the development literature and *narration* because of the powerful relationship between narrative skills and literacy. Data demonstrate that using consistent topics can produce extremely robust results.

Basis for Comparison   Since 1984, a reference database (RDB) has been developed that includes more than 250 children from 3 to 13 years of age in two speaking conditions: conversation and narration (Miller & Leadholm, 1992). Children included in this sample were of diverse socioeconomic status (SES) and ability levels. Equal numbers of children were from high, average, and low SES backgrounds, and equal numbers of children represented high, average, and low classroom performance as judged by their teachers when compared with all children whom they have taught at that grade level. Children were sampled from urban and rural schools from the state of Wisconsin. Age groups were targeted at plus or minus 3 months of 3, 4, 5, 6, 7, 9, 11, and 13 years of age. Equal numbers of males and females were included in each age group. Statistical analyses reveal that performance is very consistent both within and across age groups. Variables expected to be related to advancing age confirmed not only the validity of the database but also its utility in making judgments about individual performance. These variables included MLU, number of different words, total words, and words per minute, all of which correlated with age at $r = .65$ or greater. Other variables have proved to be excellent descriptors of performance differences including rate and timing measures, measures of verbal fluency (mazes), and general measures of syntax and semantics. The SALT Profiler basic report is shown in Table 1. These SALT Profiler measures provide the first step in describing disordered language performance.

Observations About the LSA Process

Reference Database   The solutions to the three factors that limit implementing LSA into clinical practice—time, consistency, and basis for comparison—are considered progress but not final by any means. Additional improvements can be made in all stages of the process—sampling, transcription analysis, and interpretation. Analysis of the RDB (Miller & Klee, 1995) documents the function of some individual variables—the frequency of mazes in utterances, for example. Children in the RDB produced more mazes in narrative samples than in conversational samples at all ages, and they produced more mazes when attempting longer utterances than in shorter utterances, confirming the hypothesis that mazes are an indication of formulation load on the speaker (Miller, 1987). Another example important for interpreting LSA data suggests that missing data cannot be interpreted as absent knowledge (e.g., if a form like wh- questions does not appear in an individual sample, it does not mean that the child lacks the knowledge to produce wh- forms, only that the sampling condition did not elicit questioning behaviors).

Language Sample   Recording the language sample is the cornerstone of the LSA process. The RDB data demonstrate that if consistent sampling conditions are followed, then the data that result will show the consistent trends that previous research has led researchers to expect. There is a relationship between age or developmental level and the sampling contexts available. Children cannot be expected to produce consistent narratives until they are at least 3 years of age, and topics must be introduced absent of time and space in order for children to make past and future references. The sample contexts chosen for the RDB were selected for two reasons. Conversation as a sampling context is the foundation for research on language development and therefore would provide data for comparison. Narration was selected because of its relevance to school perfor-

Table 1. Salt Profiler basic report

Category	Measure	Description
General	CA	Current age of target speaker (if available)
	Total utts.	Total number of speaker attempts
Syntax/ morphology	MLU (morph)	Mean length of utterances in morphemes
Semantics	TTR	Type-Token Ratio (# of different words/total words) calculated in the first 50 C&I utterances
	Diff. word roots	# of different word roots (excludes mazes)
	Tot. m. body words	Total # of main body words (excludes mazes)
Intelligibility	% Intelligible utts.	Percentage of the verbal utterances that are complete and intelligible
Mazes and overlaps	Utts w/mazes	Number of utterances containing mazes
	# of mazes	Total number of mazes
	# Maze words	Total number of maze words
	% Mz wds/tot wds	Percentage of total words that are in mazes
	Utts w/overlaps	Number of utterances containing overlapping speech
Verbal facility and rate	Number complete wds	Total number of completed words (includes mazes)
	Elapsed time	Transcript duration in minutes if timing information is found in transcript (elapsed time is estimated from surrounding timing lines)
	Utts/minute	Total number utterances/elapsed time
	Words/minute	Total number words/elapsed time
	Betw. utt pauses	Number of pauses between utts (: and ; lines)
	Betw. utt time	Total pause time (minutes) of between-utterance pauses
	W/in utt pauses	Number of pauses within utterances, including pauses within mazes and within incomplete and unintelligible utterances
	W/in utt time	Total pause time (minutes) of within-utterance pauses
Omissions and error codes	Omitted words	Number of omitted main body words
	Omitted b. morphs	Number of omitted main body bound morphemes
	Abandoned utts	Number of abandoned utterances (ending with a ">")
	Error codes	The following four error codes are totaled. The equal sign (=) at the end of the code is the SALT "match any" symbol and stands for any or no characters in that position. Specifically, [EO=] would count all codes that begin with "EO."
	[EO=]	Total number of overgeneralization error codes
	[EP=]	Total number of pronoun error codes
	[EW=]	Total number of other word-level error codes
	[EU=]	Total number of utterance-level error codes

mance in which oral narrative skills have been linked to reading success. Narratives also are more demanding of the speaker than conversations, requiring the speaker to formulate the story or event without the aid of the conversational partner. The contrast between the two can be illuminating for many children.

Some additional features of the language sample are important for understanding the analysis and interpretation stages of LSA. Comparing a sample with a database requires that sampling conform to the constraints of the database relative to sample type (conversation or narration) and sample length (number of utterances or the time duration of the sample). Attention to these features will help prevent comparing "apples" and "oranges" when making clinical decisions.

Analyzing the Language Sample Analysis is viewed as a hierarchical process whereby general measures can point the way to more detailed and time-consuming analysis. The SALT Profiler variables should be considered general indicators of performance. The initial goal is to determine the pattern of performance across categories to document areas of impairment; once those areas have been identified, follow-up with the detailed analysis specific to the child's problems can be carried out. For example, if MLU is low, then a detailed syntactic analysis using the Language Assessment, Remediation and Screening Procedure (LARSP) (Crystal, Fletcher, & Garman, 1976) or the Assigning Structural Stage (ASS) (Miller, 1981) may be desirable to develop a specific description of the forms available because this is an efficient use of time. Part of the descriptive problem is to determine the ability of the SALT Profiler general analysis to identify disordered performance, requiring additional analyses to develop an intervention plan. Several types of SALT variables are reviewed as indicators of 1) delayed development (e.g., MLU, number of different words, total words); 2) indicators of disordered performance or intrusive variables like mazes (e.g., filled pauses, repetitions, revisions), abandoned utterances, errors at the word or utterance level, and omissions of words or morphemes; 3) rate variables including transcript duration, pauses within or between utterances, and total pause time. Words and utterances per minute are discussed in detail with examples from individual children.

General Measures to Describe Disordered Performance Exploring the language samples of hundreds of children with language disorder and discussing the primary communication problems of these children revealed several areas that would benefit from specific measures. Three categories of measures were added to the SALT program in an effort to quantify behaviors that seemed to occur frequently among school age children The first category involves time or rate issues. All clinicians and researchers have had the experience of collecting a language sample from children with language disorder for whom the first and foremost problem encountered is that they do not talk very much. Obtaining a sample is like "pulling teeth." If the amount of talking is that prominent a feature of disordered performance, then it should be quantified. Perhaps if frequency of talking could be increased, then communication would improve. To capture the rate variable, a measure of transcription duration was added to document how long it took, in minutes and seconds, for the child to produce a transcript of 100 complete and intelligible utterances. To complete the rate evaluation, the number of words and utterances that the child produced per minute were calculated to explore how these measures quantified speaking rate. Pause data were added to account for pauses greater than 2 seconds, both within and between utterances, to help interpret the rate data and to document how pauses were distributed among the various disorder types. The second category of behaviors—mazes—was added to capture the verbal fluency of these children. The form and frequency of these behaviors in typical children was of interest in determining the degree to which these behaviors could be used to document word-finding or utterance-formulation problems. The third category of behaviors—errors—was added to alert clinicians to individual words or utterances that may require further analysis. Errors and omissions are added at the time of transcription to aid in the interpretation. The coding of errors recognizes that school-age children do produce word-choice or morphological errors of syntax, semantics, or pragmatics that are not developmental. Adding these variables to the analyses offered the opportunity to quantify several new categories together with the old.

Summarizing the Data Across Measures There are two parts to how the SALT analyses categories describe language disorder. First is a taxonomy of topologies of disordered language performance generated by SLPs working in public school settings (Miller, Freiberg, Rolland, & Reeves, 1992). This taxonomy includes the following types: utterance-formulation impairments, word-finding problems, rate problems (slow talker or fast talker), semantic/referencing problems, pragmatic problems, and language delay. These are not exclusive categories but are descriptive of areas of impairment. Second, the SALT Profiler can provide insight into four of these six categories: utterance-formulation impairments, word-finding problems, rate problems, and language delay (see Table 2). Table 2 also lists the variables associated with each category. These general variables are calculated automatically, and the program identifies those variables that are 1 or more standard deviations from the mean for the age group and speaking context from the RDB. Semantic/referencing problems and pragmatic impairments will require hand-calculated indices requiring human judgment of context.

Profiler data from 256 children ages 2;9–13;8 years of age with disorders of language production were evaluated to determine the validity of the measurement categories in describing the diversity of disordered performance (Miller & Klee, 1995). The data clearly document that no single variable will identify the range of problems displayed in this sample (see Table 3). Children showed impairments in distinct groups of variables, showing patterns of performance impairments that were descriptive of their unique production problems as well as identifying areas that will require further analysis. The data in Table 3 are illustrative of several points. First, the taxonomic categories are not mutually exclusive, as indicated by the overlap in the number of children with impairments in

Table 2. A clinical typology of language disorders

Clinical types	Characteristics
Utterance formulation	Maze revisions at word- and phrase-level units; increased MLU; pauses within and between utterances; word-order errors
Word finding	Maze revisions and repetitions at word- or part-word–level units; pauses within utterances; word omissions; word-choice errors
Hypo-verbal rate	Decreased number of utterances and words per minute; pauses within and between utterances
Hyper-verbal rate	Increased number of utterances and words per minute, which may be combined with reduced semantic content
Pragmatic or discourse	Noncontingent utterance; pronominal reference errors; problems with topic maintenance, new versus old information, and narrative structure
Semantic or reference	Overgeneralization, word-choice, and NP-VP symmetry errors; abandoned utterances; redundancy
Delayed development	Decreased number of different words and total number of words; delayed syntactic development as measured by MLU and other detailed syntactic analyses

each category. Second, the number of children in each category is not related to age, given the consistency of the mean age for each measurement category. This is somewhat surprising because language delay might be expected to be more evident in younger children than in older children. Third, only 20 children were not identified by at least one category. This level of sensitivity is far greater than past research in which standardized measures identified slightly more than 50% of the children with language disorders, and MLU identified 71% of the children (Aram et al., 1993). The combined measure derived from the language sample using the SALT Profiler identified 92% of the sample of 256 children. These data confirm the descriptive power of language-sample analysis as a measurement system of disordered language performance. Clearly the types of analysis discussed in Chapters 1, 4, 5, 6, 9, and 12 will be necessary to complete detailed descriptions of the different types of disordered language performance.

Table 3. Number and percentage of subjects with performance ± 1 standard deviation from the group mean on any of the measures of the five categories using conversational samples

Measurement category	Number of subjects	Percentage of subjects	Mean age (years)
Language delay	147	57.4	7.9
Increased mazes	97	37.9	8.2
Slow rate	98	38.3	8.2
Fast rate	19	7.4	7.7
Increased pauses	127	49.6	8.5
None of the above	20	7.8	8.5

Adapted from Miller and Klee (1995).

ASSESSING LINGUISTICALLY
AND CULTURALLY DIFFERENT CHILDREN

To explore the SALT Profiler measures' ability to identify disordered language performance among linguistically and culturally different groups of children, language samples were evaluated from more than 90 African American children and 60 Hmong children from Wisconsin. As Gutierrez-Clellen (see Chapter 2) discusses in detail, measuring and interpreting the language performance of children learning English as a second language (ESL) or of children whose culture is different from the mainstream culture presents a significant challenge because language is a major expression of every culture. Language-sample analysis provides an opportunity to examine language performance, taking culture and language differences into consideration when interpreting the results. Specific measurement categories to document African American English vernacular can be implemented, for example, to document the features of the dialect that are different from standard English. The first task was to evaluate the language samples of typically developing African American children ages 7, 9, and 11 years, with at least 30 children in each group. Children were selected to represent the range of SES, school ability, and sex distribution found in the RDB. A conversation and a narrative sample were recorded for each child. The SALT Profiler program was used to analyze the transcripts. The results for the 7- and 9-year-old children revealed few differences relative to the RDB. The only consistent difference was for the 9-year-olds, who had MLUs consistently longer than the RDB sample. These data would suggest that when SES and ability are controlled, race is not a factor in overall language performance. The data for the 11-year-olds showed a different trend. The 11-year-olds were different on almost every variable, particularly those documenting the amount of language produced. It was difficult to explain this outcome. Each transcript was reexamined, and the results could not be attributed to a few outliers. More than 70% of the children in this age group had scores 1 standard deviation or more below the mean on more than half of the variables. It appeared that the 11-year-old children were not talking as much as their younger peers. The only explanation that seemed plausible was that most of the examiners were Caucasian and that when children reached adolescence, they were more sensitive to the social differences and simply were not interested in interacting with a Caucasian adult.

The Hmong children were selected from graduates of ESL programs. Two groups were evaluated: 1) 30 children who were 9 years of age and who were attending second grade and 2) 30 children who were 11 years of age and who were attending fifth grade. Each of these children provided a conversation and a narrative sample that were analyzed using the SALT Profiler program. The results revealed that developmental variables such as MLU, total words, and number of different words were not different from the RDB for either age group in either sample context. Significant differences were found in the number of mazes produced, the number and length of pauses, and the speaking rate of both age groups. The Hmong children all produced significantly more mazes, more pauses, and fewer words per minute than the RDB sample. Because the children had graduated from their ESL programs within the previous year, the lack of difference between age groups is not surprising. The mazes, pauses, and speaking rate data describe the word-finding and sentence-formulation difficulties experienced by these children as they work toward verbal fluency in English. These variables were sensitive to the children's difficulties with English in both conversation and narration. The SALT Profiler variables characterize the Hmong children learning ESL as having vocabulary and basic sentence formation skills similar to their age-matched native-speaking peers but experiencing difficulties with proficient use of the language as measured by their frequent use of pauses, repetition, and revision of word and phrase segments. This is exactly the picture expected of this group of language users, thus demonstrating the power of these general variables to capture language proficiency.

EXPLORING DIFFERENCES IN SAMPLE SIZE

Finding the optimum size for a language sample has preoccupied researchers since the 1950s. Early work used 50 utterances (Templin, 1957). Other studies used even smaller samples. Loban (1976), for example, proposed 30 consecutive narrative utterances. Length of sample determines the amount of material available to evaluate; the goal is to collect a sample that provides sufficient breadth of utterance type and vocabulary diversity so that the sample reflects total language abilities without constraint. Studies over the years have consistently pointed out that shorter samples are not as stable as longer samples for specific measures, but not all measures require long samples to be stable. Because length of sample reflects cost, it is important to evaluate how long a sample must be to derive consistent values from the SALT Profiler measures. To evaluate sample length, transcripts of different lengths were created from the RDB at 50, 75, 100, 125, and 150 utterances for conversation and narration. This created 2,520 transcripts. Each transcript was analyzed using the SALT Profiler with the results sent to a rectangular data array for statistical analysis. The results show consistent trends. MLU was consistent across transcript length in both speaking conditions. There were no differences between samples of 50 utterances and samples of 150 utterances. Using clear segmentation rules in transcription likely contributes to this outcome by limiting any variability introduced by vague or inconsistently applied segmentation rules. The words-per-minute measure of speaking rate also did not change for transcripts of different sizes. Apparently, 50 utterances provide enough data to sample speaking rate. Measures of utterance content, like the number of different words, changed as a function of transcript length, as would be expected. The number of different words increases linearly over transcript length for each age group. Although the slope of each line was not calculated, visual inspection of the curves would indicate that the slopes are equal for the 5- to 13-year-olds, and the 3- and 4-year-old children had a somewhat flatter curve for the longer transcripts, though the difference is not dramatic for these data. It would be possible to create prediction tables for the number of different words expected by transcript length. The maze measures all increased linearly with increasing sample size suggesting that mazes are distributed equivalently across utterances in transcripts.

Together, these data make a strong statement about sample length when comparing performance across samples or across children. Samples must be of the same length for frequency and time variables if accurate comparisons are to be made. Variables that are averages, such as MLU, seem to be stable over transcript lengths from 50 to 150 utterances because all of the utterances are used in the calculations. Other variables, like question or past-tense use, require that children be given the same number of opportunities (e.g., 100 utterances) in order for comparisons to be meaningful. Additional research would be advised to consider sample length relative to speaking context and type of measure to find the optimum sample size.

STATEWIDE IMPLEMENTATION OF LSA

In 1990, the state of Wisconsin sought to improve diagnostic consistency in identifying children with language disorders who qualify for services in the public school system. There had been a spiraling increase in children enrolled for speech and language services statewide of more than 21% over 3 years. The Wisconsin Department of Public Instruction pursued using LSA as an assessment tool that would improve the consistency of decision making, describe intervention targets, and provide documentation of intervention progress. The three barriers that had limited the implementation of LSA in clinical practice—time, consistency, and comparison data—had been overcome as a result of a long-term project with the Madison Metropolitan Public Schools (Miller & Lyngaas, 1995) that paralleled the development of SALT. The statewide implementation of LSA began with the development of a written guide to LSA, *Language Sample Analysis Guide: The Wisconsin Guide for the Identification and Description of Language Impairment in Children* (Miller & Leadholm, 1992), which was distributed to all SLPs working in the schools in the state. This was followed by a series of workshops to assist SLPs in implementing LSA. The workshops have provided training for more than 1,000 SLPs in the state and have resulted in implementing LSA with thousands of schoolchildren in Wisconsin.

CONCLUSION

This chapter has pointed out five major long-standing issues about the progress that has been made in understanding child language disorder. First, the failure of the field to invest in adequate descriptive work to characterize disordered language performance has resulted in a lack of agreement on the definition of language disorder. Another way to express this is to suggest that unidimensional theories have provided unidimensional descriptions of language disorder (e.g., SLI as a grammatical impairment). This volume addressed these issues, pointing out that measures follow theory on the one hand and contribute to theoretical development on the other hand. Researchers and clinicians are caught in a catch-22 in which using the most recent definitions requires using old measures. The SALT Profiler data suggest that a multidimensional approach to description improves sensitivity, identifying 92% of the children in the sample of children whom clinicians had identified as having a language disorder. These data fit the theoretical model proposed by Evans; the next step is to perform the statistical analyses using the multidimensional modeling techniques discussed in Chapter 10.

Second, there is considerable agreement that standardized tests of language performance need to be reexamined relative to what aspects of language performance they test. Many children with significant language impairment are not identified by these measures, particularly those children with high performance IQs. The question remains: What do norm-referenced tests measure?

Third, researchers appear to be satisfied with their description of typical language development, but should they be? Research is producing new insights into developmental processes by adding new explanations for old concepts or adding features to the map of the child's developmental progress to adult competence. The model of development is the foundation of the description of disordered performance. Can researchers trust the developmental database? Consider for a moment that most of what is understood about language development comes from cross-sectional studies of single variables like syntax. It is time to develop longitudinal data sets across all aspects of language so that researchers can examine issues of synchrony of development between language processes (i.e., comprehension and production) and among linguistic levels (i.e., vocabulary, syntax, semantics, pragmatic skills).

Fourth, not having an agreed-upon definition of disorder means that there is no gold standard for documenting the validity of measurements of disordered language performance.

Fifth, researchers and clinicians both could use tools that assess disordered language performance more efficiently. Many of the best measures (e.g., LSA) still require a great deal of time and effort. As a result, clinicians and researchers often choose not to use them. Frequently, measurement procedures are used because they are easy, not because they produce the best data. The detail of assessments must be improved without requiring more time and training to gather the data.

Despite these issues, the future holds a great deal of promise based on the major breakthroughs of the early 1990s: parent report measures of early language development (see Chapter 8) and the advances in computer analysis of language samples. Parent report measures have provided access to the wealth of information that parents have about their children's language behavior and perhaps will open the door to other measures exploiting this rich data source. Using computers to evaluate a variety of analyses simultaneously, to construct databases or transcript files for children at different ages, and to automatically compare an individual child with the database will provide the descriptive power needed to characterize language disorder in children.

REFERENCES

Aram, D., Morris, R., & Hall, N. (1993). Clinical and research congruence in identifying children with specific language impairment. *Journal of Speech and Hearing Research, 36,* 580–591.

Brown, R. (1973). *First words.* Cambridge, MA: Harvard University Press.

Crystal, D., Fletcher, P., & Garman, M. (1976). *The grammatical analysis of language disability: A procedure for assessment and remediation.* London: Edward Arnold.

Loban, W. (1976). Language development: Kindergarten through grade twelve. *National Council of Teachers of English, 18.*

Miller, J. (1981). *Assessing language production in children.* Needham, MA: Allyn & Bacon.

Miller, J. (1987). *A grammatical characterization of language disorder. Proceedings of the First International Symposium on Specific Speech and Language Disorders in Children.* London: AFASIC Press.

Miller, J.F., & Chapman, R.S. (1981). The relation between age and mean length of utterance in morphemes. *Journal of Speech and Hearing Research, 24*(2), 154–161.

Miller, J., Freiberg, C., Rolland, M.-B., & Reeves, M. (1992). Implementing computerized language sample analysis in the public school. *Topics in Language Disorders, 12*(2), 69–82.

Miller, J., & Klee, T. (1995). Quantifying language disorders in children. In P. Fletcher & B. MacWhinney (Eds.), *Handbook of child language* (pp. 545–572). Cambridge, MA: Blackwell.

Miller, J., & Leadholm, B. (1992). *Language sample analysis guide: The Wisconsin guide for the identification and description of language impairment in children.* Madison: Wisconsin Department of Public Instruction.

Miller, J., & Lyngaas, K. (1995, June/July). A successful collaboration: A behind the scenes look at a research/clinician pairing. *Asha, 47*–49.

Templin, M. (1957). *Certain language skills in children: Their development and interrelationships.* Minneapolis: University of Minnesota Press.

Tukey, J. (1977). *Exploratory data analysis.* Reading, MA: Addison-Wesley.

Author Index

O'Connor, R., 264, 277
Oetting, J., 4, 24, 26
Oetting, J.B., 190, 191, 204, 205
Ogura, T., 175, 181
O'Hanlon, L., 169, 181
Oller, D.K., 41, 55, 59, 74
Oller, J.W., 43, 46, 52, 55
Olson, R.K., 148, 159
Olson, S., 12, 25
Olswang, L., 64, 74, 232, 254, 293, 297, 301, 305, 306
Olswang, L.B., 270, 277, 305
Oroz, M., 16, 17, 27
Ortiz, A.A., 29, 53, 55
Osgood, C.E., 209, 210, 211, 254
Osterhout, L., 161, 181
Overton, T., 65, 74
Owens, R., 146, 159

Pace, S., 216, 246
Pae, S., 190, 191, 205
Palin, M., 230, 253
Palincsar, A., 265, 270, 277, 306
Palinscar, A.S., 286, 302
Palmer, C., 230, 253
Palmer, F., 180
Papousek, M., 59, 74
Pappas, C.C., 124, 140
Paraskevopoulos, J., 181
Parisi, D., 220, 221, 225, 246
Parker, T.S., 235, 236, 254
Parker, W., 32, 51
Paul, R., 6, 7, 14, 15, 20, 25, 63, 73, 156, 159, 193, 195, 204
Peach, R., 222, 254
Pearson, B.Z., 41, 55
Peitgen, H.O., 236, 254
Peña, E., 32, 46, 53, 55, 295, 296, 304, 305, 306
Penn, C., 227, 254
Pennington, B.F., 148, 159
Perez, C., 127, 140
Perkins, M.N., 32, 55
Peters, C., 13, 24
Peterson, C., 124, 125, 126, 129, 131, 132, 133, 134, 139, 140
Peterson, S., 161, 181
Pethick, S., 73, 180
Piaget, J., 62, 74
Pickering, D., 269, 276

Pierce, P., 268, 278
Piercy, M., 12, 26
Pindzola, R., 292, 304
Pinker, S., 146, 159, 213, 230, 254
Piredda, L., 122, 139
Plante, E., 30, 31, 33, 55
Pliner, C., 26
Pollio, H., 209, 211, 218, 254
Pond, R.E., 63, 75, 129, 141, 296, 307
Posner, M.I., 161, 181
Postal, P., 220, 254
Prather, E.M., 73, 77, 95
Preece, A., 124, 140
Prelock, P., 3, 27
Prigogine, I., 235, 236, 238, 240, 254
Pritchard, R., 128, 140
Prizant, B.M., 57, 64, 75
Propp, V., 128, 140
Provine, K., 175, 181
Prutting, C., 3, 26, 61, 75, 225, 227, 228, 230, 232, 254, 266, 278
Puckett, M.B., 270, 278

Quinn, R., 32, 45, 53, 55, 127, 138, 263, 270, 275, 295, 304, 306

Radford, A., 107, 115, 120
Raichle, M.E., 161, 181
Ramsey Musselwhite, C., 32, 55
Ramstadt, V., 3, 23, 223, 251
Rand, Y., 282, 284, 291, 298, 303, 304, 306
Raphael, T.E., 270, 275
Rapin, I., 5, 25
Raven, J.C., 286, 306
Records, N.L., 190, 206
Redmond, A., 223, 247
Reeves, M., 318, 324
Reichle, J., 57, 74, 221, 253
Reid, K., 150, 158
Reilly, J., 22, 179
Reilly, J.S., 73, 175, 180, 181
Reinharth, B.M., 292, 306
Rescorla, L., 3, 11, 14, 16, 25, 26, 166, 167, 170, 172, 181, 193, 204
Resnick, J.S., 22
Retherford, K., 222, 254
Rey, 283
Reynell, J., 10, 26, 74, 129, 140, 216, 254

Subject Index